The Health Policy Agenda for the American People

Editor
E. Jill Hirt, Ph.D.

Editorial Consultant
Robert W. Riley

Design
Kym Abrams Design

Production Consultant
Lisa Brenner

Illustrator
David Lesh

Typesetting
Master Typographers

Printer
Great Northern Design and Printing

Primary Health Policy Agenda Staff
Bruce E. Balfe, M.A.
Vice President, Issue Planning and Management

Kathleen R. Lane, Ph.D.
Director, Health Policy Agenda

Severine J. Brocki, Ph.D.
Associate Director, Health Policy Agenda

Gail Bieber, M.A.
Senior Policy Analyst, Health Policy Agenda

Jan Sugar-Webb, M.Ed.
Research Assistant, Health Policy Agenda

Brenda Elliott
Administrative Assistant, Health Policy Agenda

Pauletta Reid
Administrative Secretary, Health Policy Agenda

The Health Policy Agenda for the American People is published in three publications. This publication includes an introduction to the Health Policy Agenda, followed by discussion of specific health care issues, recommendations, and implementation plans. The two other publications are the Summary Report, which lists all of the recommendations, and the Reference Report, which contains background material developed during the course of the project.

The products of the Health Policy Agenda are the result of the collective decision-making of the representatives of participating organizations. This does not imply that any individual organization has adopted these products in whole or in part.

The Steering Committee expresses its gratitude to all of the participants of the Health Policy Agenda for the American People. Working with the multiplicity of individuals and organizations involved in the Health Policy Agenda over the past five years has been an invaluable experience that has brought many challenges and rewards. A project of this magnitude could not have been accomplished without the expertise, time, and patience that each participant brought to this undertaking. Although diverse in background, the participants came to share an unusual degree of mutual respect and understanding for each others' opinions and perspectives during the course of their endeavors.

We also extend our thanks to the organizations that provided support for this effort, and to their staffs, who spent many hours researching the issues, compiling background information, and reviewing the reports.

Joseph F. Boyle, M.D.
Chairman, Health Policy Agenda Steering Committee

Joseph F. Boyle, M.D. (1982-1986)

Chairman of the Steering Committee

Judith Barr (1985-1986)

Edmund McTernan, Ed.D. (1984-1985)

American Society of Allied Health Professions

John L. Bomba, D.D.S. (1985-1986)

Burton H. Press, D.D.S. (1982-1985)

American Dental Association

Robert A. Carpenter (1985-1986)

Member at Large

John E. Chapman, M.D. (1982-1986)

AMA Section on Medical Schools

Eunice R. Cole, R.N. (1982-1986)

American Nurses' Association, Inc.

John A. D. Cooper, M.D. (1984-1986)

Association of American Medical Colleges

Theodore R. Cooper, M.D. (1982-1986)

Member at Large

John J. Coury, Jr., M.D. (1982-1986)

American Medical Association

Donald K. Crandall, M.D. (1984-1986)

Joseph T. Painter, M.D. (1983-1984)

John J. Ring, M.D. (1982-1983)

Chairman, Work Group on Payment for Service

Edgar G. Davis (1982-1986)

Business Roundtable

William R. Felts, Jr., M.D. (1982-1986)

Chairman, Work Group on Delivery Mechanisms and Processes

E. E. Gilbertson (1982-1986)

American Hospital Association

William E. Golden, M.D. (1982-1986)

AMA Medical Student and Resident Physician Sections

Robert B. Helms, Ph.D. (1984-1986)

Robert J. Rubin, M.D. (1982-1984)

U.S. Department of Health and Human Services

William S. Hotchkiss, M.D. (1983-1986)

American Medical Association

Frank J. Jirka, Jr., M.D. (1983-1984)

American Medical Association

Louis J. Kettel, M.D. (1982-1986)

Chairman, Work Group on Education

Gene Kimmelman (1984-1986)

Consumer Federation of America

Sister Irene Kraus, R.N., M.B.A. (1982-1986)

Chairman,

Work Group on Health Resources

Frederick J. Krebs (1986)

Eric J. Oxfeld, J.D. (1985-1986)

Frank W. Armstrong (1984-1985)

Robert A. Carpenter (1982-1985)

U.S. Chamber of Commerce

The Honorable Scott M. Matheson (1983-1986)

Member at Large

Robert B. Maxwell (1986)

Clarice C. Jones, M.S.W. (1983-1986)

American Association of Retired Persons

William E. Mayer, M.D. (1984-1986)

John M. Beary, III, M.D. (1982-1984)

U.S. Department of Defense

Diane B. McCarthy (1982-1986)

Member at Large

James L. Moorefield (1982-1986)

Health Insurance Association of America

Gerald J. Mossinghoff (1986)

C. Joseph Stetler (1984-1986)

Lewis A. Engman (1982-1984)

Pharmaceutical Manufacturers

Association

Beverlee A. Myers, M.P.H. (1984-1986)

American Public Health Association

Russel H. Patterson, Jr., M.D. (1982-1986)

Specialty and Service Society

Paul C. Reinert, S.J. (1982-1986)

Member at Large

William Y. Rial, M.D. (1982-1983)

American Medical Association

Harrison L. Rogers, Jr., M.D. (1984-1986)

American Medical Association

James H. Sammons, M.D. (1982-1986)

(Ex-Officio Member)

American Medical Association

Richard T. F. Schmidt, M.D. (1982-1986)

Chairman, Work Group on Medical Science

Frank E. Staggers, M.D. (1983-1986)

Lucius C. Earles, III, M.D. (1982-1983)

National Medical Association

Paul M. Starnes (1985-1986)

James R. Tallon, Jr. (1983-1985)

National Conference of State Legislatures

Bernard R. Tresnowski (1982-1986)

Blue Cross and Blue Shield Association

Robert M. Vanecko, M.D. (1982-1986)

Chairman, Work Group on Evaluation,

Assessment, and Control

David M. Worthen, M.D. (1984-1986)

Donald L. Custis, M.D. (1982-1984)

Veterans Administration

Victor M. Zink (1984-1986)

Council on Employee Benefits

Contents

Introduction

The decade of the 1980s is a critical turning point for every facet of the nation's health care system. Dramatic advances in biomedical science and technology are changing health care practices and procedures. New technologies such as organ transplants, genetic engineering, dialysis, and other life-saving treatments that were nonexistent 10 to 20 years ago are now part of accepted medical practice. New technologies are often used prior to a full and clear understanding of the financial and social consequences involved, but it is usually not long before cost-benefit questions and ethical issues arise. Scientific discoveries and the complex issues that accompany them will no doubt continue into the next decade and the next century.

Efforts to control costs and stimulate competition are also causing changes in health care delivery, financing, health manpower, and education. A bewildering array of public and private schemes for the delivery and financing of care are being implemented rapidly. And the move toward competitive corporate health care is altering traditional health care roles and relationships.

Surveys indicate that most Americans believe that the health care they receive is good and that they have adequate access to health care. However they also believe, as do many health professionals, that costs are a serious problem. Many observers fear that the changes now being implemented will, to some degree, reduce the accessibility and quality of care available to the public and that Americans will be paying more out-of-pocket costs for their health care.

Particularly during times of rapid change, short-term and piecemeal decisions are made by both the public and private sectors. This can be counterproductive and often results in laws and policies that are ineffective in guiding the future direction of health care. An issue-by-issue approach is no longer adequate, considering the scope and complexity of the decisions that are required. What is needed is a reexamination of the basic values upon which the health care system is based and the development of a long-range comprehensive and cohesive policy to guide government, the health professions, and the public through these complex issues.

To this end, the Health Policy Agenda for the American People was initiated in 1982. Over 425 representatives from 172 different health, health-related, business, government, and consumer groups have met over the past five years to develop the Agenda. Their mission was to examine the immediate concerns of today, as well as the issues that will be confronting the health sector into the next decade and the next century. Other reports have addressed such specific components of health care as medical education, health manpower requirements, and the cost of health care. But none included such a diverse group of participants and none is as comprehensive as the Health Policy Agenda.

The Structure and Process of the Health Policy Agenda

From its inception, the Health Policy Agenda has functioned on the basis of one major premise—that a consensus approach among knowledgeable people would yield reasonable, workable results. The structure of the Agenda was based on this premise, and three major groups—a Steering Committee, an Advisory Committee, and Work Groups— were established to accomplish its tasks.

The work of the Health Policy Agenda was guided by a 37-member Steering Committee, representing allied health professionals, business, consumers, dentists, hospital administrators, insurance providers, nurses, physicians, the pharmaceutical industry, and state and federal government. There were also five at-large members on the committee. The Steering Committee provided overall direction for the project and was the final decision-making body. It met on 14 occasions during the five years of this project.

The primary work of the Health Policy Agenda was done by the six Work Groups, each consisting of 20 to 30 representatives from health-related, business, government, and consumer organizations. Each Work Group addressed a specific policy area: medical science; health professions education; health resources; delivery mechanisms and processes; evaluation, assessment, and control; and payment for service. Each Work Group was convened from 10 to 14 times during the course of the Health Policy Agenda.

The Advisory Committee was made up of representatives from 151 organizations with interests in health affairs. This committee performed a review function for the Health Policy Agenda, providing the project with a wide spectrum of opinion on health care issues. The Advisory Committee met five times during the course of the project to review materials developed by the Work Groups; after incorporating Advisory Committee comments, the Work Groups presented their materials to the Steering Committee for final approval.

The project placed great emphasis on building a consensus. When disagreements existed among members, they were to address their differences and come as close as they could to a true consensus position. However, there were times when individual differences could not be completely reconciled; in these cases, the consensus represented agreement short of unanimity. While some organizations may not agree with all portions of the Health Policy Agenda, their participation has given them the opportunity to understand the nature of differences between their policy positions and those of other organizations. This in itself is an important contribution to health care policy. Participating organizations that were represented on the Steering Committee were also given an opportunity to present formal comments and dissenting opinions to the Health Policy Agenda. (These can be found in Appendix I.)

The Health Policy Agenda was developed in two phases. During the first phase of the project, which concluded in mid-1984, 159 principles were developed. These principles are value statements that describe what should exist in health care; they include statements about equity, individual and professional rights and responsibilities, the role of government, and the quality and cost of health care. They provide a blueprint for the development of an optimal health care system, and constitute the long-term foundation of the Health Policy Agenda. (A list of the principles can be found in Appendix II.)

In the second phase of the project, the principles were used as the basis for the development of policy proposals by the Work Groups. In developing the policy proposals, participants were asked to challenge the conventional wisdom on health care and to propose actions that are far-sighted and relevant into the next century. These policy proposals, containing background information that was used to compile this report, can be found in the Reference Report of the Health Policy Agenda. (A guide to cross-reference material in this report to policy proposals in the Reference Report can be found in Appendix III.)

Overview of the Health Policy Agenda

Seven policy areas are addressed in separate chapters of the Health Policy Agenda: supplying the professionals, providing the technology and facilities, organizing the resources, communicating health information, ensuring quality, paying the bill, and preparing for the future through research. In each chapter, specific problems are identified and specific solutions are recommended. The responsible agents or organizations and initial steps required to implement the recommendations are also discussed. (The recommendations themselves are highlighted in each chapter.)

A number of themes underlie the Health Policy Agenda and serve to integrate the Agenda as a whole:

□ The ultimate goal of the health care system is to serve the public interest, individually and collectively. This includes a societal obligation to improve access to health care services for those who face social, cultural, and financial barriers to adequate health care.

□ Both the public and private sectors should participate in defining health care needs and in the delivery and financing of health care services. A balance between public and private sector involvement is essential to an effective health care system.

□ For the health care system to function effectively, there must be clear communication among all participants. The availability of information is a hallmark of a progressive, high quality health care system.

□ When possible, health care decisions should be made at the local level. Except where direct federal government involvement is necessary—e.g., in fulfilling societal obligations to special populations—the government role should be restricted to one of oversight to ensure that the private sector is functioning properly. A centralized system cannot make the numerous and diverse decisions required on an everyday basis at the local level.

□ The success of the health care system depends on a clear delineation and understanding of the roles and responsibilities of key participants, including consumers.

□ Because of the costs of educating health professionals, incorporating new technology, and administering sophisticated facilities, pressure will always exist to contain overall health care expenditures. The cost of health care must be addressed in conjunction with the improvement of the quality of care and the availability of services. There should be incentives for all key participants to control costs.

These themes are addressed in each chapter and serve as a framework for the recommendations.

In Chapter I, "Supplying the Professionals," the education of health professionals, minority representation in the health professions, boundaries of practice among and within the health professions, and the supply and distribution of health professionals are discussed. The quality of health care is dependent on the quality of the educational process and programs, both of which are in turn dependent on adequate financial support; recommendations concerning the financing of undergraduate and clinical graduate educational programs are made. Representation of minorities in educational programs and in the health professions has not markedly changed during the past 15 years, and recommendations to increase their representation are proposed. Recommendations are presented to ensure that graduates of foreign health professional schools who choose to take advanced professional education or to practice in this country meet the same or equivalent standards of competence required of graduates of accredited U.S. health professions programs. Increased specialization, technological innovations, and the need to control the cost of health care have contributed to a more depersonalized type of health care, and recommendations are made for educational programs to recognize the need to educate health professionals who are both competent and caring. The increasing supply of health professionals is likely to result in more practice disputes among and within the various professions, and recommendations to resolve

these disputes are proposed. Recommendations are presented to achieve and maintain an adequate supply and distribution of health professionals to meet the health care needs of all of the American people, including the needs of those presently underserved or inappropriately served by the current system. The chapter concludes with recommendations to ensure the continued competence of all health professionals.

Chapter II, "Providing the Technology and Facilities," includes a discussion of moral and ethical issues in the use of health care technology and the allocation of privileges to use technology. The definition, licensure, and supply and distribution of health care facilities are also addressed. Recommendations concerning the application or withdrawal of health care technologies and the acquisition of expensive or resource-intensive technologies are made. The rapid development of new health care technologies has raised some questions concerning who should be allowed to use them and what criteria should be used to make these decisions, and recommendations are proposed regarding the responsibilities of health professionals and facilities. Considerable changes have occurred in the past 20 years in the numbers and types of health care facilities offering services to the public and it is recommended that a new definition of health care facilities be adopted. There is little uniformity in the approaches taken by individual states in determining which health care settings should be licensed, as well as concern about the supply and distribution of facilities. Recommendations are presented to address these areas so that the health care needs of all individuals in all parts of the country can be met through the delivery of quality health care services.

In Chapter III, "Organizing the Resources," the planning and delivery of health care services, access to health care services, and technology transfer are discussed. Although centralized planning efforts have not been considered to be highly effective in the past, the health care delivery system must be responsive to changing societal needs and be able to provide for the health care needs of special populations. Recommendations for local planning efforts to meet these needs are made, as are recommendations that the public and private sectors meet their responsibilities in providing access to needed health care services. It is recommended that the transfer of health care technology be influenced by the safety, efficacy, potential for societal benefit, and cost of the technology. Recommendations regarding the responsibilities of all of the participants in the technology transfer process are also proposed.

Chapter IV, "Communicating Health Information," includes discussion of health information and education, informed consent, the confidentiality of health care records and information, and public health care needs. The collection of individual decisions to adopt healthy lifestyles and to be prudent users of the health care system will have a significant effect on the overall health status of the country. Recommendations to facilitate individual decision-making through the provision of health information and education are presented, and specific responsibilities of all of the participants in the health care system are delineated. Clear communication and shared decision-making between patients and health professionals provide the foundation for optimal health care treatment, and recommendations concerning informed consent, the use of surrogate decision-makers, the maintenance of privacy of health care records and information, and access to health care records are made. The chapter concludes with recommendations to address public health care needs in health professions educational programs.

In Chapter V, "Ensuring Quality," the quality of health care services is addressed. The assurance of quality has evolved to the point where it is now one of the central policy issues in health care. Many different mechanisms have been developed to measure the quality of health care, and recommendations regarding the assessment of quality, the factors to be considered in the assessment process, quality assurance mechanisms, and the licensure and certification of health professionals are proposed. The issues of patient injury, compensation for injury, and professional liability are very complex and recommendations concerning the professional and societal responsibilities for patient injury are presented. It is recommended that ethical considerations be an integral part of the decision-making process in providing quality health care. Recommendations are also made to improve the quality of health care through the assessment of health care technology and through health services research and evaluation activities.

In Chapter VI, "Paying the Bill," the design of a cost-effective payment system and the role of government in the health care delivery system are addressed. The unabated increases in health care expenditures necessitate a reexamination and reformulation of the existing health care system. Recommendations concerning the health care payment system, which does not currently operate in a comprehensive and consistent manner to contain costs, are proposed. The recommendations regarding the role of government as provider, payor, and regulator of health care services are based on maintaining an appropriate balance between the public and private sector so that public safety, access to health care, cost containment, and fair competition are maintained.

Chapter VII, "Preparing for the Future through Research," includes discussion of the availability of funding and health professionals for research, university-industry cooperative research ventures, ethical and societal considerations in research, the use of animals in research, and communication among the research community, the media, and the public. Biomedical research contributes to the economic well-being and the scientific preeminence of the country, and support of research activities is essential to the continued improvement in the health of the American people. Recommendations are presented to continue and strengthen the nation's long-term commitment to research.

A complete list of all of the recommendations of the Health Policy Agenda follows Chapter VII.

Implementation of the Health Policy Agenda

A project of this magnitude, which has brought together a diverse group of individuals and organizations, has not previously been attempted by the private sector. The Health Policy Agenda provides a national basis for responding to social, economic, scientific, educational, and political issues as they affect the health care system.

An Implementation Committee has been appointed by the Steering Committee to oversee the implementation of the Health Policy Agenda recommendations. Coalitions that are interested in particular policy areas will be an important part of the implementation process, and the Implementation Committee will play a key role in organizing and coordinating coalition activities.

If the recommendations contained in the Agenda are implemented, the participants of the Health Policy Agenda envision a health care system that will provide cost-effective, quality health care to all individuals in the nation. There will be open lines of communication between participants in the health care delivery system, enabling everyone to use health care resources in an effective manner. Clarification of the roles and responsibilities of patients, payors, providers, government, and business will also result in more efficient use of health care resources. There will be less overlap and duplication of services, and hence more efficient health care. The Health Policy Agenda provides a framework for policy-making in which there is concern for the nation as a whole.

The challenging issues addressed by the Health Policy Agenda confront all Americans, individually as recipients of health care and collectively as members of society. Many entities—from local health care facilities to federal agencies—are struggling with health care access, quality, and costs. The objective of the Health Policy Agenda is to provide enduring guidance on these issues, guidance so compelling that it will have a major impact on the health of the American people.

2 DISTRIBUTION

1 Increased Funding Support

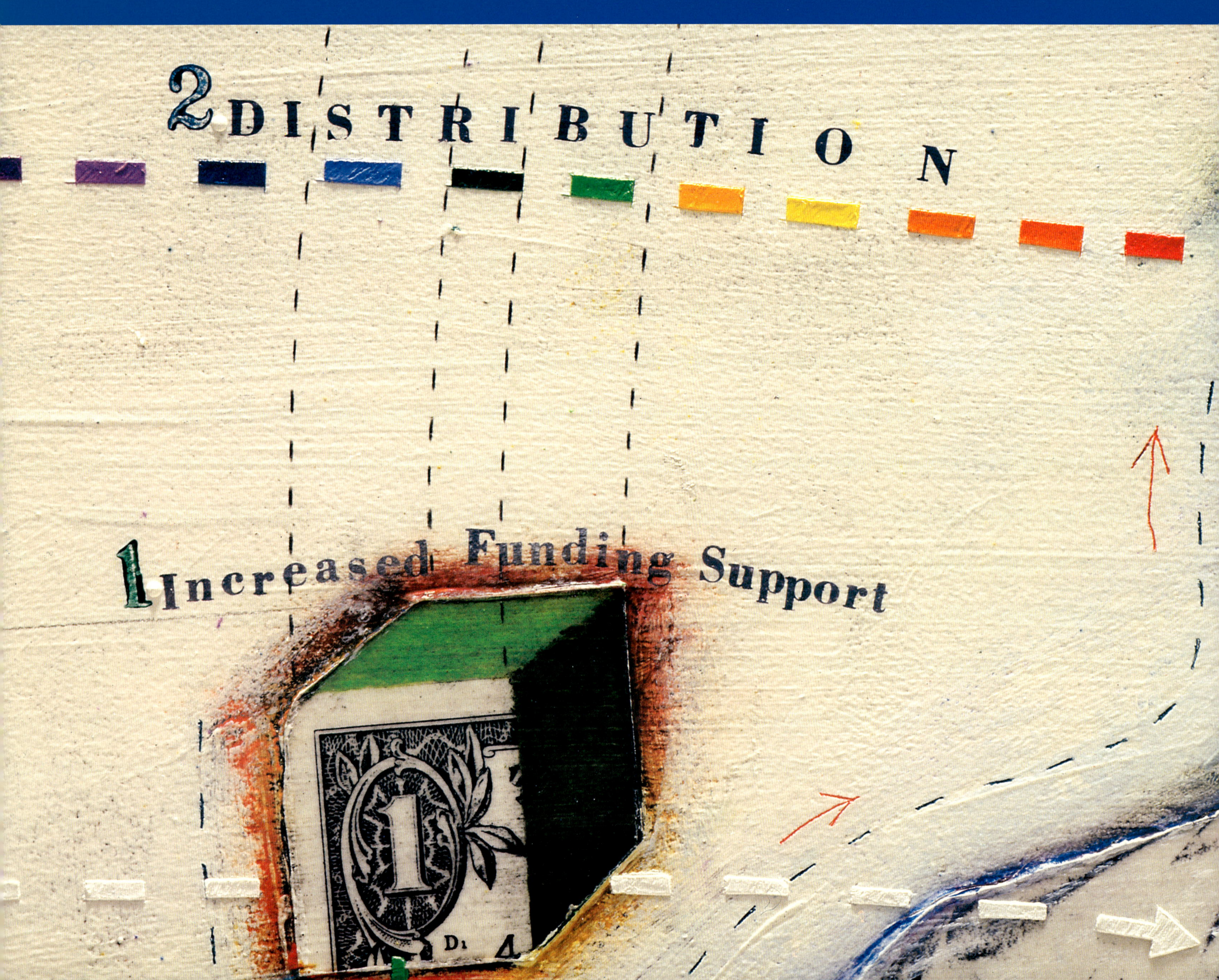

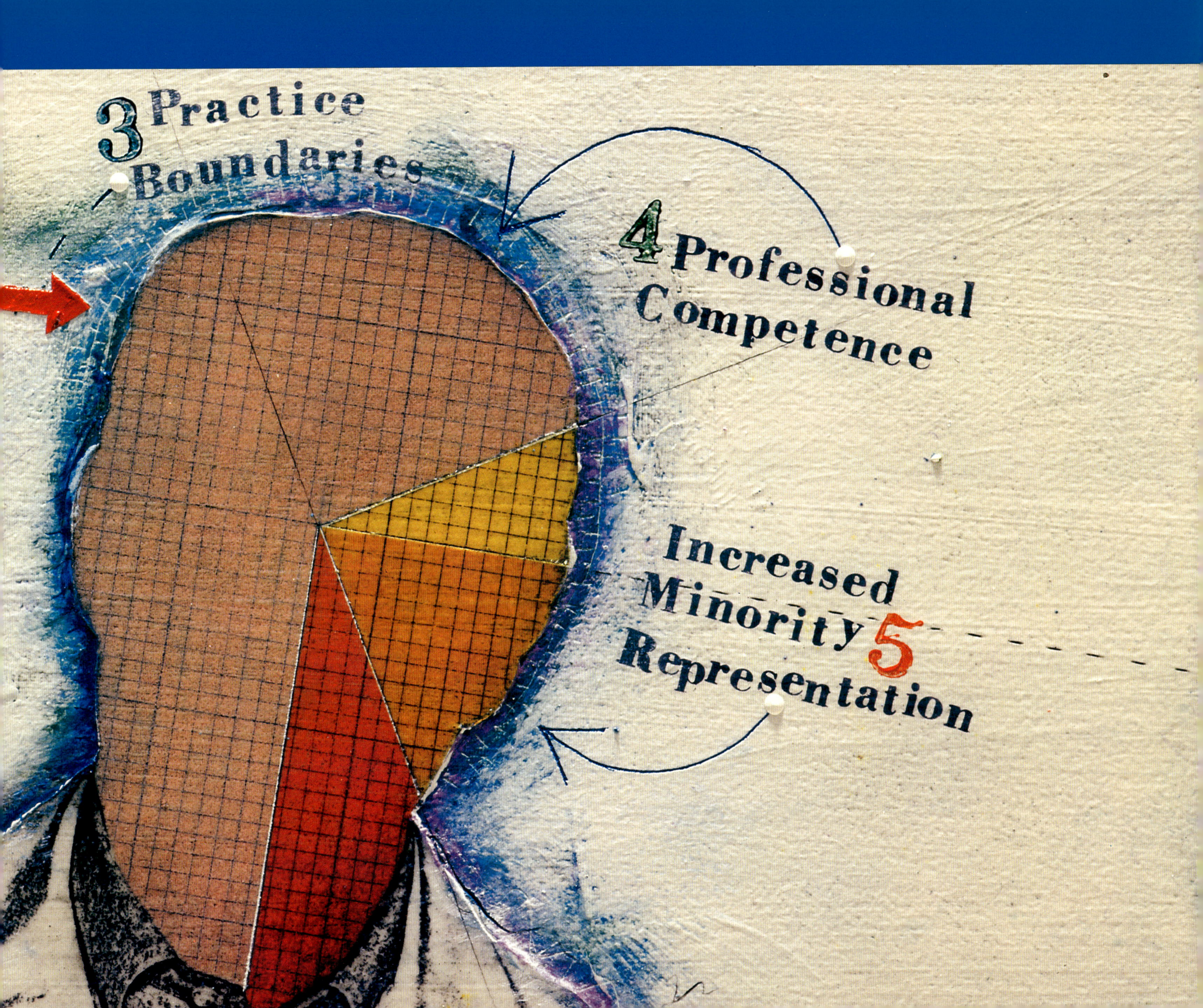

3 Practice Boundaries
4 Professional Competence
Increased Minority 5 Representation

Education for the health professions in the United States is thought to be the best in the world. The concentration on education, research, and patient care ensures that health professionals have a sound theoretical basis, a continuing interest in the advancement of knowledge, and practical experience. The cooperation between teaching institutions and the research community has led to new technology and new treatments that are of inestimable benefit to our society.

The quality of health care depends on the quality of the education professionals receive. We must ensure that competent and caring professionals meet the demands of our society.

To maintain this high quality, a number of issues related to the education, supply, and distribution of health professionals need to be addressed. The quality of health care depends upon the quality of the education of those who provide care. And the education of health professionals is, in turn, dependent upon adequate financing of both undergraduate and clinical graduate programs. Since 1980, total spending to train professionals has dropped sharply. Much of this reduction occurred through the elimination of capitation grants (grants that were established in the early 1970s to encourage professional schools to increase their enrollments) and institutional assistance, as well as through significant reductions in National Health Service Corps grants. The question of how to provide financial support for clinical graduate education is being widely discussed at present, and much of this discussion is directed toward third-party payors' responsibilities. Educational institutions are increasingly reliant on income from patient-care revenues and tuition fees paid by students. It is important that decreased financial support not lead to deterioration in the high quality of the nation's health professions' educational system.

Representation of minorities in the health professions has not markedly improved during the past 15 years. Efforts must be renewed to provide equal access to educational programs, and to provide financial and other support services to enable under-represented groups to stay in and graduate from school.

The role of foreign medical graduates (FMGs) is changing. In the early 1970s, FMGs accounted for one-third of all students in training in the United States, but FMGs are now filling only 18% of all residency positions. There has also been a marked change in the composition of the FMG pools—in 1979, 35% of FMGs in residency programs

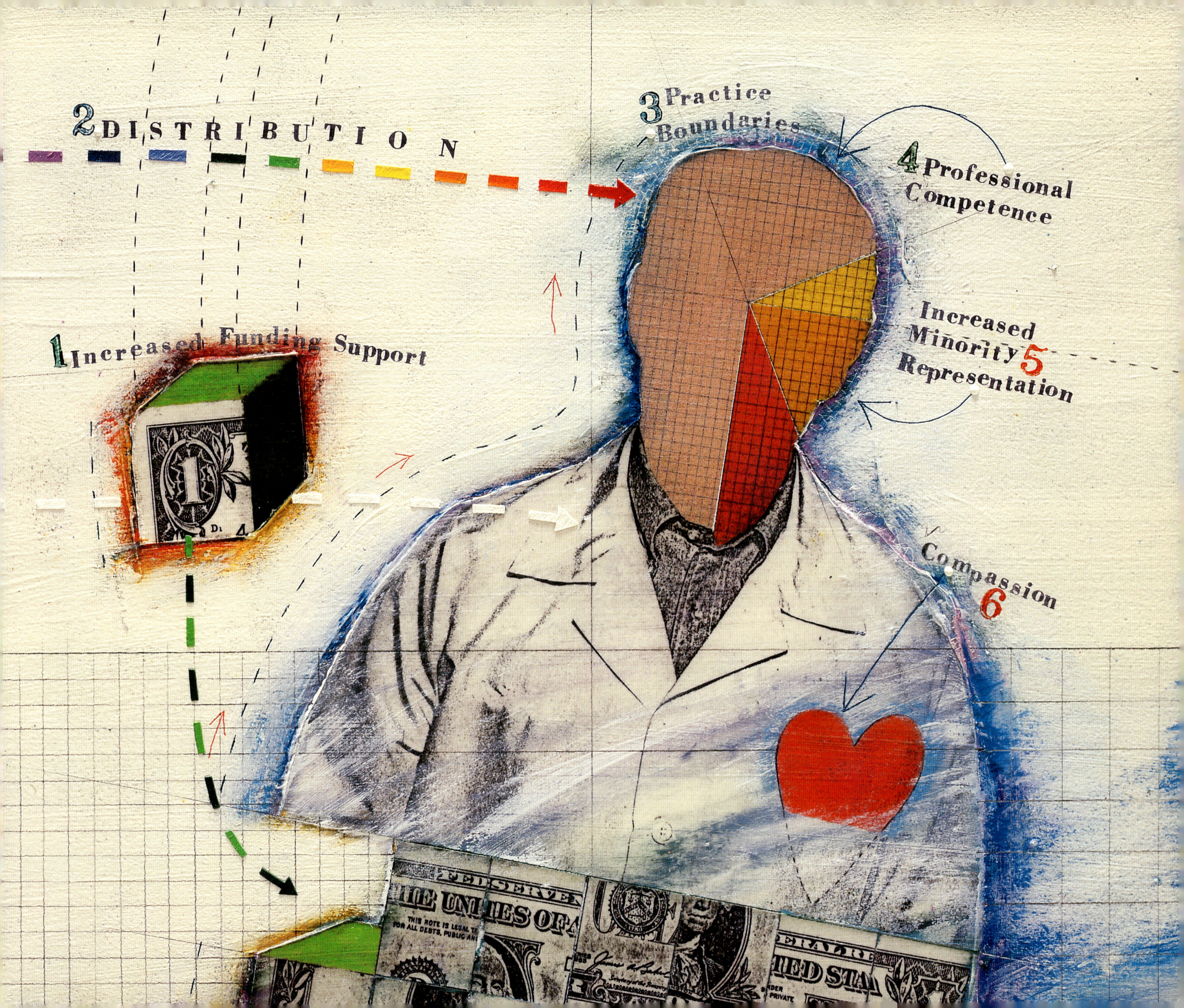

2 DISTRIBUTION
3 Practice Boundaries
4 Professional Competence
Increased Minority Representation 5
1 Increased Funding Support
Compassion 6
THE UNITED STATES OF
THE FEDERAL RESERVE
THIS NOTE IS LEGAL TENDER FOR ALL DEBTS, PUBLIC AND PRIVATE

were U.S. citizens who attended medical schools abroad; the comparable percentage in 1984 was 55%. Mechanisms are needed to ensure that FMGs who choose to take advanced professional education or to practice in this country meet the same or equivalent standards of competence required of graduates of accredited U.S. health professions programs.

One of the most frequently cited complaints about health care, aside from its cost, is that health professionals do not exhibit the degree of compassion for their patients that they did in the past. Increased specialization, technological innovations, and the need to control the cost of health care have no doubt contributed to a more depersonalized type of care, and increased emphasis needs to be placed on the need to prepare practitioners who are not only competent but also compassionate in their attitudes toward their patients.

The supply of health professionals has grown in the past few decades, and it is expected to grow into the next century. There are many who are concerned that the United States is heading into an era when it will have too many health professionals. But there are others who believe that the marketplace will ensure that an excess will never exist and/or that there can never be too many health professionals. The ultimate goal, of course, is to achieve and maintain an adequate supply and distribution of health professionals to meet the health care needs of all of the American people, including the needs of those presently underserved or inappropriately served by the current system.

The increasing supply of health professionals is likely to result in more disputes over practice boundaries among and within the various professions. Health professionals should be allowed to provide those services for which they have trained and which they are competent to perform. Furthermore, individual members of the public should be able to exercise free and informed choice among the diverse qualified health professionals who provide similar or identical services.

The rate at which scientific knowledge is expanding makes the maintenance of professional competence a matter of concern both to health professionals and to the public. Health professionals must ensure that the best possible care is being provided to patients, and the public is legitimately concerned about the necessity for health profes-sionals to maintain competence over the course of their careers. To maintain competence, health professionals have an obligation to participate in continuing education programs, and these programs should be designed to meet changes in the field of health care delivery.

Specific recommendations concerning educational needs and requirements, supply and distribution, and boundaries of practice as they affect health care professionals are discussed in this chapter.

Financing Undergraduate Education

For purposes of this discussion, the term "undergraduate education" refers to education leading to the first professional degree. Even though most physicians earn BA degrees before entering medical school, the MD is considered an undergraduate or first profes-sional degree.

Financial support of health professions education historically has come from varied sources, including federal and state government appropriations, alumni and foundations, university budgets, patient revenues, and tuition. In the 1960s and early 1970s, institutions sponsoring health professions education received increased governmental support; since that time, federal training and research grants have been sharply reduced and federal capitation grants have been phased out. Coupled with this curtailment of federal support, many states and localities are reappraising their financial commitment to both public and private institutions. Forced to adjust to these economic realities, educational institutions have generally reduced expenditures and are increasingly reliant upon income from patient-care revenues and tuition fees paid by students.

The rising cost of education is a matter of concern to educators and to the public. Increases in tuition in both public and private institutions have made health professions education less desirable for some prospective applicants (particularly minority applicants), and have contributed significantly to the debt burdens of all students who lack private sources to finance their educations. In addition, although practice by full-time faculty has always been viewed as desirable in the educational process, the dependence on practice revenue in teaching programs is of concern to many educators because the larger amount of time spent earning fees from practice leaves less faculty time available for direct teaching responsibilities.

An important issue is preserving the high quality of the health professions educational system and assuring equal access to educational opportunities for qualified students. A pluralistic system of financial support for health professions education should be continued, because the multiple bases of support reduce the consequences of exposure to economic pressures or to fluctuations of individual funding sources. Ideally, the system for funding undergraduate education for health professionals will ensure high standards, minimize the cost of quality education, and allow the enrollment of a diverse group of students.

The participants of the Health Policy Agenda believe that financial aid should be based on demonstrated need, and as it cannot be assumed that funding will always be sufficient to cover the costs of education, the issue of reducing costs should be addressed.

Pluralistic Financial Support for Undergraduate Education

Educators are concerned about relying on a single source of income to support undergraduate education of health professionals because the source of income can affect the educational program. Financial support must be adequate to maintain the quality of educational programs, and the pluralistic system of financial support for undergraduate education for the health professions should be maintained. Both the public and private sectors have roles to play in contributing to the financing of undergraduate education; specific recommendations are outlined below.

Federal, State, and Local Government Support for Undergraduate Education

In light of the value that society places on quality health care, the federal, state, and local governments have an obligation to continue their support for the education of health professionals. The federal government should continue its support of undergraduate education for the health professions, especially to enhance access to the professions for minority and disadvantaged students and to supply professionals to underserved areas. The role of the Armed Forces, the Public Health Service, and the Veterans Administration in health professions education is important and should be continued. The federal

government's role as guarantor of loans and provider of research grants should also be maintained. Activities that publicize the need for continuation of appropriations for health professions education are essential. In addition, the federal government should monitor its spending on health professions education and make the data available on an annual basis.

Traditionally, state and local governments have provided a greater percentage of the support for health professions education than has the federal government, and this support has become even more important as some sections of the federal government reduce funding. In some ways this may be a desirable shift because the states and localities are in a better position than the federal government to judge the local nonfederal manpower requirements and to determine the educational resources that will be needed for these programs.

State and local governments should continue to support undergraduate programs of education for the health professions. The legislative staffs of health professions organizations must join with the faculty of teaching institutions in justifying support for health professions education. When preparing their plans for legislative activities every year, health professions organizations should consult with health professions schools in order to include information about education in those plans.

Faculty and administrators in programs of health professions education already provide state governments, including state legislatures, with information on the health education needs within the state. These efforts must continue.

Additional Support for Undergraduate Education

Alumni have a continuing responsibility to provide support for health professions education. Whether through voluntary participation in direct educational endeavors or through financial support of institutions, the practicing professional concerned with the welfare of the nation should actively support the educational system.

The commercial segments of the health care sector also bear responsibility for the education of health professionals. The long-term viability of the health care delivery system depends on the education of new professionals, and all providers should accept a part of this responsibility. Health maintenance organizations, which provide care to an increasing portion of the population, should work to facilitate the educational process. Some of these organizations already recognize and act on these responsibilities, affiliating with professional schools to provide educational opportunities in their facilities. Similarly, for-profit enterprises in the health care sector should accept that their role in the provision of care carries with it some responsibility for the system as a whole.

Public and private programs of undergraduate education for the health professions should actively solicit contributions from alumni and from private foundations. Organizations representing health professionals should mount fund-raising campaigns to aid programs in their discipline, seeking funds both from foundations and alumni. Health professions schools and the organizations that represent them should widely publicize the support received from commercial segments of the health care sector.

Voluntary teaching by practitioners in a variety of settings is an important contribution to a school, and studies should be conducted to determine the feasibility of providing additional incentives for volunteer teaching activities. Specifically, studies should be made of the feasibility of introducing tax deductions or credits for practitioners who volunteer their time for educational purposes. Current regulations prohibit tax deductions for the value of time devoted to charitable purposes. Permitting such deductions should encourage involvement of additional volunteer faculty and significantly enhance the current system.

Patient Care Income and Undergraduate Education

In many health professions, undergraduate training for nursing, pharmacy, and allied health education occurs in a hospital setting. Hospitals have been able to recover a portion of these educational costs through third-party reimbursements and in fact there is growing institutional reliance on income derived from providing health care services through medical and dental training programs. Recent changes in the reimbursement system may threaten the viability of these teaching programs. Teaching hospitals in particular can be dramatically affected by changes in reimbursement regulations, and because the educa-

tional process is heavily dependent upon access to patients, the financial stability of teaching hospitals is crucial.

While income from patient care should be used to support undergraduate education programs for the health professions, disproportionate reliance on this source of funding should be avoided. Health professions organizations, including organizations of health professions schools, should monitor the effect of the introduction of new reimbursement systems and the growth of alternative health care delivery systems on undergraduate education programs. When the educational system is adversely affected, steps must be taken to assure the financial viability of educational programs.

A related concern is that faculty may have to devote more of their time to patient care than to teaching in order to provide revenue for the support of the teaching institution. As faculty devote more of their time to practice, there are risks and benefits for educational institutions that must be carefully assessed. The teacher/practitioner provides a different role model from that of the teacher/academician. Further, the energy devoted to patient care may detract from an institution's educational mission.

Student Tuition and Fees for Undergraduate Education

Student tuition payments constitute an increasing fraction of the revenues of many educational institutions. The cost of educating health professionals is high because of the intense one-on-one clinical experiences that are essential to producing qualified professionals. These costs influence tuition rates. Recently there have been substantial increases in tuition in both public and private institutions, increases which have made health professions education less desirable for some prospective applicants and have contributed significantly to the debt burden of all students who lack the private resources to finance their educations.

Undue reliance on tuition and fees to support undergraduate education for the health professions should be avoided. Health professions organizations and organizations of health professions schools should monitor on an annual basis changes in tuition rates and the proportion of total revenues of health professions schools that is derived from tuition. Appropriate action should be taken to ensure that excessive tuition and fees do not prevent qualified students, especially underrepresented groups, from obtaining an education.

Financial Aid and Undergraduate Education

Concern about the impact of rising tuition makes it important to raise additional funds for financial aid. The current practice of charging all students the same tuition rate and deciding financial aid on a case-by-case basis should be continued.

Student financial aid at the undergraduate level for health professionals should be based on demonstrated need. Programs of health professions education should review student financial aid programs. Legislative staff of associations of health professions schools and of associations representing practitioners should provide legislators with information about the need for financial aid. Regulations setting limits on the amount of aid available based on parental income should take into account the size of families and other limitations on parental abilities to assist children.

Financial Aid Trust Funds for Undergraduate Education

Undergraduate programs for health professions education should consider financial aid trust funds as a means of increasing funding for student financial aid, including scholarships. These trust funds can be financed in two ways. As schools raise tuition levels, a fraction of the increased revenue should be earmarked for financial aid to qualified students from disadvantaged backgrounds. Alternatively, future tuition receipts could be used as the base for revenue bonds to support an investment portfolio. In either case the interest income from student loans could finance educational aid. For this reason, and because students benefit from the educational investment, the trust fund proceeds should finance loans rather than scholarships.

The argument in favor of the financial aid trust fund concept is that relatively low tuition levels could be raised without precluding access to education for individuals with limited financial resources. However, a drawback to financial aid trust funds is the degree to which they may limit the flexibility of school administrators. When feasible, schools should establish trust funds using income from tuition payments. When desirable, health professions schools and associations representing practitioners should encourage legislators to establish the means for issuing tax-exempt bonds for support of these trust funds.

Cost Containment in Undergraduate Education

There is limited potential for reducing the real cost of educating health professionals. However, when possible, the costs of undergraduate education should be reduced; cost-containment measures include eliminating duplication of classes and facilities, controlling the length of education programs, reviewing the use of preceptorships as a teaching strategy, and contract education.

Eliminating the duplication of classes and facilities in academic health science centers is probably the most promising avenue for cost savings that will not impair the quality of the educational enterprise. For example, rather than teaching basic science courses in each of the health professions, common courses should be devised when possible.

Savings also may be effected by preventing the lengthening of educational programs and by altering teaching strategies. Medical schools have experimented with a six-year combined premedical and medical curriculum, and this strategy is one that is recommended as a means of reducing costs. It should be acknowledged, however, that educational programs may need to be lengthened when new treatment modalities are introduced or when the knowledge base for a profession expands.

Much of the health professions education is provided as preceptorships, which require a low student-teacher ratio. Attention can be given to whether the imperative to reduce costs requires higher student-teacher ratios than is possible through widespread use of preceptorships.

Contract education is, on occasion, a cost-effective alternative to the development of entirely new educational programs. It can also be considered an appropriate alternative to controlling costs through reduction in the size of existing educational programs. (Reducing the size of classes in programs of health professions education would probably have only a marginal effect on the cost of educational programs, since it would still be necessary to maintain faculty in all subject areas and to retain library, laboratory, and other facilities for the smaller-sized classes. Per-student costs would assuredly increase. Economically, it would be preferable to close one program or institution rather than to reduce enrollments in several.) Contract education is especially useful when local conditions warrant only small-scale involvement in health professions education. For example, a state government may enter into a contract with an educational institution in another state to provide for student enrollment in educational programs. Once enrolled, the student may pay a lower tuition because of the state's financial contribution. Contract education cannot substitute for a public higher education system. It can, however, supplement that system when the need for greater educational capacity is transitory, or when a state is too small to support an efficient educational program. The use of existing or new contract education programs should be examined by health professions educators and administrators if there is a need to reduce the costs of education.

Financial Data on the Costs of Undergraduate Education

A basic step in making sound financial policy is to understand the current environment, but financial data for many health professions educational systems are not regularly collected. A consistent, comparable data collection strategy on the costs of undergraduate education should be used by all health professions. Collecting financial data is a costly and difficult undertaking. Resources should be donated by the schools themselves or their organizations. Medicine and dentistry already have roughly comparable systems of data collection that could be used as models for other professions.

Financing Clinical Graduate Education

The high quality of clinical graduate education programs for the health professions in this country ensures that patients are provided with excellent care. While the specific content of programs differs from one profession to another, "hands on" patient care experiences are a part of all professional training programs, and most of this experience occurs in hospitals. Clinical trainees benefit both from the didactic education they receive and from the practical experience they gain in providing care to patients under the supervision of experienced faculty.

Funding for clinical graduate education, including the payment of stipends to trainees, also varies considerably among the health professions. For example, there are few graduate-level programs for allied health professionals, and clinical trainees are rarely provided with stipends. However, hospitals may request payment from undergraduate institutions based on the hospitals' involvement in training allied health professionals. Dentists, podiatrists, and pharmacists may receive stipends as a result of their involvement in clinical graduate education programs, but nurses enrolled in graduate programs that are clinical in nature do not get stipends and, for the most part, services rendered to patients are not reimbursed.

For example, most professional entry-level education in the allied health professions is offered at the baccalaureate, associate, or hospital certificate level, and there are only a few entry-level graduate programs. Dental graduates are able to enter practice after completing graduate training in one of eight dental specialties, or they can receive post-graduate training in general practice or advanced general dentistry. Clinical education in nursing for initial licensure is offered at the baccalaureate, associate, and hospital diploma levels. There are three areas of functional concentration in masters level nursing programs—clinical specialization, nursing education, and nursing services administration. Pharmacy degrees can be obtained at either the baccalaureate or graduate level. Pharmacy programs for residents include general hospital pharmacy, clinical pharmacy, or a specialized pharmacy residency. Podiatric medical training is offered at the post-baccalaureate level, and upon graduation and completion of national examinations, the podiatric resident is eligible for licensure.

Although there are variations among the health professions regarding the payment of stipends to graduate trainees, increasing requirements for graduate education in professions such as dentistry, nursing, pharmacy and podiatry will increase the number of programs and trainees that seek monetary assistance. At the same time, clinical graduate education, like undergraduate education, is being affected by attempts to contain costs. Most of the debate over the financing of clinical graduate education has focused on insurance and government—especially Medicare—contributions.

Patients in a teaching hospital benefit directly from graduate programs— because trainees are always on duty, care is provided very quickly upon admittance, and continuous monitoring of care is also possible. Additionally, a major part of clinical graduate education occurs in tertiary hospitals in which very highly specialized care is provided to severely ill or injured patients. Specialists are called as needed, but it would be very expensive for these specialists to provide the extensive amount of care that is now provided by trainees.

However, concern over the rising costs of medical care has resulted in efforts by third-party payors to limit their financial liability for medical services, and the definition of community obligation has begun to change. Third-party payors are questioning the hospitals' traditional practice of subsidizing services deemed worthy of the community but not explicitly financed by it, such as the costs of education and care for the poor.

Certainly programs of clinical graduate education add to the costs of teaching hospitals and the specialized and uncompensated care provided in these hospitals tends to make these hospitals less competitive in terms of per-patient treatment costs. But when compared to the total increase in health care costs, increases in the cost of graduate education have been modest—in fact, costs of graduate education constitute a smaller percentage of total health care costs at present than in earlier years.

The welfare of the public requires continued support for clinical graduate education, and these programs should be funded by the public and private sector, trainees, patients, and third-party payors. There are two major cost components in clinical graduate education—stipends for trainees and other educational costs such as faculty time, classrooms, libraries, and facilities. While changes in the method of financing clinical graduate education are inevitable, these changes should not adversely affect the high quality of programs or access to care.

Because clinical graduate education occurs at the same time as the treatment of patients under supervision, separating the educational costs from total health care costs in the hospital and ambulatory setting is extremely difficult. Efforts have been made, but the results have not been widely accepted and therefore this issue remains quite controversial. The participants of the Health Policy Agenda believe that patient care costs associated with educational programs should continue to be included in payments made by Medicare and by insurance carriers. Teaching hospitals that engage in patient care activities—including research, tertiary care for severely ill patients, and uncompensated care—should be reimbursed by all payors. Stipends should be paid to clinical graduate trainees because they do provide services to patients, but they should be paid at a lower rate than practitioners. However, payments should not be made twice for the same services; i.e., hospitals should not bill for services provided by both residents and the supervising physician. When calculating the value of services, the teaching responsibilities of clinical graduate trainees should be considered. To control the costs of clinical graduate education, professional organizations should undertake a study of potential cost-savings innovations, including the shortening of educational programs. Finally, medical residency training programs and subspecialty training programs require continued support.

Support for Clinical Graduate Education

To maintain the current quality of educational programs, compensation arrangements that depend on all payors for patient services, as well as specific private and public programs for direct educational support, must be continued. A system of financing clinical graduate education that includes support from patient care revenues, including payments from Medicare and major insurance carriers, as well as specific subsidies, should be maintained. Because all of the costs of clinical graduate education cannot be paid from patient care revenues alone, federal, state, and local governments, as well as private foundations and private industry, should provide some share of support for clinical graduate education as part of their support for health professions education. The role of the Armed Forces, the Public Health Service, and the Veterans Administration in clinical graduate education should be continued.

Reimbursement for Education Program Costs in Teaching Institutions

Because of their limited experience and as part of the learning process, clinical graduate trainees at times order diagnostic tests that would not be ordered by an experienced practitioner. Additionally, supervising faculty must prepare their trainees to treat patients with diseases not previously encountered, and they must also review the work performed by trainees. These activities have traditionally been reimbursed as indirect medical education costs, and additional patient care costs associated with educational programs should continue to be included in payments made by Medicare and by insurance carriers. Direct patient payments should also pay for these costs.

Reimbursement for Special Functions of Teaching Institutions

At present, Medicare payment procedures treat the costs of providing uncompensated care and the care for severely ill or injured patients as indirect medical education costs. However, there is some question as to whether these are educational costs per se. For example, although teaching hospitals as a group provide a substantial proportion of care to patients who cannot pay and although clinical graduate education is provided primarily in tertiary hospitals, such care may or may not be related to the educational mission of the hospital. The fact that provision of such care is considered to be an indirect medical education cost may, at times, seriously overstate the true cost of clinical education. Teaching hospitals that engage in patient care activities including research, tertiary care for severely ill patients, and uncompensated care, should be reimbursed by all payors in both the public and private sectors. In other words, the costs of performing such activities and functions should not be considered as an indirect medical education cost, and should be borne by all payors. If reimbursement cannot be provided for treating patients who cannot pay, the responsibility for treating these patients should be shared among all hospitals, both profit and not-for-profit.

Payment of Stipends to Trainees in Clinical Graduate Education Programs

Clinical graduates treat patients under the supervision of experienced practitioners and should be paid for their work. The modest stipends and benefits paid to clinical graduates can be viewed as contributions to cover the value of their services in excess of their educational costs. Stipends should be paid to trainees in professions requiring lengthy education when the trainee provides patient care services.

Clinical graduate trainees often perform other important services. For example, advanced trainees often serve as instructors. In the university setting it is a common practice to pay graduate assistants for their teaching services. Similarly, when calculating the value of services, the teaching responsibilities of clinical graduate trainees should be considered. Salaries and stipends should be viewed as payment for teaching as well as for patient care services.

Controlling the Costs of Clinical Graduate Education Programs

In some cases, the time required to complete clinical graduate education is being lengthened because of the development of new and complex diagnostic and treatment procedures. Nevertheless, the possibility of limiting or even reducing the length of training time must not be neglected as it is a major means of controlling the present cost of clinical graduate education. A study of potential cost-saving innovations in programs of clinical graduate education, including, when feasible, the shortening of the duration of education, should be undertaken by professional organizations responsible for such training. While the value of the services provided by trainees should be considered, subsidized training should not continue beyond the point when the trainee is able to practice without supervision. The review of educational programs should ensure that the length of training is justified by the need to master clinical knowledge and skills. Other methods to control the costs of training, such as better supervision, should be considered as well.

Support for Residency Training and Subspecialty Training

Unlike the other recommendations in this section, these recommendations deal exclusively with *medical* residency training.

Physicians represent the largest group of health professionals seeking clinical graduate education. In 1985, for example, there were slightly over 78,000 residents on duty. In the same year, about $1.6 billion was spent on their stipends and benefits, and most of these funds came from Medicare, Medicaid, Blue Cross, and commercial insurance payments for patient care. An amount at least equivalent to the cost of stipends is spent on other educational costs, and most of these costs are also paid from patient care revenues.

About 28% of the hospitals that participate in Medicare have programs for training physicians after medical school graduation. Under Medicare's hospital payment system based on diagnosis-related groups (DRGs), teaching hospitals receive two kinds of special payments—one for "direct" medical education costs and one for "indirect" medical education costs. Direct medical education costs include stipends for residents, salaries for teachers, and classroom costs. Until recently, direct costs for graduate medical education were based on a "reasonable cost" reimbursement system; i.e., they were paid in proportion to the share of each hospital's total cost generated by Medicare patients. Under the newly enacted Consolidated Omnibus Budget Reconciliation Act of 1986 (COBRA), Medicare payments will be made on the basis of each hospital's average cost per resident, with adjustments for general economic inflation. Indirect medical education costs represent the added costs for patient services borne by teaching hospitals as a consequence of their educational mission; Medicare pays for indirect costs associated with teaching programs such as increased diagnostic testing, increased numbers of procedures, higher staffing ratios, and treatment of severely ill patients. Medicare pays for those indirect costs through an add-on to the DRG payment rate—hospitals with approved medical education programs receive an additional payment based on the ratio of full-time-equivalent residents to the hospitals' number of beds. In 1988, Congress is expected to conclude its study on the advisability of providing additional payments to hospitals serving a large number of indigent patients, and further modifications in the payment for indirect costs may be made. Medicare currently provides about $2.5 billion to teaching hospitals for both the direct and indirect costs of approved medical education programs.

Under COBRA, a limit was placed on the number of years of residency training that Medicare will finance. Under this act, Medicare will not recognize costs for an intern or resident whose training exceeds five years or the minimum number of years of formal training necessary to satisfy initial board eligibility in his or her specialty. Medicare and other third-party payments should be made for the number of years of residency training required for admission to basic specialty board examinations or for five years.

Also under COBRA, residents assigned to hospital outpatient departments will continue to be counted in determining the indirect teaching adjustment. Despite the fact that a considerable amount of residency training is provided in large teaching hospitals, there are sound educational reasons for increasing the amount of residency training provided in ambulatory settings. Primary care physicians in particular see more patients in office and clinical settings than in hospital settings, and training in these settings would be beneficial. Rules concerning payments for residency training should be changed to permit payments for such training provided in ambulatory settings. The trend toward providing more patient care in outpatient settings reduces the number of patients in hospitals. Residents may need to work in outpatient settings simply to ensure that there see an adequate number of patients and receive a comprehensive training experience.

The welfare of the public requires continued training of medical and surgical subspecialists. Inadequate financial support for subspecialty training may lead to a decline in the number of physicians seeking such training, the accumulation of large debts for those who do, or in the entry of only those individuals with unlimited financial resources. For these reasons, subspecialty training should be supported. Medicare and third-party payments should not be used to pay for the training of subspecialists, but subspecialists should be supported with stipends that might be derived from budget revisions, program economies, or other funds. As at present, foundation grants and private industry should provide some of the support for such training.

Minorities in the Health Professions

For a variety of reasons, the diversity of the population in this country is not adequately represented among students enrolled in programs of education for the health professions nor, as a consequence, among health care practitioners themselves. Specifically, "underrepresented groups" are defined as including certain ethnic and racial minorities, students with low incomes, students from rural areas, women students in some professions, and disabled persons. Some increases in minority enrollment in health professions education

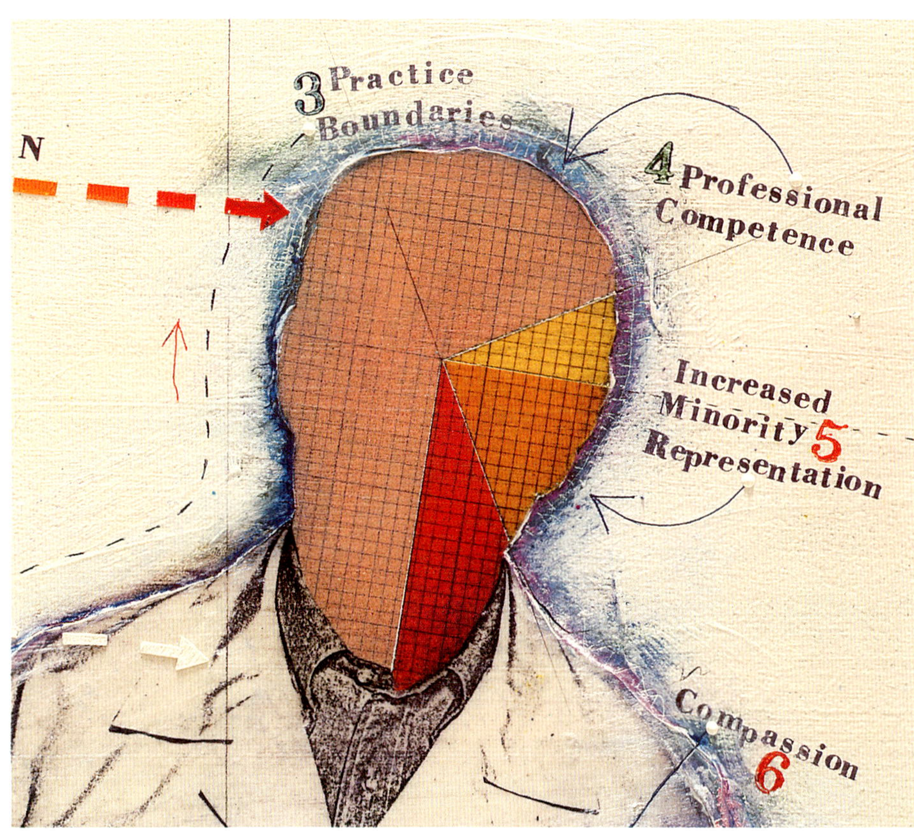

We must increase our efforts to provide equal access and financial support for underrepresented groups in health professions education.

have occurred over the past 30 years, but these increases are insufficient.

Cultural, social, economic, and personal factors have all played a role in limiting the enrollment of underrepresented groups in programs of health professions education. In particular, the absence of role models, lack of knowledge of career opportunities within the health professions, inadequate preprofessional preparation, and stereotyped views of faculty, administrators, and counselors serve to discourage participation in health professions education. In addition, economic considerations can discourage prospective applicants and cause qualified persons to choose other careers with shorter training periods and less educational indebtedness.

The importance of this issue extends beyond the principle of equal opportunity for individuals. A major concern is the need for improvement in the health of minority and rural citizens, and the quality of care provided them. The incidence of disease is much higher among minority groups, the poor, and rural residents than it is in the general population. While the participants of the Health Policy Agenda do not subscribe to the position that good care can be provided only by persons of the same racial and social background, there are times when an understanding of cultural and social circumstances can help a practitioner in providing good care. Furthermore, there is some evidence that students from minority groups are likely to return to their original communities after their education is completed.

Disabled individuals are frequently overlooked when discussing the issue of equal opportunity. However, federal legislation forbids discrimination against disabled persons in programs receiving federal financial assistance. Some progress has been made in encouraging the entry of disabled persons to the health professions, but there is a need for continued support for them during the educational process.

An immediate goal in the near future is to increase the enrollment and graduation of persons traditionally underrepresented in programs of education for the health professions, and as a consequence to increase the number of persons from such groups practicing in the health professions. A broader goal is improved health for those groups that suffer a higher incidence of cancer, heart disease, and other diseases than the population as a whole. Efforts must be renewed to provide equal access to health professions education programs, and to provide financial and other support services that will enable underrepresented groups to stay in and graduate from school. In addition, health professionals must devote some of their resources to improving the educational system at all levels.

Minority Enrollment in Health Professions Education Programs
Each educational institution should accept responsibility for increasing its enrollment of members of underrepresented groups. Educational institutions have the major responsibility for increasing the enrollment of minority and other underrepresented groups in their programs. Considerable effort has been devoted to improving educational opportunities for students from minority groups, from rural areas and from the inner city. These efforts must be continued. Successful recruitment programs have been established at some schools in all health professions, and the performance of students in minority professional schools provides ample evidence that minority students are able to complete these programs.

The associations of health professions schools should monitor the efforts in schools to admit students from underrepresented groups. Institutions should give attention to the use of nontraditional criteria for the admission of students; criteria that place less emphasis on grade point averages and performance on standardized tests and more emphasis on practical experience and nonacademic measures of ability should be considered. The objective is not to admit persons of lesser ability, but to find different means of assessing ability.

Health professions organizations must provide unequivocal support for equal access to education and must support activities undertaken by the government and private agencies toward this end. These organizations are encouraged to reexamine their stated positions on the admission of students from underrepresented groups in educational programs. Existing statements indicating support for the entry of these students to professional education should be reaffirmed, and organizations that have not adopted such statements should do so.

Accrediting bodies are urged to review recruitment and admissions procedures, to consider the success of programs of health professions education in enrolling women, minority students, and students from underrepresented groups, and to share their expertise as part of the accreditation process.

Retention of Minority Students in Health Professions Education Programs
Having gained access to health professions education programs, many minority students find themselves confronting problems in the classroom, including lack of adequate preparation for the curriculum, lack of role models, lack of peer support, and other academic and social problems related to being in a new and unfamiliar environment. Experience to date indicates that educational programs that are successful in graduating significant numbers of previously underrepresented groups provide support through tutorial programs, advisory and counseling services, and peer support programs. These services and programs provide assistance to students to enable them to remain in and ultimately graduate from health professions education programs.

Programs of education for health professions should devise means of improving retention rates for students from underrepresented groups. Students should be given precise information as to who can provide assistance and who can provide advice on the circumstances under which assistance can be sought. Faculty should be alerted very early about the need for remedial or supplementary tutorials. Students may need additional time to complete a prescribed course of study; and even though permitting additional time for completion of a course will increase educational costs and student indebtedness, it should be allowed. However, all courses should have a maximum period of time for completion of studies leading to graduation.

Studies of retention activities should be undertaken and published in professional journals. In addition, accrediting agencies are requested to review arrangements for support of minority students and students from underrepresented groups as part of the accrediting process.

Financial Aid for Minority Students in Health Professions Education Programs
The problems of high educational costs and student indebtedness affect all health professions education programs. However, individual students are affected to different degrees

and in different ways. For many students, particularly minority students, the barrier to education in the health professions is financial. Not only is tuition high in many programs, but scholarship aid is not widely available and loans are expensive. Compounding the problem for many students from minority families is a lack of the financial experience needed to manage extensive indebtedness. Thus, some able students enter the work force as soon as possible, believing that they must begin earning money immediately upon graduation and without fully realizing that additional education will result in increased income. Other qualified students from underrepresented groups choose careers other than the health professions to avoid educational indebtedness.

The need for additional financial aid may be perceived as conflicting with efforts to reduce health care costs. However, funds are needed to increase the proportion of students from underrepresented groups.

Financial assistance, including scholarships, and financial counseling should be provided to minority students who are in need; financial aid should be based on a demonstration of need. Programs of education and the national health professions organizations must support the appropriation of federal and state monies for scholarships and educational loans, but must seek funds from other sources as well. Educational programs must reinforce their efforts to augment institutional funds which can be used for financial assistance. Because of the extent of financial need, scholarships rather than loans are needed for many members of underrepresented groups.

Program administrators should make certain that current information about financial aid is readily available to students, and that financial aid offices are easily accessible. As part of the accrediting process, accrediting bodies are requested to determine that appropriate programs of financial aid have been developed.

Educational loans should be repaid in a timely fashion, and if not in cash, then in kind. Health professions organizations should discuss the feasibility of developing loan forgiveness programs for students who engage in social service programs following completion of their education. These social service programs could be established at both state and federal levels. If a social service plan can be developed, legislative staff of health professions organizations should draft appropriate model legislation.

Entry of Disabled Persons to Health Professions Education Programs
Progress has been made, but disabled persons continue to be underrepresented in programs of education for the health professions. Educational institutions have received information about their responsibilities under the Rehabilitation Act of 1973. In addition, under recently adopted standards for accreditation of medical schools, each health professions school needs to address the standards for the admission of disabled individuals.

Health professions organizations should support the entry of disabled persons to programs of education for the health professions, and programs of health professions education should have established standards concerning the entry of disabled persons. Professional organizations should review their policies on the entry of disabled persons with appropriate ability to the professions. Organizations that do not have a policy of this kind should adopt one. Organizations of health professions education should prepare statements regarding standards for entry to educational programs and to the practice of the professions, which can guide programs of education in developing their own standards.

Financial and Support Services for Disabled Persons in Health Professions Educational Programs
Disabled persons deserve the same consideration for financial support and advisory services as other individuals in health professions educational programs. There may be a need for additional services to support disabled persons, ranging from special equipment to the removal of physical barriers in buildings, rooms, and doorways, to transportation to and from classes.

Financial support and advisory services and other support services should be provided to disabled persons in health professions education programs. Assistance to the disabled during the educational process should be provided through special programs funded from public and private sources. Periodic reviews of educational facilities should be conducted to ensure that disabled persons have free and unencumbered access to all buildings and rooms. Periodic surveys should also be conducted to ensure that special needs of disabled persons are being met or can be addressed. Health professions educators should ensure that adequate support services and financial support are available to disabled persons.

Collection of Data on Minority Students in Health Professions Education Programs
Extensive data are available on minority students in dental, medical, and pharmacy schools, but better data on enrollment and graduation are needed for other health fields. Data must be collected about underrepresented groups in health professions education as a means of improving recruitment and educational activities. Steps need to be taken to arrange available data in forms that permit comparison among the professions, and professional organizations need to cooperate in standardizing collection efforts.

Representatives of the associations of health professions schools should meet to discuss the need for information about student enrollments in general and the enrollment of students from underrepresented groups in particular. The associations should agree on the general categories for which information will be collected and should discuss the format in which information will be published. To the extent possible, a standard format for publication should be used.

Health professions organizations, including the organizations of health professions schools, should collect information about applicant pools and about the enrollment and graduation of underrepresented groups. Schools should track students after graduation as a means of collecting information about their practices, particularly about where the practice is established, what communities are served, and what the experience is in career advancement. Attention is directed to the excellent information concerning minority students in medical schools provided by the American Association of Medical Colleges, and to the reporting activities of the Association of Minority Health Professions Schools.

Educational Outreach Programs in Health Professions Education
Programs of health professions education should join in outreach programs directed at providing information to prospective students and at enriching educational programs in secondary and undergraduate schools. Minority graduation rates at the high school level must be improved. Students must learn of careers open to them, and of the educational requirements for entry into these careers. State departments of education and local school districts must be supported in efforts to strengthen graduation requirements, so that students will be prepared to enter health professions or other science-based education.

School administrators and faculty must also be supported in efforts to improve graduation rates. The stereotypes that relegate women to literature courses instead of science, and minority students to the manual arts instead of mathematics, must be eliminated, and students must be encouraged to achieve their full capacity as individuals. Students should be encouraged to study the sciences.

Programs of health professions education should join in outreach programs directed toward enriching the curricula of neighboring schools. Outreach programs can include work/study activities, high school summer programs, and visits to schools and colleges by students and faculty. Faculty and students from programs of health professions education are encouraged to provide volunteer services to local schools directed at enriching educational programs. Government initiatives should be encouraged to foster these outreach activities.

In addition, health professions organizations, especially the organizations of professional schools, should establish regular communication with counselors at both the high school and college level as a means of providing accurate and timely information to students about health professions education. Many programs of health professions education have established liaisons with high schools and colleges as a means of recruiting students. Frequently, however, student advisory offices in high schools and colleges are inadequately staffed, and advisors may not have the information they need to advise students properly.

Relationships with high schools and colleges should be expanded and attention paid to recruiting students from underrepresented groups. Preprofessional counselors should encourage students to prepare for health professions education. In addition, the organizations of professional schools are urged to prepare information concerning entry requirements, costs of education, financial assistance, and the practice of the

Students must study math, science and communication skills beyond the minimum required for graduation from high school if they are to be prepared for entry into programs of health professions education.

profession for distribution to preprofessional counselors.

Educational institutions should recognize the importance of preprofessional counseling and should provide adequate support and funding. Efforts should be made to advance counseling as an educational profession, to raise the status of counselors, and to encourage retention of experienced counselors in their profession. The associations of professional schools are urged to inform the regional scholastic accrediting organizations of the important services provided by counselors and to request that accreditors assure that preprofessional counseling is adequate.

Support of State and Federal Legislation to Strengthen Education
Health professions organizations must support programs directed at strengthening preschool, elementary, and secondary education legislative activities at state and federal levels. Students must study mathematics, science and communication skills beyond the minimum required for graduation from high school if they are to be prepared for entry into programs of health professions education. Every educator can provide examples of promising students who are hampered in professional education as a result of inadequate or late preparation.

Health professions organizations should support legislation proposed at state and federal levels to strengthen preschool, elementary, and secondary education, especially for students from minority and disadvantaged groups in rural and inner-city schools. Increases in teacher salaries, the maintenance of buildings and facilities, and opportunities for continuing education are needed.

Officers of health professions organizations and their legislative staffs should meet annually with national education organizations to discuss and adopt positions on educational legislation before Congress. National organizations should organize similar meetings of state and local organizations to review pending legislation at state and local levels. A particular objective is to assure adequate funding for elementary and secondary education.

Graduates of Foreign Health Professional Schools

The quality of health care is highly dependent on the quality of the education of those who provide care. Quality control mechanisms exist for United States and Canadian health professional schools, but comparable mechanisms cannot easily be applied to schools in other countries, and there is uncertainty surrounding the quality of care that graduates from foreign health professional schools provide.

Graduates of foreign health professional schools practicing in the United States include dentists, nurses, pharmacists, physicians and other health professionals. A major difference between the physician and nonphysician groups is that the former contains a significant number of U.S. citizens, whereas the latter is composed almost entirely of foreign nationals. Only a negligible number of U.S. citizens go abroad to receive training in dentistry, nursing, and pharmacy. In medicine, however, large numbers of U.S. citizens do go abroad for their medical education.

Changes in immigration rules have affected the flow of graduates of foreign health professional schools into this country. For example, until 1965, physicians entering the country as immigrants were subject to the Quota Act of 1921, which favored countries in the Western Hemisphere. In response to a perceived shortage of physicians during the 1960s, the Immigration Act of 1965 established two occupational preference categories: those having an exceptional ability and those with skills in short supply. These preference categories, both applicable to physicians, led to a rapid increase in foreign medical graduates (FMGs). However, in 1976, federal legislation eliminated these preference categories, and since then the percentage of FMGs has remained stable at approximately 20% of the total physician population. Foreign Nurse Graduates (FNGs) were governed by the same immigration laws as FMGs, and the most recent estimate is that about 4% of registered nurses in the country received their primary nurse education in foreign schools. Foreign Dental Graduates (FDGs) have faced immigration policies that are more restrictive than than those faced by either FMGs or FNGs, and less than 1% of pharmacists are foreign-trained.

Changes in the mechanisms to assess the competency of graduates of foreign health professional schools have also affected the supply. As of July 1984, the Foreign Medical Graduate Examination in the Medical Sciences replaced the previous examinations administered by the Educational Commission for Foreign Medical Graduates. The new examination is recognized to be more difficult than previous ones, and FMGs must pass it before they can apply for an Exchange Visitor visa or take a residency position. In fact, FMGs in residency programs have declined from about 32% in 1970 to about 18% in 1985, and with the more difficult exam, fewer FMGs may be eligible for U.S. residencies. FNGs must pass a screening examination before taking the state board licensing exam in most states, and about 20 states will accept FDGs for licensure only if they pass a national examination.

Graduates of foreign health professional schools will continue to come to the United States for their residencies and to practice. Even though there is a perceived surplus of some health care professionals, supply is not the issue here. The Health Policy Agenda's goal is to ensure that graduates of foreign health professions programs who choose to take advanced professional training or to practice in the United States meet the same or equivalent standards of competence as those required of graduates of accredited U.S. health professions programs.

Graduate Education and Practice Requirements for Graduates of Foreign Health Professional Schools

Over the years the United States has made significant contributions to world health and world medicine by making graduate medical education available to foreign national FMGs who have returned to the country of origin upon completion of their training. However FMGs, both foreign nationals and Americans, have experienced considerable difficulty in entering practice or obtaining graduate training here. In 1984, for example, only 22% of foreign nationals and 48% of American FMGs matched with residency positions. And only 24% of foreign nationals and 17% of American FMGs passed the national examination administered in January of 1985. Since 1978, about 38% of FNGs have passed both the nursing and English parts of the examination of the Commission on Graduates of Foreign Nursing Schools. Foreign dental graduates often have serious difficulties meeting the licensure requirements; the failure rate of FDGs on state and regional boards ranged from 31% to 75% between 1970 and 1982.

Among all groups of licensed health professionals, there has been a general trend of strict examination of both academic and clinical qualifications. Dentistry requires supplemental education in a U.S. accredited dental school as the entry-level determination of competence. With the current emphasis on public information and utilization review, more uniform standards and requirements are needed for foreign-trained health professionals seeking to practice in the United States. Two specific concerns are the assessment of the adequacy of the education of foreign or U.S. graduates of foreign health professions programs who desire to practice in this country, and the evaluation of the competency of such graduates for practice.

Any United States or alien graduate of a foreign health professional educational program must, as a requirement for entry into graduate education and/or practice in the United States, demonstrate entry-level competence equivalent to that required of graduates of United States' programs. Agencies recognized to license or certify health professionals in the U.S. should have mechanisms to evaluate the entry-level competence of graduates of foreign health professional programs. The level of competence and the means used to assess it should be the same or equivalent to those required of graduates of U.S. accredited programs.

The Council of State Governments should be invited to establish a task force of representatives of agencies that license health professions to assemble information regarding standards and processes that licensing agencies use at present to evaluate graduates of foreign programs. The task force should then formulate recommendations for mechanisms to evaluate entry-level competence of health professionals based on the experience of agencies that have a record of licensing graduates of foreign programs.

The task of evaluating clinical skills as distinct from clinical knowledge is difficult, and no totally satisfactory method has been devised to date. However, the expertise of the Educational Commission for Foreign Medical Graduates, which has developed the new Foreign Medical Graduate examination in the Medical Sciences, and of the Commission on Graduates of Foreign Nursing Schools, should be called upon by the task force in formulating recommendations regarding eligibility to enter graduate training or to stand for licensure. The means used to assess competence will necessarily vary according to the nature of the specific health profession under consideration, but the processes employed by all states for individual health professions should be uniform.

The National Commission for Health Certifying Agencies should be invited to establish a broadly representative task force to gather information and make recommendations for health professions' certifying agencies similar to those that the Council of State Governments' task force, cited above, is charged to formulate for licensing agencies.

To further strengthen the education of foreign health professionals, foreign health professional schools that graduate students who wish to practice in the United States are encouraged to seek voluntary accreditation of their programs. Agencies recognized to accredit health professions educational programs should convene a series of meetings to explore the development of mechanisms to evaluate foreign health professions programs which have graduates who seek to pursue graduate training or to practice in the U.S. Initial emphasis could be on developing a means to evaluate programs in medicine and nursing, since these have the largest number of graduates seeking further education or practice privileges in the U.S. The accumulated experience and knowledge of all accrediting groups should be used in arriving at appropriate evaluative mechanisms. Consideration should be given to developing ways to recognize the approval given to programs by foreign national approval bodies as well as to ways to evaluate individual programs. The assembly of accrediting agencies should establish task forces to deal with costs, implications for international relations, legal liability and other issues that need resolution before an effective evaluation program for foreign health professions programs can be begun.

Licensure and Credentialing Requirements For Employment in Health Care Facilities

To protect the health and safety of persons being served, all health care facilities, including governmental facilities, should adhere to the same or equivalent licensing and credentialing requirements in their employment practices. Exempting some state and/or federal governmental health care facilities from such requirements is not in the best interest of the populations being served.

Educating Competent and Caring Health Professionals

Probably the most frequently cited complaint about health care, aside from its cost, is that health professionals are not sufficiently compassionate. As the American health care system has grown in size and technological sophistication, it has also grown more impersonal. Many people long for an earlier time when treatment was perceived as being more personal.

Practitioners can make changes in procedures to combat this perceived problem. Efficiency, rather than being measured solely on the basis of cost, can be measured from the point of view of the patient. This can pose a dilemma, of course, in that time spent with patients increases costs. However, a balance must be found between the need for economy and the need to provide for a patient's comfort and sense of well-being. In fact, experience suggests that personal attention aids the healing process.

Providing care that is perceived by patients as compassionate is not an easy task. Compassion is not only a matter of being sympathetic or empathic. Curing disease and caring for the needs of a patient are the best services that a professional can render. The first and major ingredient of compassion is unquestionably professional competence. Professional judgment is an integral part of compassionate care as well. Furthermore, practitioners' attitudes reflect the attitudes of society as a whole, and they will not all demonstrate compassion in the same manner. While it is reasonable to expect health professionals to adhere to somewhat higher standards of behavior, they are members of society and are representative of it.

Although it is the physician who is most frequently criticized, all health professionals share in the responsibility for providing competent and compassionate care.

Inattentiveness on the part of one practitioner serves to discredit all. The participants of the Health Policy Agenda believe that the goal of health professions education should be to prepare practitioners who will be competent to provide care and who will exhibit caring attitudes toward patients. Practitioners must be knowledgeable about the systems in which they work, and must be willing to initiate changes to make the systems operate for the comfort and well-being of patients.

Objectives of Health Professions Education

Health professions organizations and professional schools have a responsibility to provide high quality educational programs. First and foremost, health professions educators are responsible for providing students with a solid foundation of scientific knowledge and skills upon which lifelong learning and professional competence can be based. Faculty should serve as examples to students by participating in continuing education programs themselves, and by exhibiting the intellectual curiosity that ensures that each patient is provided with the best treatment and care that is available. Programs of health professions education should admit students who provide evidence of an interest in lifelong learning and for independent study of problems. A number of reports have been issued which state that educational programs should spend more time on providing students with the tools they need to solve problems when they are in practice and in encouraging a problem-solving approach to their practices. Programs of health professions education should foster educational strategies that encourage students to be independent learners and problem-solvers.

Teaching, the treatment of patients, and research activities are all primary objectives of institutions involved in health professions education, and the fulfillment of each of these objectives ultimately requires the competent and caring treatment of individuals. Faculty of programs of education for the health professions should ensure that the mission statements of the institutions in which they teach include as an objective the education of practitioners who are both competent and compassionate. Faculty can ensure accomplishment of this objective through appropriate consideration in the initial selection of students for admission, and in the education of students as they pursue their degrees. Both of these areas are discussed in detail below.

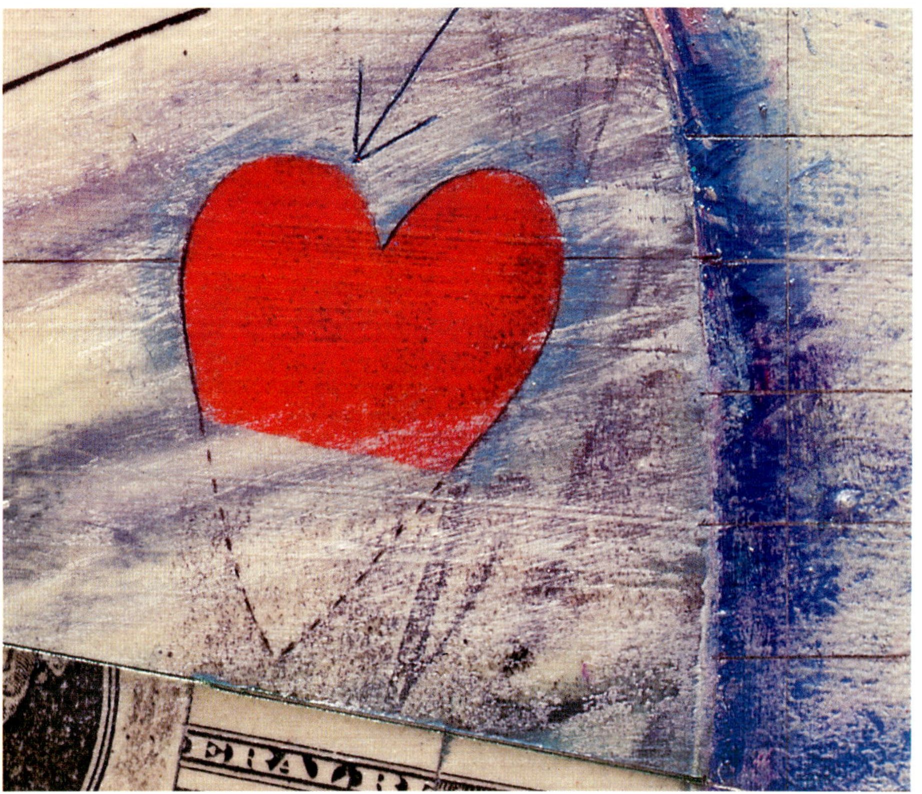

The delivery of quality health care encompasses the use of professional skills, compassionate concern for patients, effective utilization of resources, continuity in patient care, and consideration of the risks and benefits of treatment options.

Selection of Students for Admission into Health Professions Education Programs

Every educational institution seeks the entry of the best students into its programs through the establishment of rigorous academic and personal requirements for admission. Applicants must generally submit transcripts, scores on placement tests, letters of reference and biographical essays, and be interviewed by an admissions committee. However, there are certain pitfalls with each of the criteria used for admissions. For example, most educators agree that admissions should not be based on grade point averages and placement score tests alone because these are not absolute predictors of how a student will perform if admitted. Most also agree that personal attributes of applicants should be taken into consideration, but evaluation of personal characteristics is certainly subjective. Admissions committees may be misled by vague letters of reference. Interviews often are not standardized and different questions are frequently asked of different applicants.

Because of the problems involved in the interpretation of criteria that are used for admissions, it is preferable to use as many performance-related criteria as possible in the admissions process. Admission to a program of health professions education should be based on more than grade point average and performance on admissions tests. Interviews, applicant essays, and references should continue to be part of the application process in spite of difficulties inherent in evaluating them. Because applicants who have engaged in social (as opposed to solitary) activities may be better at establishing interpersonal relationships and because employment records may serve as an indicator of future employment performance, admissions committees should review applicants' extracurricular activities and employment records for indications of suitability for health professions education. It should be noted, however, that the review of extracurricular activities and employment provides an indication but not proof of an applicant's suitability for health professions education.

Admissions committees should be carefully prepared for their responsibilities, and efforts should be made to standardize interview procedures and to evaluate the information gathered during interviews. Faculty should provide admissions committees with guidelines in regard to the weight to be placed on letters of reference, applicant essays, and applicant histories. To the extent possible, interviews should be structured; i.e., committees should make certain that all candidates are asked similar questions and that the conditions under which interviews are conducted are similar.

Because there is uncertainty regarding the predictive validity of criteria that are used for admission to health professions education programs, research should continue to focus on improving admission procedures. Particular attention should be paid to improving evaluations of personal qualities. For example, it may be that some personality types are best suited for certain health professions or for certain specialty fields in the health professions. The identification of such relationships could assist not only in admissions but also in counseling, both before and during professional education.

Educating Compassionate Health Professionals

In addition to ensuring the competence of health professionals, it is equally important to select students who are compassionate. Educational programs can and should reinforce the humane qualities of students. Faculty of programs of education for the health professions must place greater emphasis than they have in the past on educating practitioners who are skilled in communications, interviewing and listening techniques, and who are compassionate and technically competent. A student's relationship with a patient should be reviewed just as his or her technical performance is reviewed, and instruction should be given as to how it can be improved.

Showing compassion involves more than being empathic with a patient's plight. It involves making the maximum effort to care for the patient's intellectual and emotional needs, as well as physical needs. It also involves having sufficient respect for the patient to provide information about the patient's condition and about the proposed treatment.

Students should be instructed in the art of eliciting and providing information in a manner that demonstrates concern for their patients. In providing this instruction, it should be remembered that relationships between patient and practitioner are complex, and that there is no single pattern that is right for all patients or for all practitioners. For instance, some patients want complete details of their condition and of the proposed treatment; other patients do not. Some practitioners enjoy providing treatment details to patients; others, equally competent, prefer to provide less information. Educators should work with students in developing an approach to patients that is appropriate for the practitioner but that permits flexibility in dealing with patients. In all cases, educators and practitioners must keep in mind that the most compassionate care is that which is directed toward curing disease and caring for the needs of the patient. This care may, at times, involve providing information and advice to patients that they may not wish to hear.

Programs of health professions education are encouraged to consider ways in which additional emphasis can be placed on the development of high ethical standards and compassion in students. All faculty should ensure that the development of compassion has a firm and respected place in the curriculum and, when appropriate, that courses in ethics and related fields be mandatory.

The attitude of faculty is important in the development of compassion in their students. Faculty of health professions education should be attentive to the environment in which education is provided; students should learn in a setting where respect and concern are demonstrated. In particular, there is a need for appropriate support activities for students and a need to reduce stress. The requirement for appropriate support activities for students is part of the accreditation requirements for a number of health professions programs, and should be extended to all programs. Support services can include the formation of interdisciplinary discussion groups or provision of counseling services; the latter should include all students to reduce the stigma attached to seeking psychological assistance.

The faculty and administration of programs of health professions education must ensure that students are provided with appropriate role models; whether a faculty member serves as an appropriate role model should be considered when review for promotion or tenure occurs. A great deal of education for the health professions is provided in clinical settings where students observe practitioners and, at advanced stages, work under the immediate supervision of practitioners. In these circumstances, role models are extremely important. Deans and administrators must ensure that rewards are provided for faculty who provide good role models for students.

Unfortunately, even the most careful selection procedures will not guarantee that only the most competent and caring practitioners will be selected for health professions education programs, and ongoing evaluation of student performance is necessary. Efforts should be made by the faculty to evaluate the attitudes of students toward patients. Where these attitudes are found lacking, students should be counseled. Provisions for dismissing students who clearly indicate personality characteristics inappropriate to practice should be enforced.

In many health professions programs, clinical education—the time at which a practitioner's attitudes and relationships with patients can be evaluated—comes after a lengthy period of theoretical education. Thus, both students and faculty may perceive that too much time and effort has been invested in a student's education to consider dismissal or withdrawal. Faculty of health professions education programs should give attention to the possibility of beginning some aspects of clinical education much earlier, perhaps during the first year of multiyear programs. Doing so would permit earlier evaluation of student clinical performance, more time for effective counseling, and, in some instances, dismissal or withdrawal at less cost to both the student and the institution.

Determining that a student does not interact well with patients does not indicate, in every case, that he or she should be dismissed. With effort and experience, the student may improve relationships with patients. Alternatively, he or she can be directed into an area of practice where personal interactions are at a minimum. In those few instances where students are found totally unfit for practice because of personal attitudes, there should be procedures for dismissing them from programs.

In addition to evaluating students' relationships with patients, faculty must be willing, when necessary, to respond to evidence of unsatisfactory ethical standards. Faculty cannot, for instance, tolerate cheating or dishonesty.

Attitudinal expectations and behavioral standards should be described in program catalogs and student handbooks. Expected attitudes toward patients should be described, as well as penalties for failure to meet expectations.

Health Professions Education and the Integration of Patient Care Services

Increases in specialization among health practitioners, the division of responsibilities among a multiplicity of providers, and the high mobility of the population in general have resulted in a certain amount of depersonalization in patient care services. It is not uncommon, for example, for patients to have their health care provided by a succession of professionals, and it is therefore necessary to address the issue of coordination of care. In spite of the high degree of specialization in health care, faculty of programs of education for the health professions must prepare students to provide integrated patient care; programs of education should promote an interdisciplinary experience for their students. Practitioners must, for instance, be prepared to transmit patient records promptly when requested to do so. Opportunities for students from various fields to work together as colleagues should be fostered, as should academic activities directed toward informing students of the responsibilities and special expertise of other health professionals.

Continuing Education in Ethics and Patient Relations

Continuing education is ordinarily thought of in terms of maintaining technical skills and scientific knowledge and in keeping abreast of new techniques and discoveries. Yet, patient relations and ethics are also important areas for individual and classroom study. Patient relations and ethics are appropriate subjects for continuing education; educational providers should increase the offering in these fields. Sponsors of continuing education programs should develop self-assessment programs to provide practitioners with an opportunity to compare their behavior with accepted standards.

Boundaries of Practice for Health Professionals

Disagreements over boundaries of practice arise periodically among health care professions and within specialties of particular professions. Some health care professionals contend that constraints imposed by other professions and various laws and regulations unfairly prevent them from providing services for which they feel they are qualified. An example is the recent Florida law which allows pharmacists to prescribe certain drugs that once required a physician's prescription. This law is the first of its kind in the nation, and has stimulated some conflict between physicians and pharmacists.

Four factors have been critical in the development of boundaries of practice: professional licensure, voluntary certification programs, health care facility rules delineating clinical privileges, and third-party payor coverage restrictions. Each of these mechanisms, however, has inherent limitations and has fallen short in defining the scope of practice. The acceptance of licensing began to wane in the late 1960s and 1970s as several federal agencies issued reports that were critical of the way in which licensing had been used in certain occupations. Determining scope of practice by licensure and certification, though feasible when there are a small number of professions, may not be practical given the growth in the number of health providers. Finally, changes in the training and capabilities of established health professions have created problems for health care facilities in the delineation of hospital privileges and for third-party payors in determining whom to reimburse for particular services.

Problems relating to boundaries of practice probably will continue to exist because of the increasing number and types of health care providers and the growing complexity of health professions education. There is a marked degree of overlap in training, qualifications, and functions among health professionals. The problem is further aggravated by the increasing number of specialties within health care professional groups and by lack of sufficient contact and coordination between the various educational programs for health professionals. Competition among health care providers in an environment of limited financial resources, together with the desire of health care practitioners for increased training, enhanced prestige, and greater financial reward, creates the potential for continuing jurisdictional disputes among and within professions.

In addition, an increasingly informed and demanding public desires more freedom in choosing a health care practitioner. Traditionally, the patient's entry into the health care system was determined by physicians and dentists. Today, the patient's entry is through other health professionals as well. Consumers of health care are becoming better informed and many desire to have more information about the qualifications and competence of health care professionals. Patients want and need to be able to make informed choices about

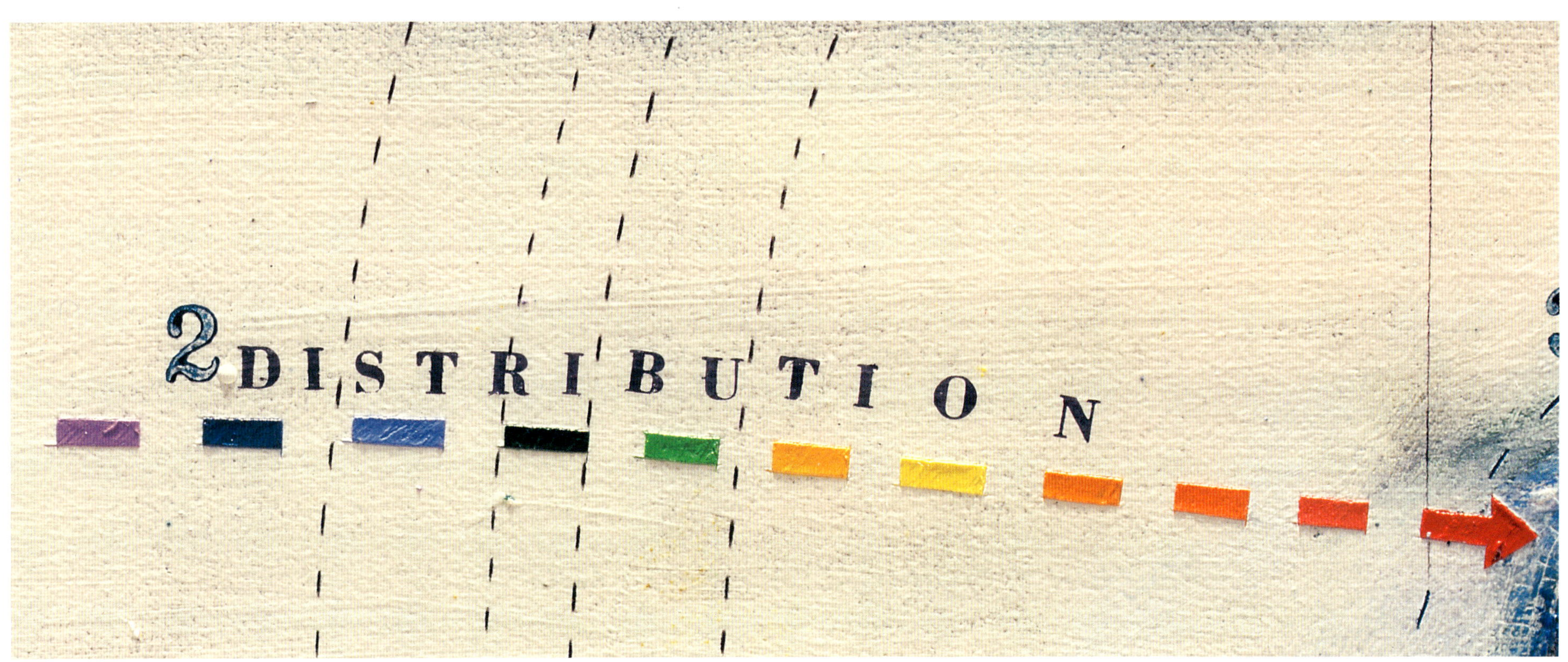

2 DISTRIBUTION

Our ultimate goal is to achieve an
appropriate supply and distribution
of health professionals to meet the health
care needs of the American people.

their health care and about who will provide it. They also want and need to know how much it will cost.

The participants of the Health Policy Agenda believe that health professionals should be allowed to provide those services for which they have appropriate training and which they are competent to perform. They should also be reimbursed fairly for providing services that fall within their scopes of practice. Furthermore, individual members of the public should be able to exercise free and informed choice among the diverse qualified health care professionals who provide similar or identical services.

Resolution of Boundary of Practice Disputes

The current system for determining boundaries of practice, though it has its merits, has some important shortcomings. The system is vulnerable to political pressure and places limitations on public input in some cases. An essential prerequisite to productive resolution of differences concerning respective practice roles among all health professions is a clear delineation of the services each profession is now performing and those it desires to perform. Several states currently have boards or commissions that incorporate some of the needed characteristics for mediating practice disputes, but more effort is needed in this area.

Each state should establish a well-staffed and adequately financed bureau of health professional licensure for the purpose of administering and coordinating the work of the individual licensure and certification agencies or boards. That bureau should be overseen by a blue ribbon commission including representatives of the professions and the general public. The commission should be charged with mediating disputes regarding the boundaries of practice permitted under certification and/or licensure, the standards of certification and/or licensure, and the appropriateness of disciplinary actions taken by the individual licensing and certification agencies or boards.

As a first step, guidelines for the development of the blue ribbon commission in each state should be developed. The commission should be appointed by the governor of the state or elected by the state legislature. It should be an independent body with broad and varied membership, and should not be dominated by any single health professional group. Membership on the commission should include representatives from many areas, including health care professions and facilities, consumer groups, labor, business and industry, government, and third-party payors.

The commission should be responsible for adjudicating conflicts over the scope of practice, standards of practice, and boundary disputes. The commission should also assist in determining which health professions should be licensed in the state. Recommendations should be consistent with the principle that a health profession or occupation should be licensed if the practice of that profession or occupation by persons who have not shown themselves to be competent and qualified to deliver health care services would pose a risk to the life, health, or safety of the public. The findings and decisions in any state should be widely disseminated, so that they may be used in the deliberations of other states.

The commission should have oversight responsibility for the state's bureau of health professional licensure. The commission would mediate between individual licensing agencies or boards and would be advisory to unlicensed groups.

Third-Party Payment Programs for Services

Reforms in delineating the services provided by different health professionals must occur concurrently with reforms in the systems that reimburse professionals for their services. Currently, services covered when rendered by one category of health professional may not be covered when performed by other types of health professionals, even though they are legally authorized to provide this service. For instance, nurse midwives are not always reimbursed through third-party payors, even though they may be licensed to perform certain obstetric care. These inconsistencies are not fair to health professionals. Nor are they in the public interest, since they unnecessarily limit the range of alternative providers from which patients can choose.

Public and private third-party payment programs for the services of health professionals are required to define which services are treated as covered benefits. (These benefit definitions appear in the contracts delineating the coverage of privately insured persons, and in the laws and regulations delineating the rights of beneficiaries under government programs.) It should be an objective for public and nongovernmental programs alike to define those benefits so that essentially identical services are covered when appropriately and legally rendered by any category of health professional.

Research needs to be done to determine what particular services can be performed safely and effectively by different types of providers. This research should be conducted by private foundations, academic institutions, and health services research organizations. Some of this research is currently occurring in studies of health care outcomes, and insurance coverage should be revised based on the results of these studies.

Payors must initiate detailed studies of their reimbursement plans to identify deficiencies in coverage for different health professionals providing essentially identical services. These deficiencies should be corrected. Any category of health professional that can document the adequate and appropriate training to perform a given service legally, safely, and effectively should be paid for that service by the payor if it is a covered benefit. This recommendation does not address the questions of whether there should or should not be direct billing for the service by that health professional, or of whether the level of payment should or should not be the same when performed by different categories of health professionals. These questions are separate from the issue of coverage per se, and should be addressed individually by the payor(s) and health professional(s) concerned.

Professional Responsibility Regarding Patient Referrals

Health professionals have an ethical responsibility to refer patients as needed, and the availability of alternative practitioners allows any number of choices to be made for care and referral. The information needed to assist health professionals in referrals, including knowledge on the qualifications and functions of various health professions, is currently lacking in most educational programs.

Because patients have the ultimate responsibility in making decisions about their health care, it follows that they are also responsible for maintaining coordination and continuity of care. Patients may decide that it is in their best interest to delegate this particular responsibility to a specific health professional, and if they do so, they have the freedom to choose who that health professional will be.

The health professional who coordinates an individual's health care has an ethical responsibility to ensure that the services required by an individual patient are provided by a professional whose basic competence and current performance are suited to render those services safely and effectively. In addition, patients also have a responsibility for maintaining coordination and continuity of their own health care.

Educational programs for health professionals should include instruction regarding the ethical responsibility to refer patients when necessary. Basic instruction about the qualifications of other types of health professionals should also be included in health professions education, both to provide a better understanding of and the basis for appropriate referrals.

The education of patients in the coordination and continuity of their own care is crucial. Both health professionals and the public must know the qualifications and training of various types of health professionals so that they can decide with whom the responsibility of developing a course of care will be vested.

An integral part of the referral process is the maintenance of adequate health care records for ensuring the coordination and continuity of patient care. Health care professionals are responsible for the maintenance of these records, and are also responsible for ensuring that these records are made available to other professionals when necessary.

Competency Assurance Programs to Strengthen State Licensure of Health Professionals

Both public agencies, such as state licensing boards, and private agencies, such as certifying agencies, are active in or concerned with the continuing and the entry-level competence of health professionals. However, there is a lack of coordination of competency assurance programs across different organizations. State programs to assure continued competence have been dominated by continuing education requirements. Private agencies, on the other hand, have attempted to use a wide variety of other continued competence assessment techniques. These include administration of mid-career examinations, proficiency testing, on-site job performance evaluations, practice audits, peer review, self-assessment exercises, portfolios, in-basket exercises, and simulation examinations. These efforts need to be integrated.

As a supplement to strengthen state licensure of health professionals, standard-setting and self-regulatory competency assurance programs should be conducted by and coordinated among health professions associations, certifying and accrediting agencies, and health care facilities. State agencies and private sector credentialing bodies must share information about, and work cooperatively on, the technical issues and problems associated with both entry-level and continued competency assurance programs for health professionals.

Supply and Distribution of Health Professionals

As a result of the dramatic growth in the supply of health care professionals over the past few decades medical care has become more accessible to the majority of the American public. From 1950 to 1983, the population in this country grew from about 150 million to almost 234 million—a 56% increase—while the physician population grew from about 220,000 to almost 520,000—a 136% increase. The physician population grew at a rate three times faster than that of the population as a whole from 1960 to 1983, and there are now about 220 physicians per 100,000 persons as compared to about 150 physicians per 100,000 persons in 1960. A comparable rate of growth has occurred in the allied health work force, which increased by slightly over 130% from 1966 to 1978. By 1990, the supply of physicians, nurses, and dentists is expected to increase by about 40%, while growth in some allied health fields may be much larger.

There has been some criticism that, as a whole, there are too many specialists and not enough generalists in medicine. Compared to other countries, the United States stands alone in the extent to which trained specialists serve as primary physicians. It is estimated that by 2010 almost all practicing physicians will be board certified in some specialty.

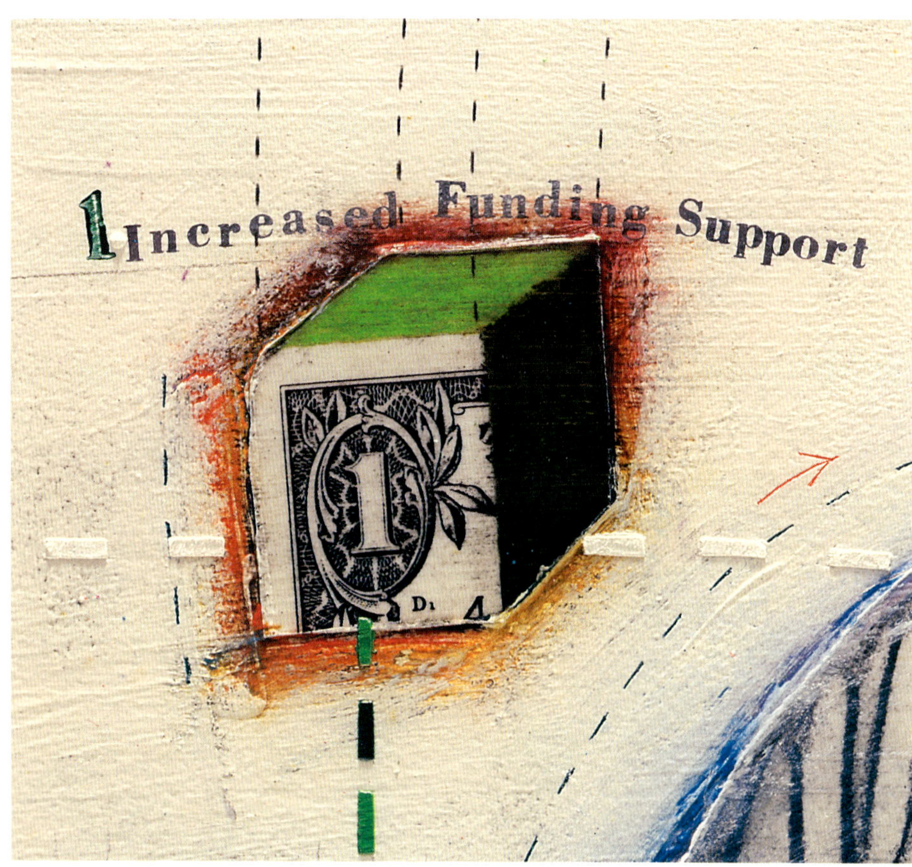

Financial support must be sufficient to preserve the high quality of our educational system for health professionals.

There has been additional criticism that the rate of growth for some health care professions or of specific specialties within some professions has been excessive in some instances and insufficient in others. Although some social benefits can arise from a plentiful supply of health professionals, an excessive surplus is undesirable because it may lead to unnecessarily high utilization, diminished skills, and accelerating expenditures. Shortages are also undesirable because they result in insufficient availability of health care services. Thus, the quality of care provided suffers if there are either too many or too few health professionals.

The ultimate goal is to achieve and maintain an adequate supply and distribution of health care professionals to meet the health care needs of the American people. To accomplish this and to have a sound basis for decision-making, there is a need for information on the supply and distribution of health professionals and on health care needs, including the needs of those presently underserved or inappropriately served by the current system.

Supply and Distribution of Health Professionals

The projected rate of growth for health professionals exceeds the anticipated rate in the general population. Per capita demand is expected to increase to some extent as the proportion of elderly individuals rises, and supply and distribution issues must be addressed to ensure proper resource development and utilization. A national consortium of concerned organizations and groups should collect, analyze, and synthesize data concerning the need and demand for, as well as the supply and distribution of, health professionals, by profession and by specialties within professions. Projections concerning the future supply of, and the need and demand for, health professionals should be developed by the consortium based on such data, and these projections should be made available to any interested parties. The consortium should be advisory rather than regulatory in nature. The term "health professionals" is not limited to physicians or physician specialists, but includes all providers of direct health care services. The consortium should be composed of representatives from consumer groups, business, labor, government, third-party payors, health professions, and educators of health professionals. Because the purpose of this group is to act in the public interest, it should not be dominated or disproportionately influenced by health care professionals or by any one professional group.

Issues related to supply should not be limited to aggregate numbers alone, but should assure adequate representation of groups that are currently underrepresented, such as minorities. For example, the percent of black entrants in dentistry, medicine, and pharmacy alone would have to double to equal the proportion of blacks in the population. According to the 1980 census, Hispanics represent about 6% of Americans. Although Hispanic enrollment in educational programs in nearly all health fields except nursing increased substantially from 1972 to 1982, the number of Hispanic students in health professions schools still falls below that ethnic group's representation in the general population.

Data analyses conducted by the consortium should rely on data collected by state and national agencies, although additional data gathering activity should be encouraged to fill information gaps as perceived by members of the consortium. Data should be collected concerning the distribution of medical specialists, the effect of the availability of medical specialty care on the use of other categories of health care professionals, graduates of American and foreign health professions programs, the needs of underserved populations, and how market forces affect the supply of and demand for health professionals. Funding for the consortium should be provided through public and private sources, with the latter being associations of health professionals, private foundations, the business community, and consumer groups.

Decisions affecting the supply and distribution of health professionals, such as public funding of health professions education, the requirements for entry to practice, or decisions to enter training for a health profession, would continue to be influenced by a variety of factors and made by the same parties and processes as at present. However, the decision-making process would be aided with the availability of data provided by the national consortium.

Licensure, Certification, and Accreditation and the Supply of Health Professionals

Licensure and certification of health professionals are intended to provide evidence of competence; the purpose of accreditation is to assess and enhance the quality of educational programs. Licensure, certification, and accreditation should not be used for the purpose of regulating the supply of health professionals. However, it is recognized that licensure and certification may affect the distribution of health professionals.

Supply and Distribution of Health Care Professionals and the Needs of Underserved Populations

Over time, the geographic distribution of health care professionals has become more similar to the geographic distribution of the general population. More physicians have begun to practice in previously underserved areas, such as small towns and cities. While there has been almost no change in the proportion of physicians serving in metropolitan areas— this figure was 86% in 1970 and 87% in 1983—by the end of the 1970s nearly every town with a population of 2500 or more had a physician or ready access to one.

Such federal efforts as the National Health Service Corps, which was developed to provide financial support for the education and training of health care professionals in return for future service in underserved inner cities or rural areas, and the Area Health Education Center Program have assisted in bringing health care to areas and populations in need. However, due to historical, cultural, and economic factors, some Americans—especially those who are in geographically remote areas or those who face language barriers—still do not have ready access to health care services.

As a first step in meeting the needs of the underserved, appropriate agencies of government, as well as business, labor, and health care professional and institutional associations should collect appropriate data on the distribution of health care professionals relative to the unmet needs of communities throughout the country. In the past, supply and distribution analyses relative to unmet needs have not sufficiently addressed the needs of the underserved. These analyses have at times led the public to believe that an ideal number of health professionals will solve the problems of underserved populations.

Methods that are used to calculate the requirements for services of health professionals should incorporate the health care needs of the underserved.

The mere preparation of more health professionals on the assumption that they will distribute themselves into the specialty settings and geographic areas where they are needed has not solved the problem to date, and there is no reason to believe it will provide a solution in the future. Rather, what is needed is a concerted effort to get health professionals into geographic areas and settings where they are needed. In the short-term, priority should be placed on funding mechanisms and organized systems of delivery to make professional practice in underserved communities more attractive than it currently is. Additionally, special attention should be directed at recruitment and retention of health care professionals practicing in underserved areas.

There are a number of long-term actions that can be taken to address the health care needs of the underserved. First, the nation's education and training programs should place a high priority on attracting students who want to serve minority and underserved populations, whether such students are from minority groups or from the general population. Second, local and national leadership groups concerned about the needs of underserved populations should advocate major changes in financing and delivery mechanisms and in education to achieve an equitable distribution of health care professionals. Finally, health care professional associations, third-party payors, and state and federal governments should stimulate grassroots pressure for modifications in financing and delivery mechanisms and in education.

Supply and Distribution of Health Professionals and Educational Programs

As noted in the previous set of recommendations, a number of issues must to be addressed relative to meeting the health care needs of underserved populations. It was specifically recommended that educational programs should place a high priority on attracting students who want to serve minority and underserved populations. Additionally, health professions' curricula should emphasize the needs of underserved populations, including the poor, minorities, the chronically ill and disabled, and the geographically isolated.

An issue that also relates to the supply and distribution of health professionals is the financing of educational programs. Decisions regarding the financing of health professions education should be based in part on the data and analyses of the national consortium on the supply and distribution of health professionals. The need for improving access to health care for the underserved should be considered, and continued emphasis should be given to linking educational assistance to service in deprived areas.

Maintaining Competence of Health Professionals

The rate at which scientific knowledge is expanding makes the maintenance of professional competence a matter of acute concern both to health professionals themselves and to the public. Health professionals must ensure that the best possible care is being provided to patients, and the public is legitimately concerned about the necessity for health professionals to maintain competence over the course of their professional careers. Maintaining competence improves the quality of care provided to patients and reduces the incidence of nonstandard treatment and professional liability complaints.

There are a variety of educational experiences that are available to health professionals to ensure their continued competence. Continuing education is not only classroom activity; it also includes a substantiation of knowledge and the refinement of skills that come from practice. The kind of learning that occurs from individual inquiry and research for the proper treatment of a patient with an unusual or a serious disorder are also forms of continuing education. (Maintaining professional competence through peer review and other activities is discussed in Chapter V.)

In the late 1960s and early 1970s, continuing education was looked upon as the means of assuring competence. During this period a number of state licensing boards and a number of professional societies developed mandatory continuing education requirements. Some of these rules are still in force, although in general, confidence within the professions in mandatory continuing education as a means of assuring competence is declining. The link between having knowledge and putting that knowledge into use is a tenuous one, although knowledge certainly is a necessary part of effective behavior change. The selection of educational programs is also problematic; frequently, professionals may choose to attend programs about subjects that they know instead of attending courses in a new subject. Far too frequently, continuing education programs are not built around carefully undertaken assessments of needs. There are, unfortunately, also examples of outright abuse of educational programs, with, in some instances, vacations masquerading as tax-deductible learning experiences. In spite of these problems, some form of continuing education is an indispensable part of all programs directed toward maintaining competence among health professionals.

Professional Responsibility for Participation in Continuing Education
Health professionals are individually responsible for maintaining their competence and for participating in continuing education; all health professionals should be engaged in self-selected programs of continuing education. Specific requirements for continuing education should be imposed by the professions rather than by licensing boards. Participants should be required to demonstrate mastery of the subject matter of the programs through examinations or other appropriate means.

While participation in continuing education is not in itself an assurance of continued competence, it is certainly related to it. Health professionals can participate in a number of continuing education activities: journal reading, participation in staff meetings devoted to reviewing and evaluating patient care, attendance at scientific meetings, and the use of audiovisual materials. Continuing education occurs in the preparation of scientific reports and journal articles, in consultations concerning unusual cases, and in case reviews of various kinds.

The cost of continuing education activities should be kept as low as possible. It is reasonable for employers to provide continuing education for employees, since such education enhances the knowledge and skills of employees and their value to the institution. However, in the absence of other financial support, individual health professionals

Development of Continuing Education Programs

Professional schools and health professions organizations should develop additional continuing education self-assessment programs, should prepare guides to continuing education programs to be taken by practitioners throughout their careers, and should make efforts to ensure that acceptable programs of continuing education are available to practitioners. Continuing education does not currently receive the degree of support that is needed from professional schools. Programs are generally not planned with the lifelong needs of practitioners taken into consideration, and far too often continuing education programs reflect the interests of only a few faculty members.

A variety of means of continuing education is desirable because different persons respond to different kinds of educational programs, and skills and knowledge can be imparted in a number of different ways. The effort to improve continuing education might well begin with a consideration of adult education theory and the ways in which it differs from formal professional education. The value of individualized instruction programs must not be overlooked. Reading is a prevalent means of continuing education. Additionally, as access to computer data banks becomes more widespread, routine reference to these sources of information will become more common, with immediate benefits to knowledge and to improvement in care. However, self-instruction cannot totally replace group learning.

Association with peers and the discussion of scientific subjects of mutual educational interest also are important. Small hospitals are less able than large ones to institute complex educational programs, but cooperative efforts can provide some degree of programming. Hospitals can also provide for educational programming which deals with the issues of the cost of care; itemized bills for hospitalization in these institutions offer opportunities for careful analysis of the treatment provided to various patients.

Professional societies should ensure that programs of both self-assessment and continuing education are available to members and nonmembers. Self-assessment programs can be useful in determining the educational needs of practitioners. Attention should also be given to developing outlines of the needs of practitioners in lifelong learning programs; these outlines should provide a review of the knowledge and skills needed for practice as well as the introduction of new knowledge and skills as they are accepted by the profession. As only a small percentage of practitioners are represented by health professions organizations, employers also have a responsibility to ensure competency through continuing education.

Licensure and Continuing Education Reporting Requirements

Many states have laws that require the reporting of continuing education in connection with reregistration of licenses to practice. However, monitoring of continuing education is best done by health professions organizations, and state legislatures should place the responsibility for monitoring with these organizations. Only those health professionals who fail to meet the requirements of a recognized health professional organization should be required to report participation in continuing education directly to a state licensing board.

Standards of Competence for Health Professionals

A number of professions have adopted definitions of competence. Because each profession deals with a subset of health care needs, definitions and standards of competence must be developed in reference to the boundaries of the scope of practice.

The development of standards of competence is basic to undertaking the assessment of competence of practitioners, and the responsibility for developing these standards belongs to the professions rather than to governmental agencies. Health professions organizations and faculty of programs of health professions education should develop standards for competence. Such standards should be reviewed and revised periodically. There are regional and institutional differences in standards of practice, and competence should be measured against the standard that applies in the community or environment where the practice occurs.

Assessing the Continuing Competence of Health Professionals

While there is little disagreement concerning the need to assess continuing competence of health professionals, there is little agreement as to how to accomplish this task. Methods to assess continuing competence include examinations, continuing education, peer review, and patient outcome; but valid and economically feasible means of assessing competence have not yet been devised. For the most part, there is considerable disagreement as to whether evaluation instruments measure competence in practice or knowledge that may or may not be used in practice. Opinion scales that are commonly used to evaluate courses are certainly not valid indicators of whether learning has occurred. Formal tests may indicate immediate gains in knowledge but are not always predictive of improvements in clinical practice. Evaluation of changes in clinical practice as a consequence of continuing education is expensive and difficult to undertake, as are evaluations of the patient's health as affected by continuing education.

Clearly, additional research is needed on how to measure competence and the outcomes of continuing education. In the absence of a cost-effective and practical means of assessing continuing competence, monitoring is best accomplished by health professions organizations. However, when reliable and cost-effective means of assessing continuing competence are developed, they should be required for continued practice.

Summary

In this chapter, the educational and professional requirements to ensure the delivery of health care services were discussed. Topics addressed included the financing of undergraduate and clinical graduate education, the enrollment and retention of minority students in the health professions programs, quality assurance measures for graduates of foreign health professional schools, educating competent and caring health professionals, the supply and distribution of health professionals, boundaries of practice for health professionals, and maintaining competence of health professionals through continuing education.

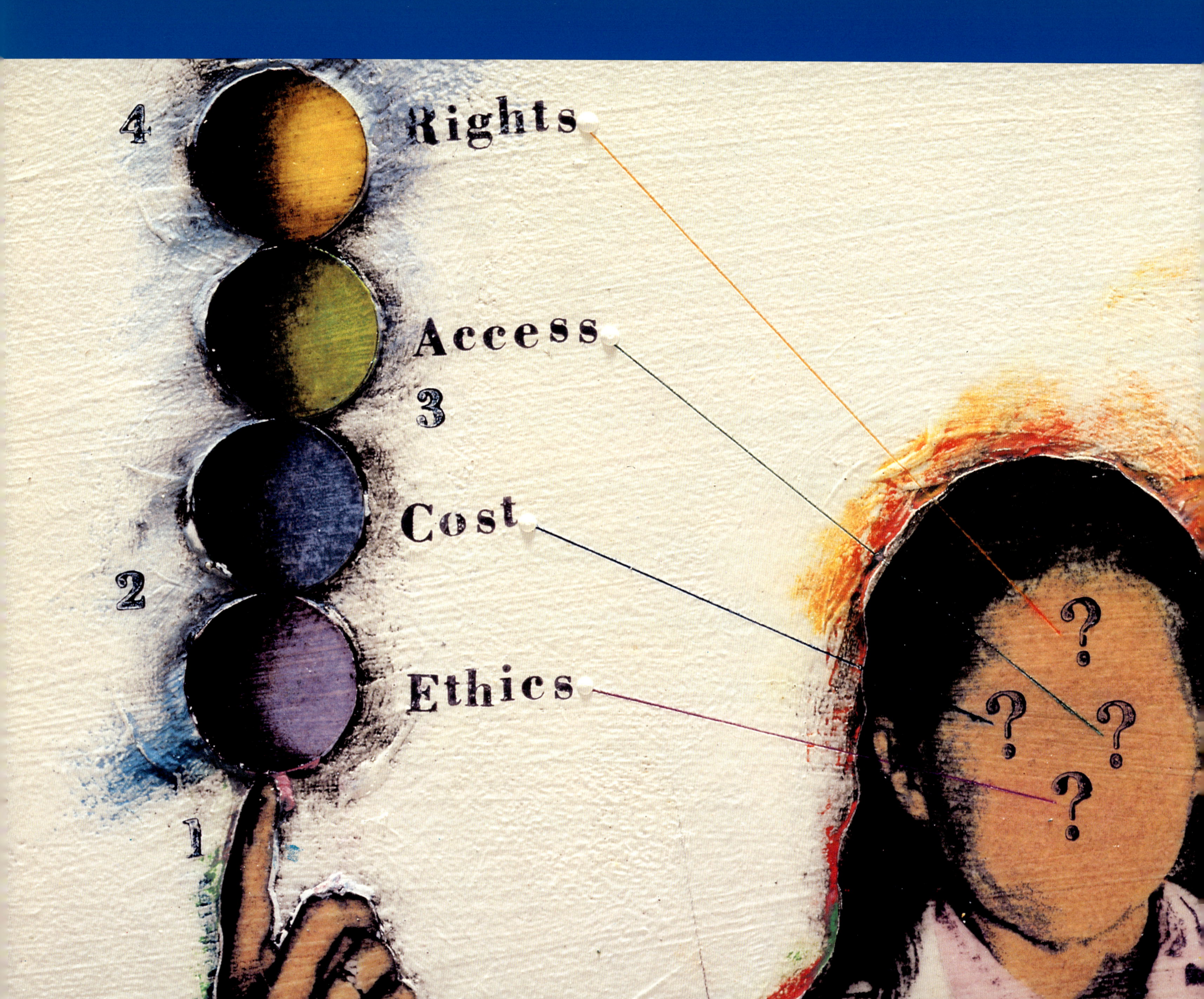

4
Rights
Access
3
Cost
2
Ethics
1

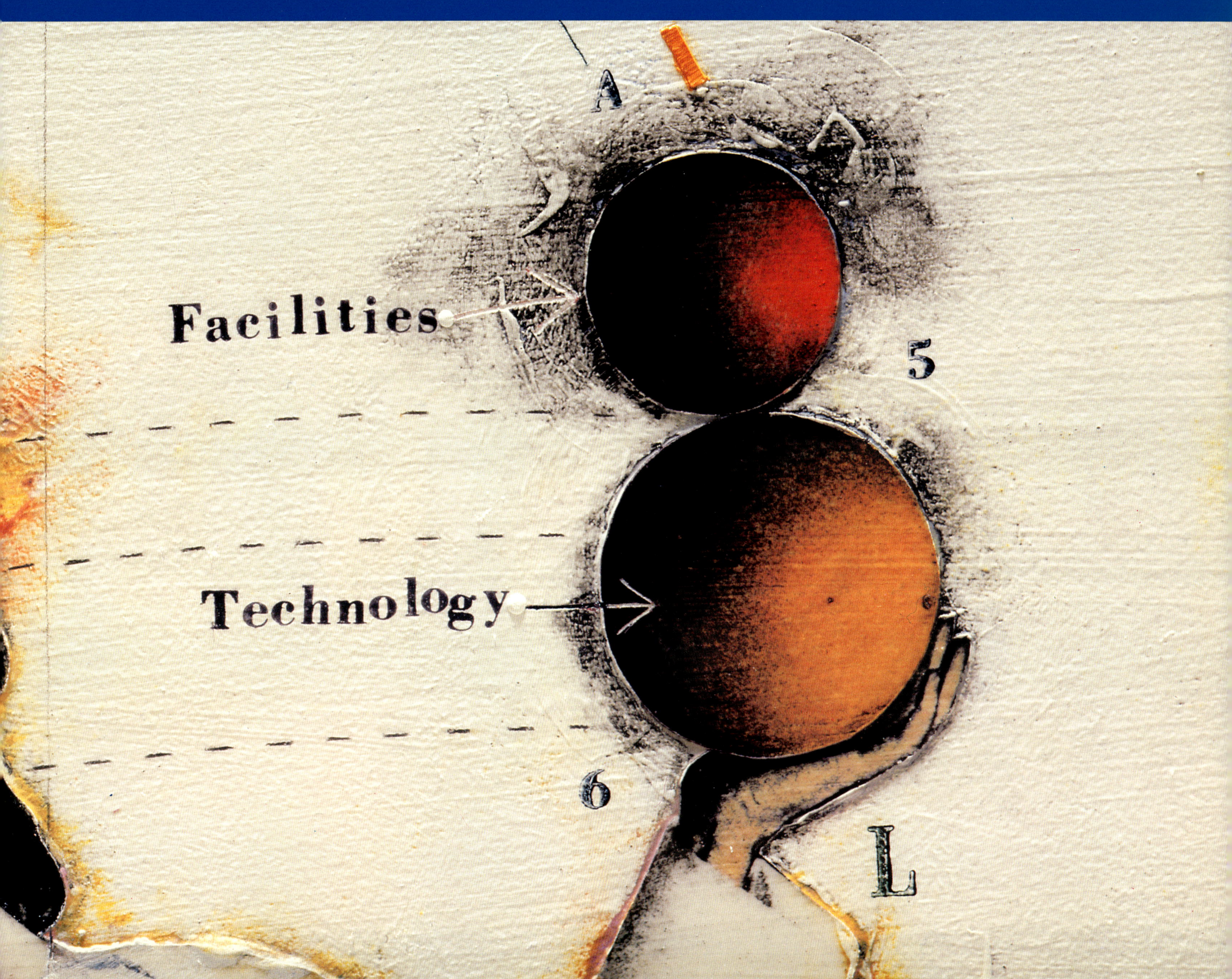
A
Facilities
5
Technology →
6
L

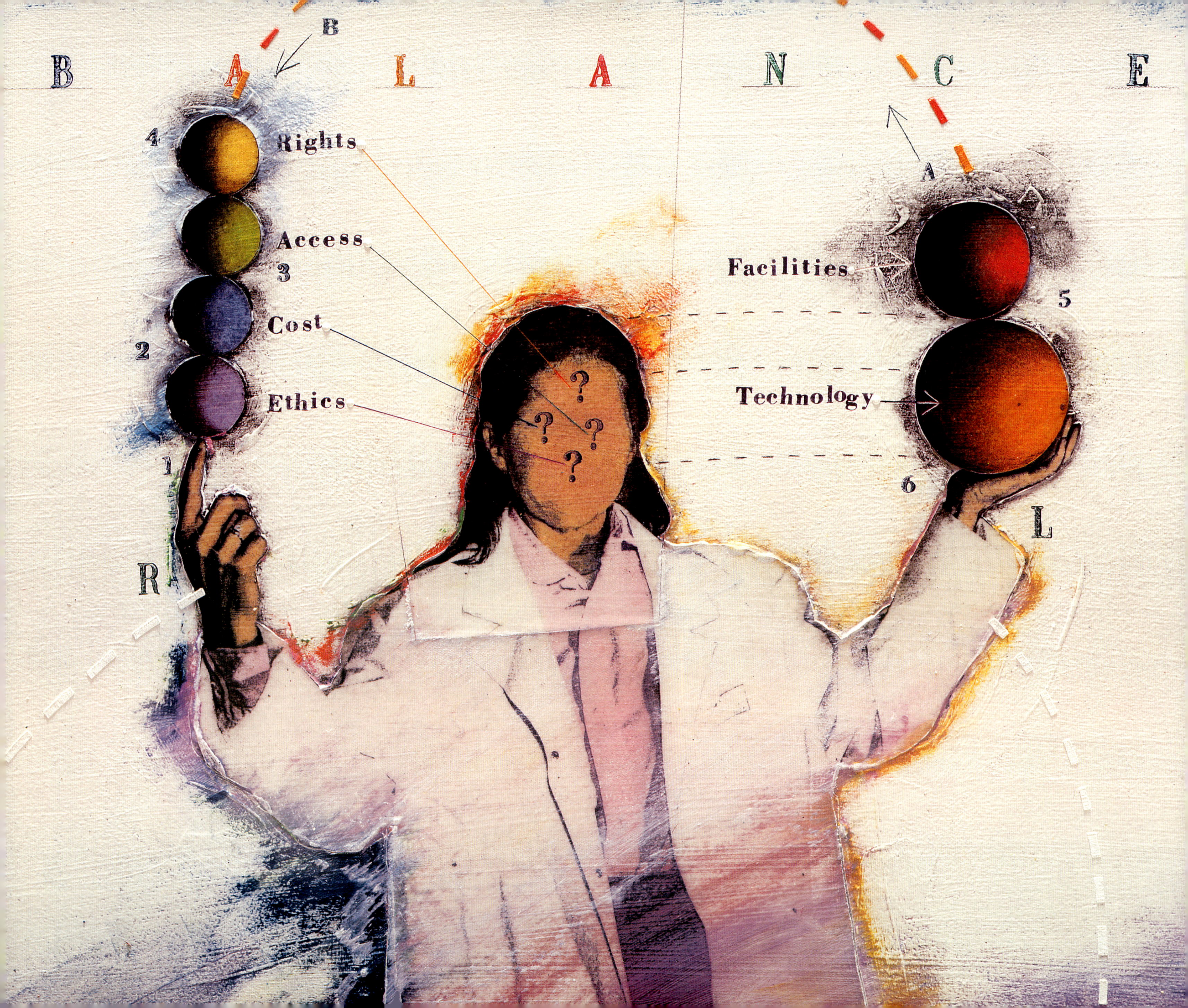

B A L A N C E
B
Rights
Access
Cost
Ethics
Facilities
Technology
4
3
2
1
A
5
6
R
A
L
?
?
?
?

The fast-paced development of health care technologies has outstripped, at least in some instances, the ability to consider thoroughly the ethical and moral consequences of using such technology with respect to individual treatment decisions. There are a number of cases to illustrate this point, including the financing of treatment for end-stage renal disease, the treatment of minors whose parents have refused them medical intervention, and the development of institutional "do not resuscitate" policies. In addition to decisions that must be made concerning the application of a particular technology, there is the issue of the allocation of finite technological resources. In decisions related to allocation, there are necessary trade-offs to be made between costs, access, individual rights, moral principles, and societal values. Society has yet to come to a resolution of these issues.

The development of these new technologies has raised questions concerning who should be allowed to use them and what criteria should be used to make these decisions. The federal government, state governments, health facilities, third-party payors, and health professionals have all played a role in the allocation of privileges to use health care technologies. Further clarification of their roles and responsibilities will help to ensure that access to technology is readily available to those who can use it in a medically appropriate and cost-effective manner.

In the past 20 years considerable changes also have occurred in the numbers and types of health care facilities offering services to the public. Traditional settings, such as hospitals, long-term care facilities, and practitioners' offices, now compete with such newer settings as urgent care centers, ambulatory surgical centers, "walk-in" clinics, and home health care agencies. There has been a shift in the provision of services from inpatient to outpatient settings, a development of multifacility systems, and increased facility specialization.

As these and other diverse health care delivery settings develop, there is a need to ensure that a reasonable degree of quality and safety is maintained in the provision of services to the public. With the development of new settings, distinctions between what does and does not constitute a health care facility have become blurred.

As a first step, then, there is a need for a definition of a "health care facility." This definition can then be used to address issues relating to quality of, access to, and payment for services.

Once a health care facility is defined, it is also possible to address the licensure of such facilities. States are responsible for the licensure of health care facilities, and they are experiencing some difficulty in determining which settings should or should not be licensed. There is little uniformity in the approaches taken by individual states to license the various types of new entities that are delivering health care services; as a result, services offered by the "same" type of facilities vary considerably both within and among states.

Finally, there is some concern about the supply and distribution of health care facilities. Market forces now play a major role in determining the supply and distribution of facilities, but market forces have not resolved access problems for those who cannot pay or who are located in remote areas. Furthermore, experience has shown that unrestricted competition can result in excess capacity and wasteful duplication that add unnecessarily to the costs of health care that a community must bear. There is a continuing need for some type of health planning to ensure that the health care needs of all individuals in all parts of the country are met.

All of these issues—moral and ethical considerations in the application of technology, the allocation of privileges to use technology, and the definition, licensure, and supply and distribution of health care facilities—are discussed in this chapter.

Moral and Ethical Issues in the Use of Health Care Technologies

Two examples—the financing of treatment for end-stage renal disease (ESRD) and the introduction of "do not resuscitate" (DNR) policies in institutional settings—can be used to illustrate the different ways in which society has tried to resolve moral and ethical issues in relationship to treatment decisions. These examples also illustrate how the technologies themselves have shaped our ethical standards.

There are two treatments for ESRD—renal dialysis and transplantation. Renal dialysis is a method for externally cleaning waste products from the blood of a person with irreversible kidney failure. The procedure was perfected in the 1960s, when it became possible to avoid the destruction of a patient's accessible blood vessels. Kidney transplants are limited by the number of suitable surgical candidates, the number of donors, and the tendency of the human body to reject donated organs; only recently have immunosuppressive agents been developed to reduce organ rejections. Without dialysis or transplantation, death is certain for a person with ESRD.

Demand for both of these treatments grew, and when demand threatened to overwhelm the supply of dialysis machines and compatible donated kidneys, a number of allocation mechanisms were tried. Initially, treatment was given to those patients for whom dialysis or transplantation was likely to be the most successful; however, selection criteria were subject to criticism because they were altered depending on the availability of kidneys or dialysis machines. A first-come-first-served approach was then tried; this failed, of course, because some early patients were in poor medical health, and there were many doubts about making medical decisions on this basis. In several areas, community-wide groups composed of medical experts and lay representatives chose who would receive treatment; in some cases neither the criteria nor the final decisions were subject to review, and the process itself seemed to be heavily influenced by personal biases of the members.

Because of the public's reluctance to make determinations of this kind and because of the high cost of treatment, the Social Security Act was amended in 1972 to extend Medicare benefits to all ESRD patients. When the ESRD program was being debated and the statute was being drafted, there was agreement among nephrologists and the government that dialysis would only be used for patients who had high potential for receiving a transplant. That position soon gave way to a situation in which almost all end-stage renal crisis results in dialysis. About 70,000 patients are now receiving dialysis and 6,000 patients are undergoing kidney transplants each year. Renal patients, who represent only 0.25% of the Medicare population, consume nearly 10% of the Medicare

Part B budget. The costs of this program necessarily imply trade-offs in the availability of other services to Medicare and Medicaid recipients.

Resuscitation, or "the revival of a living being from apparent death," has been one of the major accomplishments in health care. Advances in surgical techniques, anesthesia, and medical instrumentation have dramatically improved the ability of health professionals and lay people alike to revive individuals experiencing cardiac arrest or ventricular fibrillation. Despite these advances, resuscitation is controversial. Further complicating the issue, most of the care provided to dying patients is now delivered in institutional settings; these institutions and the health professionals working in them have an ethical orientation to preserve life, and there is considerable tension between those who wish to prolong life and those who prefer a "natural" death. A number of health care institutions have developed policies for regulating the issuance of "do not resuscitate" (DNR) orders by their medical staffs. These policies describe the conditions under which patients will not be resuscitated, and attempt to ensure that consistent decisions will be made within an institution. They also provide a formal defense in case of legal action, although there have been conflicting court decisions in this area.

Most hospitals base their DNR policies on three criteria—self-determination, well-being, and equity. The informed choice of the patient is a key element in the decision-making process. In most cases, once the patient is adequately informed about the consequences of applying, foregoing, or withdrawing resuscitation procedures, the institution or responsible health professional is obligated to ascertain the patient's preferences. Second, the health professional responsible for the patient's care must make the ethical determination as to whether resuscitation will promote a patient's welfare. In cases where self-determination conflicts with well-being (objectively and subjectively defined), further discussion typically takes place between patient and provider, with the presumption in favor of resuscitation. Finally, the policies have tried to treat patients equitably by avoiding the creation of explicit categories of patients based on non-medical characteristics, such as income or family status. While DNR policies may be achieving

their objectives without violating societal standards, the increasing number of court cases on both the use and withdrawal of resuscitation procedures and the growing fears of health professionals and institutions about liability risks raise the possibility that this decentralized approach to an important moral and ethical issue in health care may be abandoned.

Aside from these examples that illustrate specific decision-making problems in health care, there is the related issue of allocating finite technological resources at the community level. At the level of the community or medical service area, the acquisition of any given technology may involve capital for facilities and equipment, operating capital, staffing requirements, and resource demands on laboratories and ancillary services—some or all of which may need to be diverted from other health-related purposes. In a time of finite resources, trade-offs must usually be made. Trade-offs might have to occur between developing a transplantation capacity or the acquisition of new imaging equipment. Or, trade-offs might have to be made between availability of a neonatal intensive care unit (ICU) and better community prenatal care services which could reduce the need for a neonatal ICU in the first place.

The moral and ethical problems in the application of health care technology do not have simple solutions. Balancing the trade-offs between cost, equity of access, individual rights, moral principles, and social values is a difficult task. The participants of the Health Policy Agenda believe that a decentralized approach to these problems should be adopted. Individual treatment decisions should be made in the context of professional standards and accepted moral and societal values, and should be made jointly by patients and their representatives and the health professionals managing their care. (The phrase "and their representatives" is used because in many instances patients' families or other designated individuals, rather than patients themselves, are involved in making decisions concerning treatment.) Appropriate principles and processes should encourage the rational allocation of finite technological resources at the local level to ensure equity of access.

Development of Criteria for the Application or Withdrawal of Health Care Technologies

The financing of treatment for end-stage renal disease and the development of institutional "do not resuscitate" policies represent only two examples of how American society has addressed moral and ethical issues in the application of health care technology. Other problems precipitated by technological advances abound: legalized abortion and changing definitions of fetal viability; the treatment of newborns with severe congenital abnormalities; the treatment of minors whose parents have refused them medical intervention; and the demand by some terminally ill patients that health care institutions and professionals actively assist them in dying. These examples only amplify the need for society to develop a consensus about the application or withdrawal of health care technology to individual patients.

The decentralized tradition of the American health care system necessitates that decisions regarding the application or withdrawal of health care technology be made as close to the site of the actual delivery of care as possible, and the health care facility represents the most logical site. The criteria on which to base professional recommendations for the application or withdrawal of health care technology should be developed by the individual health care facility in which the technology is to be used, and should be consistent with professional and ethical considerations. The institution itself cannot make the clinical decisions on the use of technology for a particular patient; but as the collective representative of health care professionals, the institution can establish the standards that these health professionals should use in developing their recommendations concerning use of a technology.

Because decisions about an individual's health care cannot be made unilaterally, each health care facility should establish a permanent ethics committee, composed of health professionals and lay representatives from the general community, to develop the criteria. This will ensure that state-of-the-art medical knowledge will be applied and that societal standards will be upheld, and this ethics committee should modify criteria when appropriate. In addition to this permanent ethics committee, each facility should, on an ad hoc basis, convene ethics committees to advise health professionals and patients regarding the application of criteria to individual cases. Membership of these ad hoc ethics committees should include health professionals and lay representatives with the specific expertise and knowledge of the ethical and clinical issues involved in the particular case.

As previously noted, the care of dying patients is increasingly being provided in institutional settings, but some consideration also needs to be given to those cases in which decisions need to be made for patients who are not in health care facilities. In those cases in which a technology is used outside of a health care facility, local consortia of health professionals and lay people should be created to develop criteria governing the application or withdrawal of health care technology. These criteria should also be consistent with professional and ethical considerations.

Health care organizations should urge health care facilities to establish ethics committees, and local health care organizations should work in their own communities to establish ethics committees to address technologies which may be used outside of health care facilities. Accrediting bodies, such as the Joint Commission on Accreditation of Hospitals, should consider requiring the establishment and maintenance of an ethics committee as a condition for accreditation, although exceptions must be made for facilities that are either too small or too limited in their scope of services to warrant a formal ethics committee.

State laws may need to be amended; laws may be needed to protect members of the ethics committee from liability for the results of treatment decisions made on criteria developed by the committee. However, state laws should never preclude the opportunity for patients or others to challenge legally the relevance of the criteria established and to seek their modification. Concomitantly, state laws need to affirm the right of an individual to have ultimate control over the course of his or her health care and life.

The Use of Criteria for the Application or Withdrawal of Health Care Technology by Health Professionals

Recommendations of health professionals regarding the application or withdrawal of health care technology should be made on a clinically valid basis. These recommendations, which often influence whether a patient will live or die, should be based on the severity of the patient's illness, its probable course, the probability of recovery (both total and partial), and the resulting quality of life. Recommendations by a health professional to apply or withdraw a health care technology in the diagnosis or treatment of an individual patient must be based on clinically valid criteria consistent with professional and ethical standards. In particular, such decisions should not be based on the patient's chronological (as opposed to biological) age, sex, race, ethnic origin, current wealth or probable future income, but should take into consideration the quality of life resulting from application or withdrawal of the technology. This recommendation is not as self-evident as it may seem. Given the tentative state of much of medical science, the definition of "clinically valid criteria" is subject to interpretation. The possibility exists that nonclinical criteria can be transformed by social or economic considerations into seemingly clinical mandates. If such nonclinical criteria as a patient's chronological age or sex or race were used, health professionals and institutions would lose the trust and unique relationship that exists with their patients. Health professionals should periodically question their medical assumptions to ensure that they are not influenced by inappropriate concerns; American ethical values require that those in whom patients entrust their care make professional decisions, using appropriate criteria about the application or withdrawal of technology.

Decision-Making Regarding the Application or Withdrawal of Health Care Technology

The decision to apply or withdraw health care technology must ultimately be made by the patient and the health professional responsible for his or her care. To involve others or to bring the decision into the public arena under the judicial system destroys the intimate and critical relationship that has been created and may unnecessarily damage the care received by the patient without improving the care of others.

The health care professional responsible for managing and coordinating an individual's health care should have the responsibility for determining whether application of a technology is clinically appropriate and consistent with the criteria established by the health care facility. That health care professional is also responsible for communicating recommendations, including the rationale for such recommendations, to the patient. The decision to use or not to use the technology should be made jointly by the health

professional and the patient or his or her representative. When the decision to withdraw or deny a technology cannot be made by the patient or his or her representative and the health professional, either party should have the right to seek the counsel of an ethics committee.

Decisions of this nature are not to be made unilaterally; the patient should be consulted, and in fact has the final authority over his or her life. Both parties should have access to an ethics committee to provide advice and counsel. However, seeking legal remedies to resolve disputes is not encouraged; the legal system itself is not large enough to handle these issues on a case-by-case basis, and perhaps more importantly the adversarial nature of judicial proceedings can damage a cooperative relationship between patient and health professional.

This recommendation places a substantial burden on health professionals to provide sound counsel to their patients. Patients, in turn, have a significant responsibility to participate in the planning and implementation of their own health care. Although both patients and health professionals have often professed a strong desire to assume these responsibilities, doing so will require them to forego some of their past attitudes and behaviors, such as the attitude of unquestionable authority on the part of health professionals and the desire for unlimited access to the legal system by patients.

Self-Determination of Treatment Decisions for the Terminally Ill

Sophisticated technology permits the prolongation of life for many individuals with terminal illnesses. A mechanism is needed to guide individuals, their families, and health care professionals and facilities in making decisions regarding termination of treatment or decisions not to treat. With such a mechanism, decisions can be based on relatively uniform and lawful criteria.

Competent terminally ill individuals should have the freedom to make their own decisions regarding the withholding or withdrawal of treatment. Appropriate individuals should be encouraged to develop guidelines for the withholding or withdrawal of treatment and state legislatures should be encouraged to pass "right to die" legislation. Currently, 35 states and the District of Columbia have "right to die" legislation, which upholds the validity of living wills. A living will provides a legally recognized way for competent adults to express their wishes concerning life-sustaining medical treatment should they become terminally ill. In general, living wills state that if the person is in a condition from which there can be no recovery and will die imminently, life-sustaining treatments can be withdrawn or omitted.

At present, there are some variations in living wills from state to state. Almost all states require two witnesses to the signing, and in some cases the signing must occur in the presence of a notary public. Generally, the witnesses must not be related by blood or marriage to the person making the decision, entitled to any portion of the estate, or directly financially responsible for the declarant's medical care. Some states allow the person to designate a close relative or other proxy to make crucial medical care decisions should he or she be incompetent to make them, and others rule out decisions by anyone but the patient. Several require periodic renewal. In some states, legislation is also provided to address the procedures for termination of treatment when a living will is not available.

This type of legislation provides protection against civil liability, criminal liability, and charges of unprofessional conduct for physicians and other providers who comply with the terms of the agreements. One potential problem, however, is the definition of key terms, such as "physician," "life-prolonging" or "life-sustaining," and "terminal condition" and "imminent death."

"Right to die" legislation should stipulate the circumstances in which life-sustaining procedures can be withdrawn and the procedures to follow for the removal or discontinuance of such treatment. The legislation should confirm the validity of living wills. It also should provide for the removal of life-sustaining procedures for patients who have not signed a living will, but who are determined by the attending physician and confirmed by a committee of physicians to be terminally ill or comatose and beyond the possibility of returning to a cognitive state. In some localities effective bioethical committees already exist and legislation may not be necessary.

Acquisition of Expensive or Resource-Intensive Health Care Technologies
Some individuals would argue that a purely competitive, market-oriented approach to resource allocation produces improved service and equity of access at lower cost. However, recent studies show that costs for services may be higher in areas where there is competition than they are in areas where there are sole providers; institutions in a competitive market may add services and have larger staff-to-patient ratios, both of which may contribute to higher costs. In addition, a purely market-driven allocation process may poorly serve those who have difficulty in paying for needed care, or who live in areas where the population density is insufficient to attract and pay for on-site services. Even those who have geographic and financial access to a health care delivery system may not have available the services of providers who are proficient in the advanced technologies that would be of benefit.

Decisions by health care facilities or professionals regarding the acquisition or development of costly or resource-intensive technology should not be made solely on the basis of economics, scientific interest, or the needs of a relatively small proportion of the population. Rather, such decisions should be made in the context of balancing the rights of individuals with the needs of society. Consideration of equitable access should be a primary factor in making such decisions. In making decisions as to whether to commit resources to the development of capital-intensive technology in a given area, the appropriate balance between individual and societal rights should be considered. Such decisions should take into consideration the recommendations and findings of local and regional planning entities as to the need for such technology in relation to the need for alternate services that might be offered and the appropriate distribution of the technology itself.

State and local planning activities that address access, availability, distribution and costs of services should be continued and expanded, and mechanisms should be developed to facilitate coordination between planning agencies.

The Allocation of Privileges to Use Health Care Technologies

Three major and interrelated phenomena have focused new attention on the questions of who should be allowed to use particular health care technologies and the criteria to be used in making these decisions. First, the development of technology to prevent, diagnose, and treat illnesses has been rapid in recent years. The development of such technologies as CT and MRI scanners, neonatal intensive care units, and fetal surgery has placed an increasingly elaborate set of diagnostic and therapeutic tools at the disposal of health professionals. Also, the public has access to an expanding array of technologies for personal care, such as over-the-counter drugs, sophisticated first-aid kits, and home diagnostic tests.

A second phenomenon is the increased information available about health care technologies. The proliferation of scholarly journals in the health care field has facilitated dissemination of advances in health care technologies. This "information explosion" has been matched by a heightened interest in scientific developments on the part of the public.

A third development is the diversification in the training of those who deliver health care services. In part, this has occurred as a consequence of the growth in technology. For example, the occupations of surgical technologist, diagnostic medical sonographer, and nuclear medicine technologist have been established specifically to apply new health care technologies. For more established professional groups, roles and responsibilities have been modified in certain cases to allow access to new or existing technologies. The growth in the types of health professionals has raised the issue of the proper role for each type of professional in the use of health care technology.

The federal government has been heavily involved in regulating the products of health care technology and thus, at least indirectly, controlling who will be allowed to use the technology and under what circumstances. For example, in 1906 the Pure Food Act established the need for manufacturers to provide proof of the safety of a pharmaceutical before it could be used. In 1938, the Food, Drug, and Cosmetic Act created a

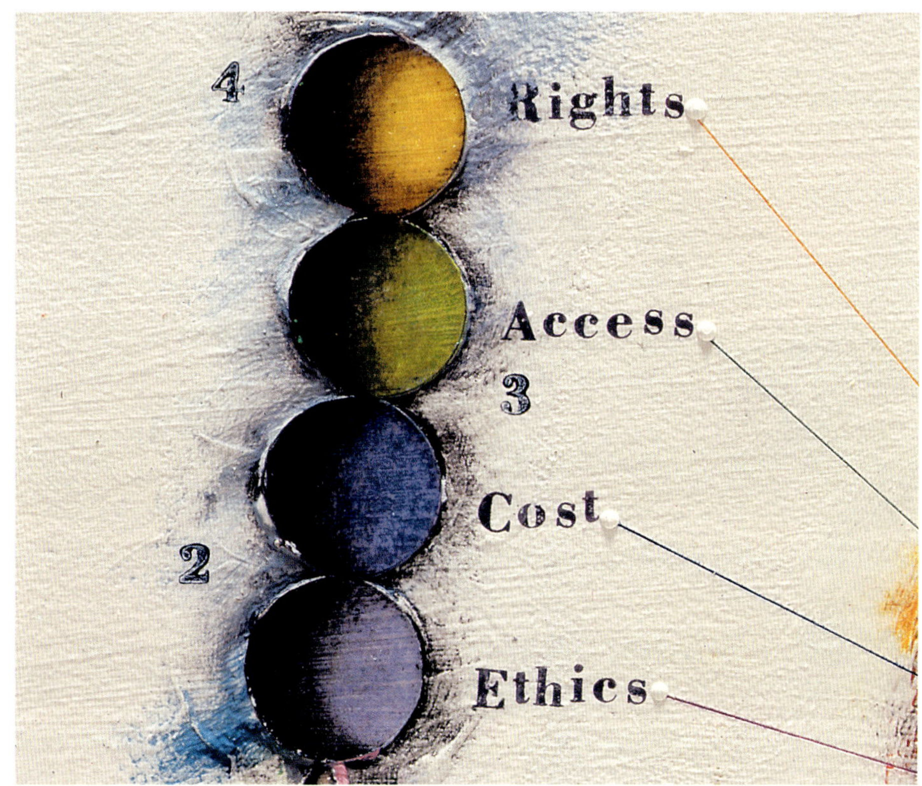

We must weigh the trade-offs between traditional moral and ethical values, individual rights, equity of access, and cost in applying new health care technologies.

distinction between prescription and over-the-counter drugs, and the public was barred from directly using certain drugs even if the drugs passed the Food and Drug Administration's (FDA) safety requirement. Amendments to the Food, Drug, and Cosmetic Act in 1962 required manufacturers to demonstrate a drug's efficacy in addition to its safety in their new drug applications to the FDA. As a result no one—neither physicians nor the public—was allowed to use a drug unless it was proven to be both safe and effective. Amendments to the Food, Drug, and Cosmetic Act in 1976 strengthened the FDA's authority over medical devices by providing for regulation according to a device's potential risk, and as a result some medical devices are now regulated to the same extent as pharmaceuticals.

State practice acts have to a large degree defined which professionals have access to which technologies. All states, for example, use practice acts to specify the extent to which health professionals can use prescription drugs. In all states, physicians and dentists have the right to use drugs for diagnostic or therapeutic purposes. On the other hand, optometrists have the right in only 40 states to use drugs for diagnostic purposes, and in only 11 states to use drugs for therapeutic purposes. State laws have also distinguished among the types of health professionals allowed to prescribe, dispense, or administer drugs. Physicians and dentists have the right to prescribe a drug for patients. In some states, pharmacists cannot prescribe or administer a drug, but they have the right to dispense. In some states, registered nurses can administer a drug but not prescribe or dispense it. Thus, practice acts quite specifically and directly determine who should be given the right to use health care technology.

Health professions associations and health care facilities also have played a major role in the allocation of privileges to use health care technologies (their roles are discussed in more detail in the recommendations contained in this section) with third-party payors exerting an influence through coverage policies and practices. Private and public payors not only decide what types of technology will be covered under their plans or contracts, but also may limit reimbursement to those instances in which the provider of the technology meets specified qualifications.

No one mechanism can efficiently determine who should have the privilege and responsibility for using particular technologies. A number of participants—the public, providers, associations, and the government—have specific responsibilities that they must fulfill to ensure that access to health care technology is readily available to those who can use it in a medically appropriate and cost-effective way.

Responsibilities of Health Professions in the Allocation of Privileges to Use Health Care Technologies

Health professional associations have played a major role in the allocation of privileges to use health care technologies. Many associations were established for the sole purpose of creating and maintaining scientific standards for the professions, and in turn they used these standards to combat quackery and to delineate their own scopes of practice. Directly and indirectly, professional associations have determined which technologies their profession has the competence and need to use. They have sponsored task analyses to profile the profession's general scope of practice and consensus conferences to discuss and recommend the efficacy of specific technologies to the profession. They have developed standards or guidelines with respect to which categories of health professionals can safely use specific technologies, under what circumstances and for which conditions, and the types of additional training that may be necessary to assure competent performance. State practice acts are based heavily on the recommendations developed by professional groups in this regard. In addition, through peer review programs, professional groups have the potential ability to monitor on a continuing basis the ability of their members to use technology safely and effectively, and to rescind or restrict professional privileges when necessary.

Each health profession has the responsibility to identify the technologies for which its practitioners have the training, competence, and need to use in delivering health care services. Professional associations should arrive at these determinations openly, based on scientifically valid standards and criteria, and should inform the public accordingly. Once these standards are adopted, the profession can evaluate whether or not it should be allowed to use a new technology, and can make recommendations as to scope of practice to health care facilities or to those responsible for developing or modifying state practice acts. This approach relies on each profession and each professional to meet the ethical responsibility to acknowledge the limits of their competence to use specific technologies. Given the costs of government regulation and the demonstrated ability of health professional groups to act responsibly, self-regulation is the most effective method for achieving an initial allocation of privileges for those technologies that the public is unable to use directly. Public information provided by professional associations should go beyond general statements as to the basic educational preparation and scope of practice common to all members of a profession by identifying additional types of specialized training, experience, or credentials that may make individual health professionals more highly qualified to use particular technologies.

Each health professional association should conduct and keep current a service inventory which delineates the activities that members of the profession perform in fulfilling the basic responsibilities of the profession. Such an analysis would identify which activities and skills are fundamental to the practice of the profession and which are peripheral. Continuing assessment of whether the profession should use a particular technology should then be made within the context of the skills, competencies, and understanding of clinical indications identified in the service inventory.

Responsibilities of Health Care Facilities in the Allocation of Privileges to Use Health Care Technologies

As the sites where most technologies are used, individual health care facilities and their professional staffs have been instrumental in allocating privileges to use technology. Many of these determinations have been made in the course of operational decisions, such as developing criteria for granting admitting privileges and restricting those privileges, deciding on individual privilege applications, making decisions to purchase technology, and planning for certificate-of-need applications. In this sense, the governing boards and professional staffs of health care facilities have taken on substantial responsibility for

allocating privileges to use health care technology, and they require a certain amount of flexibility in making decisions. For example, a health care facility may find that its mission requires it to apply more stringent regulations over the use of technology than are embodied in state practice acts or commission findings. A diversity of decisions by facilities within the context of government requirements offers individuals a choice of health care delivery modes.

Each health care facility should decide which professionals (both as a class and individually) are allowed to use each technology in the facility, subject to the facility's licensure requirements and the standards developed by health professional associations. Such decisions should be consistent with the professional practice acts in the state. Each facility should have a special standing committee, which includes representatives of all the health professions at the facility, to decide on the allocation of privileges to use health care technology. (Smaller facilities may wish to establish joint committees with other facilities of similar size.) The committee's tasks would be to establish the facility's policy regarding the classes of health professionals allowed to use a particular technology, and to review applications of individual professionals to use a particular technology. Regardless of the motivation for a facility to select the kinds of professionals allowed to use a specific technology, the facility must have established, objective criteria that it applies impartially, and these criteria must be consistent with the facility's licensure and accreditation standards.

In Chapter I, in the section on "Boundaries of Practice for Health Professionals," it was recommended that state blue ribbon commissions be established to adjudicate boundaries of practice issues. Similarly, disputes among the health professions over privileges to use a particular type of health care technology should be resolved by these state blue ribbon commissions. These commissions would ensure that disputes over the use of technology between different health professions and by different specialities within a given profession would be resolved consistently with other boundaries of practice issues. In adjudicating such disputes, however, these commissions should strive to assure that state practice acts remain broad enough so as not to impede the application of evolving new technology by qualified health professionals in the future. In carrying out their functions, the blue ribbon commissions should take into consideration the recommendations as to scope of practice developed by the concerned professional groups, and should resolve conflicts between such recommendations as they pertain to practice in their particular jurisdictions.

Given this additional mandate, the blue ribbon commissions recommended in "Boundaries of Practice for Health Professionals" should include members, both professional and public, who have demonstrated expertise in health care technology issues. In addition, the commission should be free to utilize consultants in instances where additional expertise is needed in resolving disputes.

Responsibilities for the Allocation of Privileges to Use Health Care Technologies in Health Professionals' Offices or Other Health Care Settings

A significant amount of complex and sophisticated health care technology is and will probably continue to be provided in settings that do not meet the definition of a "health care facility" proposed in Chapter II, and, as such, will not be a subject to the privilege allocation and quality assurance mechanisms that are operative in the institutional setting. In Chapter V it is recommended that voluntary quality assurance mechanisms be expanded to cover delivery of care in ambulatory settings, and that such mechanisms include attempts to evaluate and monitor the qualifications of health professionals who utilize complex and sophisticated technology on an outpatient basis.

Health professional associations should establish mechanisms to ensure that health professionals providing technology in offices or other out-of-facility health care settings are qualified to use such technology safely and effectively. Mechanisms should be based on guidelines regarding desirable training, experience, and special certification or licensure developed by the appropriate professional associations. In the ambulatory care setting, review of the qualifications of professionals to utilize technology should be conducted locally on a voluntary basis; such efforts could be monitored for validity and comparability by established peer review programs. Local health professional societies should undertake voluntary review with particular emphasis on office care. As local situations dictate, this mechanism could operate in cooperation with, or apart from, the hospital professional staff. The identity of those professionals who have subjected themselves to voluntary review should be available to the public.

Responsibilities for the Allocation of Privileges to Use Investigative Health Care Technologies

Investigative health care technologies present a unique problem in establishing criteria to govern the allocation of privileges to use a technology. An investigative technology is one for which the benefits and side effects are not well understood; i.e., the technology has progressed to limited human application but lacks wide recognition as a proven and effective intervention in clinical medicine. As a result, its use must be closely monitored, and privileges to use the technology must be more limited than for established technologies.

Privileges to use technologies classified as "investigative" should be restricted to those health professionals and facilities that can demonstrate sufficient experience in using related technologies; guarantee a critical mass of candidates for whom use of the technology is clinically appropriate; devise a research protocol that can meet recognized scientific standards; and demonstrate willingness to share data for collaborative studies, while insuring confidentiality of individual patient information. The four criteria in this recommendation are intended to accomplish two objectives. First, the use of the investigative health care technology will be limited to those providers with a demonstrated record of safety and success with related technologies. Second, those permitted to use the investigative technology will have access to enough patients to gain the proficiency necessary to realize the technology's potential. The Food and Drug Administration is already involved in the allocation of privileges to use investigative technology. Such activity should be continued, and other groups should be involved as well.

The agencies that fund clinical trials of investigative technologies, such as the National Institutes of Health and manufacturers of technology, as well as the Food and Drug Administration, should be responsible for controlling who should be allowed to use an investigative technology. Their actions should be governed by guidelines established by professional associations, accrediting agencies, and industry associations.

Definition of Health Care Facilities

In the past, health care delivery settings could be classified under one of three major categories—hospitals, long-term care facilities, and offices of individual practitioners. The first two categories have traditionally been considered to be "facilities" and therefore must be licensed in the state in which they operate. Although individual health professionals are licensed to provide specific services, the office practices of these health professionals have not traditionally been licensed because these practices have not been considered as facilities per se.

However, the emergence and rapid growth of diverse health care settings and the change in the provision of services from an inpatient to an outpatient basis necessitate a reassessment of the term "facility." Examples of new settings include urgent or episodic care centers, freestanding emergency centers, ambulatory surgical centers, hospices, birthing centers, mental health centers, drug and alcohol abuse centers, and home health care agencies. Some of these newer settings have sought exclusion from licensing or accreditation by reason of their classification as practitioners' offices, although they may or may not be providing services normally associated with practitioners' offices, such as consultation, referral, and medical record maintenance.

As the growth of alternative treatment settings continues, the lines drawn by old definitions become blurred. Ambulatory centers may be owned by hospitals, physicians, or other corporations and may be either nonprofit or proprietary in nature. Some have been reluctant or unable to provide the continuity of care normally associated with health professionals' offices. To consider them as "facilities" in the traditional sense would require their evaluation by licensure. The requirement to submit to this type of scrutiny could impair the ability of some settings to offer lower cost, more convenient alternatives to traditional institutional or professional care. At the present time, these settings and systems, such as health maintenance organizations and preferred provider organizations, have a relatively small share of the medical marketplace nationwide. However, it seems likely that the continuing concern over health care costs will lead to further expansion of such settings.

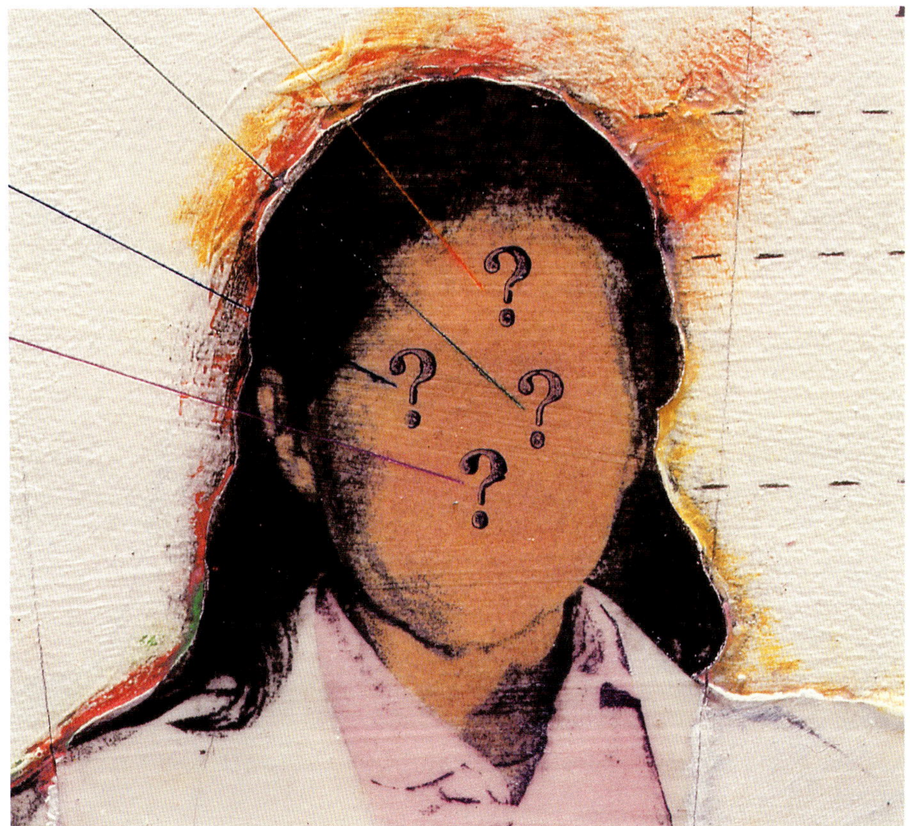

A consensus definition of the term "health care facility" will help the American public make informed choices among the array of health care delivery settings.

A definition that promotes a uniform interpretation of the term "health care facility" applicable to supply and distribution, licensure, payment for services, quality of services, and access to services will assist the American public in making informed decisions among alternatives for the provision of their health care. The implications of not using a consensus definition include lack of uniformity in the public's perception of the individual types of settings, potentially wide variations in the quality of care being delivered in diverse settings, an effect on the distribution of health care facilities, and an inability to evaluate new settings as they develop in the future.

A health care facility should be defined as "a formally organized and legally constituted entity that arranges or contracts for the provision of health care and shares public accountability for the quality, accessibility, and costs of such care with the health professionals who provide or direct the care." This definition balances the rights of individual health care professionals to provide services within the scope of their licenses in settings that may or may not be defined as facilities, and the right of the public to be reasonably assured of the quality and safety of health care provided, regardless of the setting.

Different categories of facilities are identified below; all of them have separate governance of and accountability for the health care services they provide.

Category I: Inpatient Facilities

Some examples of inpatient facilities include but are not limited to acute care hospitals, skilled nursing facilities, alcoholism and substance abuse centers, rehabilitation centers, and psychiatric hospitals. Some characteristics of this type of facility are that it has a governing body and professional staff, is subject to state incorporation laws, and provides services seven days a week, 24 hours a day.

Category II: Ambulatory Facilities (Freestanding and/or Hospital-Affiliated)

□ *Complex and/or Skilled Service Units.* Some examples of these types of facilities include but are not limited to surgery centers (including birthing centers and abortion clinics), emergency centers, and hospital emergency rooms. Some characteristics of this type of facility include the utilization of more complex skills and the provision of more complex services than usually can be provided in a health professional's office; involvement of two or more types of professional staff in the care; the potential to handle life-threatening situations; and physical facilities with specialized equipment and/or technology.

□ *Special Treatment Units.* Examples of special treatment centers include but are not limited to those that provide counseling services, toxic substance abuse treatment, rehabilitation services, home health care services, and dialysis treatment. Characteristics common to these centers include the provision of highly specialized, focused services on a continuing basis. The services are noninstitutional and may be provided by a variety of health professionals.

□ *Special Diagnostic Service Units.* Examples of special diagnostic service centers include but are not limited to independent clinical laboratories, imaging centers, and multiphasic testing centers. The primary characteristic of special diagnostic service centers is the exclusive or extensive use of technology.

Category III: Certain Health Professionals' Offices

Most offices of health care professionals are not health care facilities. However, the professional practice of one or more health professionals may become a health care facility when the scope of the practice, the utilization of technology, or the multiplicity of health professionals and allied health professionals employed reaches a level that would place it in one of the foregoing categories of facilities. Under any of the these circumstances, the community may determine that the public interest in quality, safety, distribution, access, or costs requires a particular type of practice to be classified as a health care facility.

When appropriate, distinctions need to be made between health care facilities and practitioners' offices, although in specific instances the scope of services provided in an office setting may necessitate stricter consideration of the setting as a facility. Under the recommended definition, services provided in facilities such as health and fitness centers are excluded.

It should be noted that there are cost implications for health care provided in settings classified as "facilities." These relate specifically to compliance with any city ordinances, state licensure and regulatory requirements, and voluntary accreditation standards. There is also a potential effect on reimbursement under insurance and entitlement programs. Classification of an entity as a health care facility or as an office may determine the reimbursement policies under which it operates.

Health care organizations should initiate review and approval of this definition by the policy units of their respective organizations. This definition should then be used when responding to specific initiatives by government or others that relate to licensure, supply and distribution, access, payment for services, and quality of services provided in health care facilities. This should, in turn, facilitate wider understanding, acceptance, and support of this definition by the public.

Licensure of Health Care Facilities

Having defined a health care facility, it is now possible to address the issue of licensure of facilities. Licensure helps to ensure a reasonable degree of safety and quality in the delivery of health care, and licensure requirements need to be reexamined as the number and types of facilities change over time.

Standards for licensure and regulation of traditional types of facilities, such as hospitals, long-term care facilities, and physicians' offices, have been clearly delineated. Hospitals and long-term care facilities must meet state requirements to operate. The offices of health professionals have generally not been required to comply with licensing statutes and state regulations, although some of them use equipment and technology that must meet state requirements. However, as new modes of delivery for health care have developed, distinctions between exactly what does and does not constitute an "office" have become unclear.

A few states have addressed or are attempting to address the issue of licensure or regulation of such new entities as freestanding emergency centers, ambulatory surgical centers, imaging centers, and birthing centers. To date, most of these efforts have centered on regulation (statutory authority granted to a public agency to regulate the activities of an entity that may or may not be required to obtain a license) rather than on licensure (a statutory requirement that an entity meet a prescribed set of standards and receive a license to operate). Most states, however, have no firm requirements that relate to those facilities that fall between classification as a traditional "facility" and a health professional's "office." There is also little uniformity in the approaches taken by the individual states to address the various types of new entities that deliver health care.

The participants of the Health Policy Agenda believe a reasonable degree of safety and quality in the delivery of health care in all settings should be ensured. To this end the Health Policy Agenda has addressed the question of which health care entities should be licensed as facilities, and it has provided criteria on which licensing authorities should base their decisions on compliance to licensure standards.

Uniform Principles to Govern the Development of State Licensing Acts

State governments have been addressing the licensure of hospitals, long-term care facilities, and alternative health care facilities in various ways. For example, 39 states have incorporated, in whole or in part, the accreditation process of the Joint Commission on Accreditation of Hospitals (JCAH) as part of their licensure requirements. Licenses are not granted solely on the basis of this accreditation—rather, the license is granted on the basis of an acceptable review of JCAH findings by the state licensing agency. Furthermore, the hospital must still comply with licensing laws and regulations and may have its license revoked if it is found in noncompliance with these laws and regulations. Although the JCAH also operates an accreditation program for long-term care facilities, no state has tied that accreditation to licensure.

Many health care facilities, such as freestanding emergency centers, surgicenters, and birthing centers, operate under relatively unregulated conditions. One reason for the lack of regulation is the difficulty in distinguishing many of these facilities from private physicians' offices, which are exempt from state licensure laws. For example, only two states have enacted legislation governing the licensure of freestanding emer-

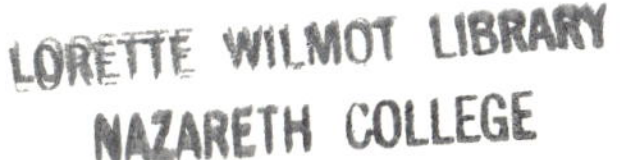

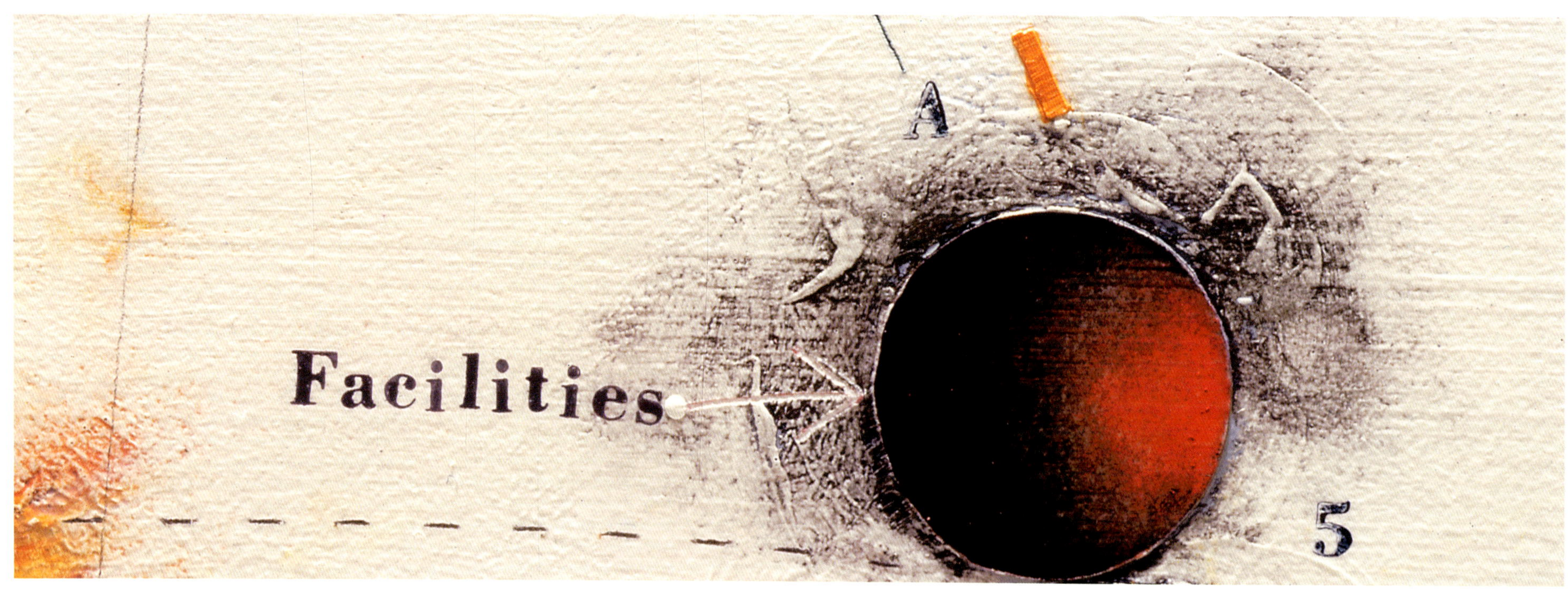

The licensing of all health care facilities can help ensure that a reasonable degree of safety and quality is delivered in all health care settings.

gency centers. Twenty-two states have specific licensure laws for surgicenters, and the other 28 either issue a letter in lieu of licensure or review the facilities under hospital licensure laws. Seventeen states license birthing centers, and 14 others have drafted regulations.

Virtually every state government is attempting to deal with the questions of the extent to which each type of facility should be subject to licensure and regulation and which services they should be permitted to deliver. In an effort to assist states, omnibus and uniform principles that incorporate minimum standards should be developed to be used by states as a basis for their individual facility licensing acts.

At a minimum the omnibus principles should include provisions for the evaluation of professional staff (qualifications, privilege assignment, performance appraisal, retention of privileges, maintenance of competence, and organization of staff); physical plant and equipment (safety, appropriateness of equipment for the services provided, environment, size, and accessibility for the disabled); services (scope of services and provision for back-up services, quality assurance, records, and contract services); and governance and administration (ownership, accountability, and financial condition).

Additionally, there should be provisions to ensure that the licensure process is fair and open, and that it is conducted in a coordinated and cost-effective manner. Multiservice facilities should distinguish among services, and like services should be evaluated by like criteria. Licensing agencies should be provided with enforcement tools—such as the authority to grant provisionary licenses, licenses with a limited duration, or licenses only for specific services—that extend beyond the traditional procedures of licensure, nonlicensure, or revocation of a license. Licensing agencies should also be granted authority to require specific types of facilities to provide minimum services. The duration of a license may vary by type of facility. There should be provisions for making information regarding licensure of a facility available to the public, and discrimination in the provision of services based on ability to pay, race, gender, religion, or national origin should be prohibited. There should be provisions for due process and appeal mecha-

nisms, and provisions for cooperation among facilities for the orderly transfer of technology. Finally, there should be provisions for reference to related statutes (e.g., certificate-of-need laws and professional practice acts).

To develop the principles, a national group composed of representatives from the National Governors Association, the National Conference of State Legislators, and the National Conference of Commissioners for Uniform State Laws should be assembled. This group should have a specific charter and lifespan.

Once principles have been developed, they can be used to guide states as they develop their own individual health care facility licensing acts. States may wish to incorporate stricter standards than those outlined in the principles in their acts, but they should not be more lenient.

State and Federal Role in the Licensure of Health Care Facilities
State governments have the responsibility to ensure that health care facilities meet minimum standards to afford a reasonable degree of safety and quality in the care that they provide. The growth in the number and types of new health care facilities has created a need to reassure the public that these minimum standards are being met. All nonfederal health care facilities should be subject to licensure by the state in which they operate. The licensure function should be carried out by the appropriate state agency. Because of their responsibility for licensing health care facilities, state governments should provide adequate staffing and funding to support the implementation and enforcement of licensure laws. To the extent necessary, sources of tax revenues and licensing fees may need to be adjusted to accommodate the increased costs resulting from implementation and enforcement of the licensing process.

Similarly, the federal government has a responsibility to ensure that minimum standards are met in its facilities. The federal government should ensure that its health care facilities meet the licensure requirements of the states in which they operate, or comparable federal standards.

Supply and Distribution of Health Care Facilities

The competitive environment of the 1970s and the 1980s has resulted in the development of many new types of health care facilities, and as utilization patterns and population demographics continue to change, so will the supply and distribution of various types of health care facilities.

During the last 15 years, two major trends have emerged which are affecting virtually every type of facility—the development of investor-owned and nonprofit multi-facility systems, and increased facility specialization. There has been a significant increase in the proportion of acute care hospitals that are managed by for-profit multihospital systems. Likewise, nursing homes have been affected by the recent trend of ownership or management by for-profit systems. Explosive growth has occurred in "walk-in" health care facilities—the first one opened in Delaware in 1973; there are now about 1,800 of these clinics, and more than 5,000 are expected to be in operation in the 1990s. Increased facility specialization is reflected in the rapid growth of ambulatory surgical centers (surgicenters), hospices, and home health care services. The first surgicenter opened in 1970; in 1980 there was 330 such centers, and this number is expected to double by 1988. There are now just over 1,400 hospices. It is estimated that the number of hospital-based home health care programs increased by 60% from 1984 to 1985 alone, and growth is expected to continue.

Future growth is expected in hospital-based alternative services and in non-hospital facilities. Many hospitals, particularly large ones, are diversifying their services to compete with nonhospital facilities, many of which are less expensive than hospitals and better able to meet specific consumer needs.

Too many or too few health care facilities in particular locations results in an ineffective health care delivery system, but results of efforts to determine an appropriate supply and distribution have been mixed.

In recent years health planning has been in a state of flux. Opposition to planning at the federal level has increased and market forces now play a major role in determining the supply and distribution of health care facilities. This trend is expected to continue in the years to come. However, market forces alone have not resolved some of the problems in health care delivery. For example, there is little or no competition to provide services to those who cannot pay or who otherwise have limited access to facilities. Moreover, experience has shown that unrestricted competition can result in excess capacity and wasteful duplication of services or facilities that add unnecessarily to the costs of health care that a community must bear. There is a continuing need for planning and regulation to ensure that the health care needs of all people in all parts of the country are met.

Community, Regional, and State Roles in the Supply and Distribution of Health Care Facilities

All segments of society, including representatives from facilities, the health insurance industry, government, business, health professionals, and consumer groups, should have a role in determining the supply and distribution of health care facilities. These individuals are familiar with local community and/or regional needs, and can work together to recommend the range of services that should be available in a given facility. Local communities or regions should exercise the responsibility for assessing their needs with respect to the type, size, scope, and location of health care facilities. The role of local communities or regions should be nongovernmental and nonregulatory.

State government involvement in the licensure of health care facilities serves as the basis for an extension of their responsibilities as planning agencies for the supply and distribution of facilities. States have the authority to regulate supply and distribution through certificate-of-need programs, and that authority should be exercised when the cost and delivery of, and access to, services will be affected by facility development or change. State governments should have mechanisms to ensure that needs of the underserved are being met satisfactorily and that wasteful duplication and costly excess capacity are minimized.

Federal Role in the Supply and Distribution of Health Care Facilities

Since the 1950s, the federal government has acted as a catalyst for state planning activities. Past attempts to centralize the planning process have not been highly successful, in part because of the federal government's distance from the needs of the populations to be served. The federal government should, however, continue to play a role in the planning process. The role of the federal government in planning the supply and distribution of health care facilities should be limited to providing planning incentives and resources to states and communities for their activities.

The Responsibility of Health Care Facilities to Serve Community Needs

As previously noted, market forces play a major role in determining the supply and distribution of facilities, but some problems in delivery cannot be met through market forces alone. It is the responsibility of the governing body of health care facilities to ensure that the primary goal of facilities is to serve community need. Individuals who are most familiar with community needs can work together to recommend the range of services that should be available.

Summary

In this chapter, the provision of the technology and facilities for the delivery of health care services has been addressed. Issues related to the moral and ethical considerations in the application of technology, the allocation of privileges to use technology, and the definition, licensure, and supply and distribution of health care facilities were addressed.

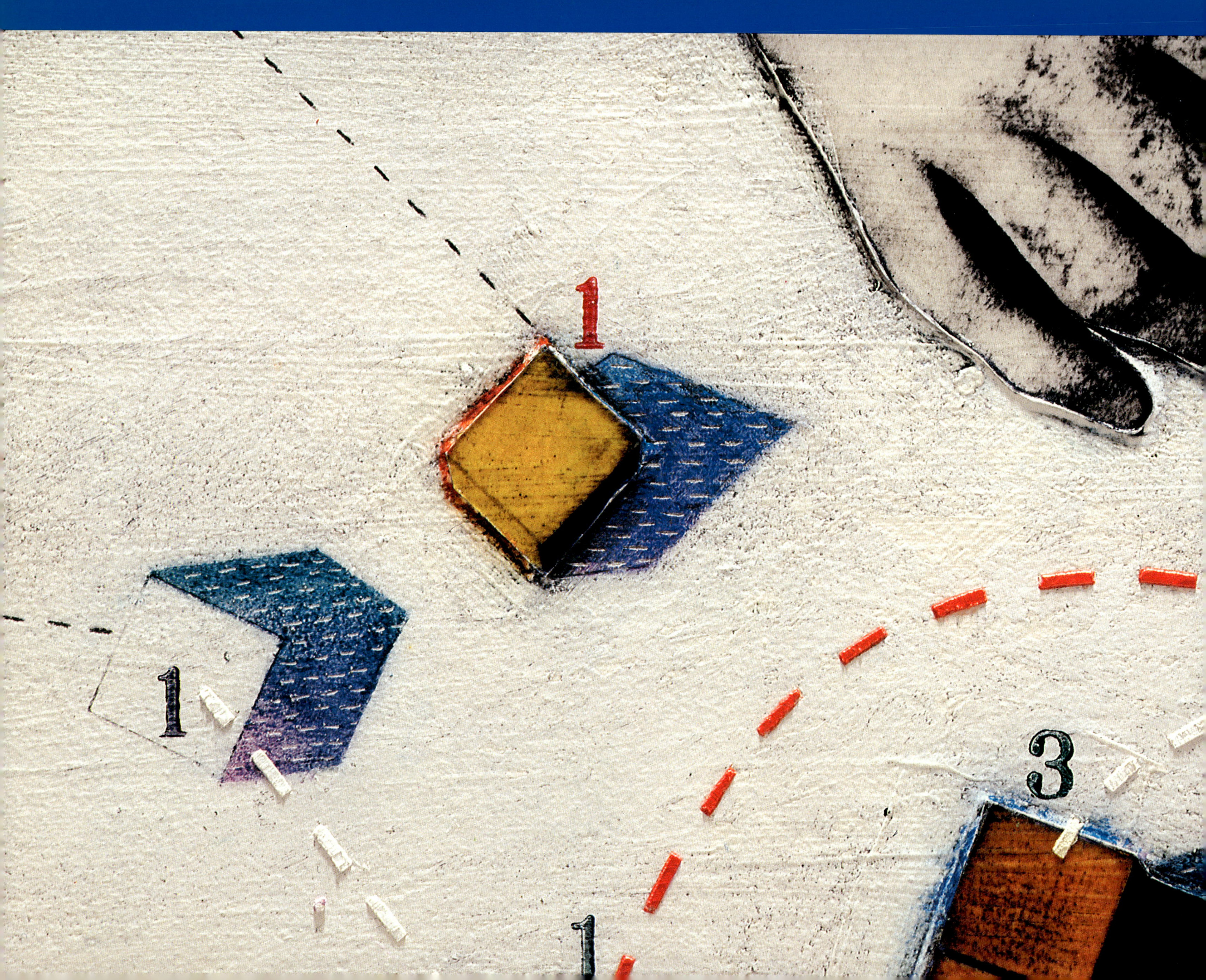

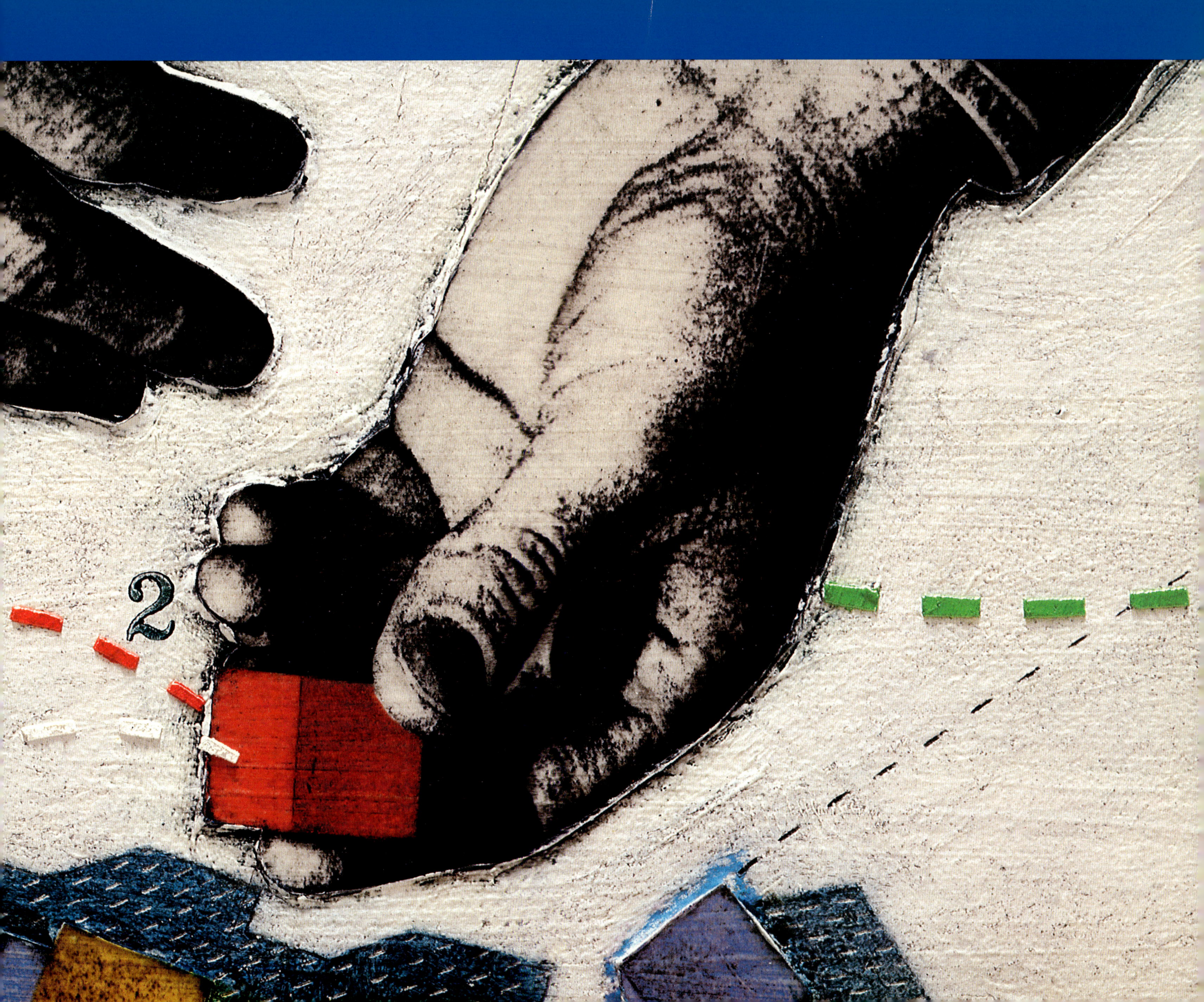
2

Chapter III. Organizing the Resources

The first two chapters addressed the need for the people, technology, and facilities to provide for the delivery of health care services. In this chapter, the organization of these resources to deliver health care will be discussed.

In planning for the delivery of health care services, it is imperative that the issues of access, cost, quality, and availability be addressed. Although planning has not been considered to be highly effective in the past, the delivery system must be responsive to changing societal needs and be able to provide for the health care needs of special populations, including the aged, the poor, the disabled, the medically indigent, and children. The participants of the Health Policy Agenda believe that planning should occur at the community level, with government at all levels ensuring that there are adequate funds and appropriate policies to facilitate the local planning process.

Both the public and the private sector have a responsibility to ensure access to health care services. Many health care professionals and facilities provide needed medical services regardless of a patient's ability to pay for those services, but as a result of the implementation of prospective payment systems and other economic pressures, some of them are reconsidering their positions. Incentives should be developed to ensure that health care services continue to be available to those who cannot pay or who can only pay at reduced rates. Mechanisms are also needed to ensure equity in access to scarce health care technologies, such as organ transplants.

In addition to the moral and ethical considerations that enter into the decision-making process regarding the use of health care technologies, the use of technology is influenced by other factors, including safety, efficacy, potential for societal benefit, and cost. The various groups that participate in the transfer of technology—manufacturers, the federal and state governments, private and public third-party payors, health care facilities, health care professionals and their associations, and consumers—must all assume responsibilities to ensure the optimal use of technologies. Issues involved in health care planning and access to health care services are discussed in this chapter, as are the factors involved in the transfer of technology and the roles and responsibilities of all constituents in the health care delivery system.

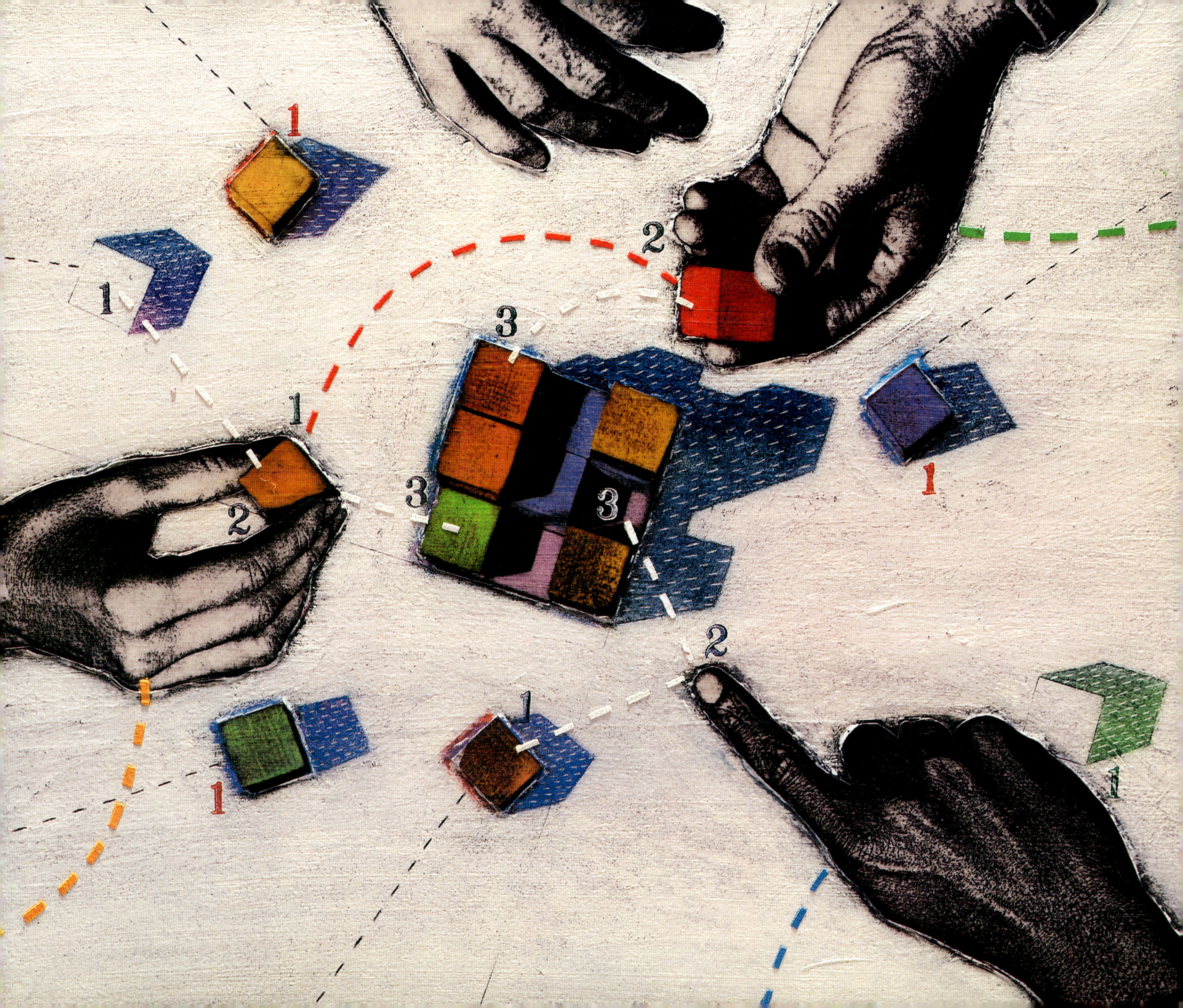

Planning and Delivery of Health Care Services

The delivery of health care must be responsive to changing societal needs. Ensuring access to and availability of high quality, affordable health care is a complicated task; a reassessment of private and public policies relating to the planning for the delivery of health care services is needed. While some argue that past health planning efforts, particularly at the federal level, have been unsuccessful, it is clear that market forces alone will not provide for all necessary health care services.

Initial health planning efforts began at the community level in the 1930s, with the first significant involvement of the federal government occurring with the passage of the Hill-Burton Act in 1946. The Hill-Burton program required health planning at the state level to guide the development of hospital facilities to meet community need, and resulted in an improvement in the geographic distribution of hospital beds. This program was considered to be quite successful, unlike subsequent federal planning activities in the mid-1960s and 1970s. The National Health Planning and Resource Development Act of 1974, as well as the 1979 amendments to this act, sought a more efficient and rational health care delivery system; specifically, it stated that "the achievements of equal access to quality health care at a reasonable cost is a priority of the federal government." However, as the program evolved, the government became less concerned with access to quality care and more concerned with cost issues. Preventing health facility expansion and purchases of new medical equipment with arbitrary caps on health care expenditures in the name of cost reduction became the primary goals of the federal program. The certificate-of-need (CON) program, for example, has primarily focused on regulatory cost-containment mechanisms without sufficient regard for the contributions that planning can make in improving the access to and the distribution of quality health care services.

As a result of past shortcomings, "health planning" has come to be interpreted by many as a process that fails to consider all of the factors necessary for the provision of quality health care, and is often equated with cost-containment and regionalization of services. The need for planning has also been questioned with the development of new and alternative delivery mechanisms, such as health maintenance organizations (HMOs),

preferred provider organizations (PPOs), walk-in health care centers, and wellness clinics. However, problems persist in the system. Millions of people in this country, particularly the underprivileged, do not have access to adequate primary health care, and despite the competitive environment, health care costs continue to escalate.

The participants of the Health Policy Agenda believe that an effective and flexible health planning system is needed to identify the appropriate mix and distribution of health care services and to promote the quality, availability, accessibility, and continuity of health care. This planning system should also address the health care needs of special populations, such as the aged, the disabled, the poor, the medically indigent, and children.

Community Planning for the Delivery of Health Care Services
No single model for the delivery of health care services can meet the needs of patients, practitioners, or other providers in every community throughout the country. However, health care planning can be an effective tool in identifying specific alternative health care services that can be responsive to local needs in an economically realistic manner. Planning for the delivery of health care services should occur and be coordinated at the community level. Factors to be considered in the planning process should include but not be limited to the health care needs of the community, the availability of health care resources, the cost of care, the quality of care, and health services research.

For a private or public sector planning agency to be effective, it must represent and have the active support of the community. The members of the planning agency should include health care professionals, provider institutions, health insurers, business, labor, government, and consumers, including minority groups. The proper mix and number of participants should be determined by the community and may vary from one area to another. Cooperation between experts in the health fields and community representatives is a prerequisite for success in addressing community health needs and priorities.

The function of a planning agency is to identify health care objectives that are responsive to the needs and priorities of the community. Data should be collected on the health status of the community, health needs, and the location of and access to facilities and manpower. The planning process must take into account current information regarding determinants of or related to mortality and morbidity. If these factors can be influenced directly by the health care system, programs can be designed and priorities established accordingly. When the factors are indirectly related to the health care system, or are related to other factors, such as accidents and drunk driving or lung cancer and smoking, health planning can be directed toward exerting as much influence as possible on these programs through health education and disease prevention efforts. Planning agencies should utilize policies, educational programs, and incentives to develop and maintain individual lifestyles that promote good health.

The degree to which the planning process should determine the appropriate mix of health care delivery mechanisms is a recent issue. Market forces currently provide for a pluralistic health care system that encourages the development and proliferation of multiple types of health care delivery mechanisms, and health planners should not prejudice the market for or against any particular mode of providing health care. Rather, the planning process should identify incentives for the providers and participants in the health care system to encourage the development and introduction of innovative and cost-effective health care services.

Currently, many types of organizations plan for health services at the local level, including health planning bodies, state health departments, individual hospitals, businesses, professional organizations, and health care coalitions. Health care coalitions are private sector initiatives that establish liaisons and systematic channels of communication among health care providers, business, labor, and others involved in the financing and delivery of care. One of their primary objectives is to constrain health care costs while ensuring access to and the availability of health care.

In those communities in which many different organizations are addressing access to and the availability of cost-effective health services on an individual basis, they should be encouraged to organize into a single entity to increase effectiveness. If a community lacks a formal structure to address these issues, it should be encouraged to organize the appropriate resources to address its health care needs. In those communities with a public sector health planning body that addresses present and future community needs, the arrangement should be continued and strengthened.

Government at all levels, as a provider, purchaser, and consumer of health services, should play an integral role in the planning process, including the provision of adequate funding and ensuring that government policies and/or regulations facilitate and do not unduly restrict the planning process. To maintain the quality, efficiency, and effectiveness of care and to maximize the use of available resources, specialized services may more appropriately be provided on a state or interstate basis. State departments of health, in many instances, may be logical organizations to assume the role of coordinator for the various planning entities. Each state should develop its own mechanisms for coordinating local planning bodies, since the needs and objectives of states vary according to population demographics, geography, and financial limitations.

While planning should occur at the community level, some mechanisms should exist for enforcing the recommendations of the planning entity. The authority to impose sanctions on those who take actions that are inconsistent with developed plans should be separated from the planning process, and each community should determine its own mechanisms for enforcement. Two appropriate mechanisms for vesting authority are (a) tying facility and provider reimbursement to compliance with planning recommendations, and (b) leaving compliance up to individual facilities or bodies but with public disclosure of those entities that do not abide by the recommendations of the planning body.

Funding for the planning process should be developed by the participants. If the planning body is a public sector entity, it should ideally be supported by both public and private funds. Whether the public funds come from the community, the state, or a combination of both will depend on state and local laws pertaining to health planning, and on the amount of money expended by the government on health care services through Medicaid, state/federal block grants, and state/community financed programs. The private funds should be provided by the other participants in the planning process with the amount determined by the planning body.

For those communities that choose to develop coalitions, a variety of alternatives for funding exist, including contributions from member organizations, member initiation fees, foundation grants, membership dues, and program activities. It is up to individual coalitions to develop the most reasonable and stable source of funding in accordance with their needs. To ensure a viable system there should be a level of financial commitment from all participants.

Community Planning for the Health Care Needs of Special Populations
Much concern has been expressed nationwide over the particular health care needs of the aged, the developmentally disabled, the physically disabled, the homeless, and the chronically mentally ill. These individuals may encounter barriers to obtaining needed medical services; these barriers include the cost of care; the availability of providers, facilities, and technologies; language; and regulations which may restrict the eligibility of needy persons to government-financed health programs. One in eight Americans, for example, has serious trouble in obtaining needed medical treatment, and one in nine has no regular source of care. The planning agency of the community should identify and plan for the needs of the aging and other special populations. The planning process should seek to ensure the availability and the coordination of a continuum of supportive health care services for special populations in senior citizen centers, day care and home care programs, supervised life-care centers, nursing homes, hospitals, hospices, and rehabilitation facilities. The planning agency should look upon "health need" as the predominant factor for determining access to health care and must plan community health services accordingly. Planners must identify barriers within the context of an overall health plan for their community, and stimulate a continuum of levels and types of quality health care in both ambulatory and institutional systems.

To plan for the health care of an aging society, it is essential to work in conjunction with mental health specialists, other health care practitioners, representatives for the aged, and representatives of the disabled, the poor, and others who are familiar with these segments of the population. There are many alternatives for the delivery of a full range of health and related services for the elderly and other special populations, and all such avenues of delivery should be addressed.

Access to Health Care Services

In spite of the increasing expenditures for health care services, certain segments of the population still do not have access to needed care. It is estimated that about 15% of Americans—35 million people—lack any type of health insurance coverage. Even with the success of programs such as Medicare and Medicaid, there are large gaps in access to health care, with a disproportionate burden falling on Hispanics, blacks, the poor, the poorly insured, and the unemployed.

State legislatures are working to develop mechanisms for allocating available resources in a manner that will provide treatment to medically indigent individuals. Thirty-three states currently participate in federal-state medically needy programs that operate in conjunction with Medicaid but allow coverage for individuals who do not fall under the minimum income requirement. In addition, many groups and individuals, both public and private, donate time and services to provide needed medical care to those who cannot pay, and for those who can only pay at a reduced rate.

In addition to the problem of general access to health care services, access to scarce health care technologies deserves consideration. Human organ transplants are now relatively commonplace—they occur, on the average, 100 times a day around the country—but in most cases the demand far exceeds the supply of available organs. Experts expect the pressures to obtain organ transplants and to have access to the best medical technologies available to increase rapidly as we approach the twenty-first century.

No single policy intervention can eliminate all of the financial strain and anxiety that accompany decisions concerning access to health care services. Nor can greatly increased public sector financing to resolve these issues be expected within the foreseeable future. The participants of the Health Policy Agenda believe that access to the health care system should be based on health needs, not on the cost for or availability of services. Both the public and private sectors should ensure that access to care and treatment is available. Mechanisms to resolve conflicts over access to scarce health care technologies are also needed.

Individual Access to Health Care Services

The health care delivery system, as it is currently designed, generally provides individuals with freedom of choice when selecting a provider or a delivery mechanism. Decisions concerning the use of health care services, including the selection of a health care provider or delivery mechanism, should be made by the individual. Payment systems and benefit designs should allow for individual choice. Some individuals are dependent on government-financed health programs, and these programs need to be encouraged to develop alternative delivery mechanisms that enable the medically indigent to attain freedom of choice among appropriate health care providers. To promote informed personal choice, guidelines concerning the options for health care should be available to the general public, employers, and other payors of health care.

Roles of Public and Private Sectors in Ensuring Access to Health Care Services

Many physicians and hospitals provide needed medical care regardless of patients' ability to pay. Such uncompensated care is defined as including charity care provided by a physician or a hospital to those who cannot afford to pay for it, as well as bad debts arising from the care of patients who presumably can pay but who do not do so. It is estimated that about three out of every four physicians in fee-for-service practice provide some form of reduced fee care. Many individual hospitals also respond to the needs of patients unable to pay for their health care. In general, public teaching and nonteaching hospitals provide the greatest proportions of uncompensated care, but hospitals with high proportions of beds devoted to obstetrics, neonatal care, and burn care also provide large shares of uncompensated care, as do hospitals deriving a large percentage of revenue from emergency and other outpatient care. Several factors are causing hospitals to reconsider their positions on uncompensated care. Foremost among them is competition; it is now less feasible for hospitals providing uncompensated care to rely on cost-shifting (i.e., raising charges to other payors to cover the costs of the free care). In addition, local governments must limit their own uncompensated care contributions. As a result of these factors,

and the institution of the Medicare prospective payment system, about 15% of hospitals have placed explicit limits on the amount of charity care they can provide.

Under the current federal Medicaid statute, individuals eligible for assistance include the "categorically needy" and the "medically needy." The current classifications of "categorically needy" and "medically needy" cover a high percentage of the population in need of assistance. However, there are others who do not meet the specified requirements for either categorically needy or medically needy. For instance, the temporarily unemployed or laid-off worker whose assets, such as a home and car, preclude participation in federal and/or state assistance programs may not have money available for health care insurance and/or minimum health care. These individuals may defer needed health care services, and postponement of needed medical attention often leads to more severe illness.

Both the public and private sectors should be encouraged to donate resources to improve access to health care services. Where appropriate, incentives should be provided for those in the private sector who give care to those who otherwise would not have access to such care. In addition, existing shortcomings in the current public system for providing access need to be addressed. Individual health care providers, institutions, and philanthropic organizations should be commended, rewarded, and encouraged to maintain, and expand where appropriate, public health services programs. Various incentives should be developed to stimulate and support increased private sector involvement as an additional source of payment for health care services; these incentives might be provided under existing or modified tax laws. There should be sustained, and where appropriate, enhanced public reimbursement of facilities and health care professionals that offer and provide voluntary care. The shortcomings and inequities in the current Medicaid system, such as the variability among states in the criteria for classification as medically needy, should be addressed.

Further, national private sector groups should address the issues of health care coverage for the unemployed who have lost health benefits and for individuals who currently "fall through the cracks" of the health care system. Because paying for the health

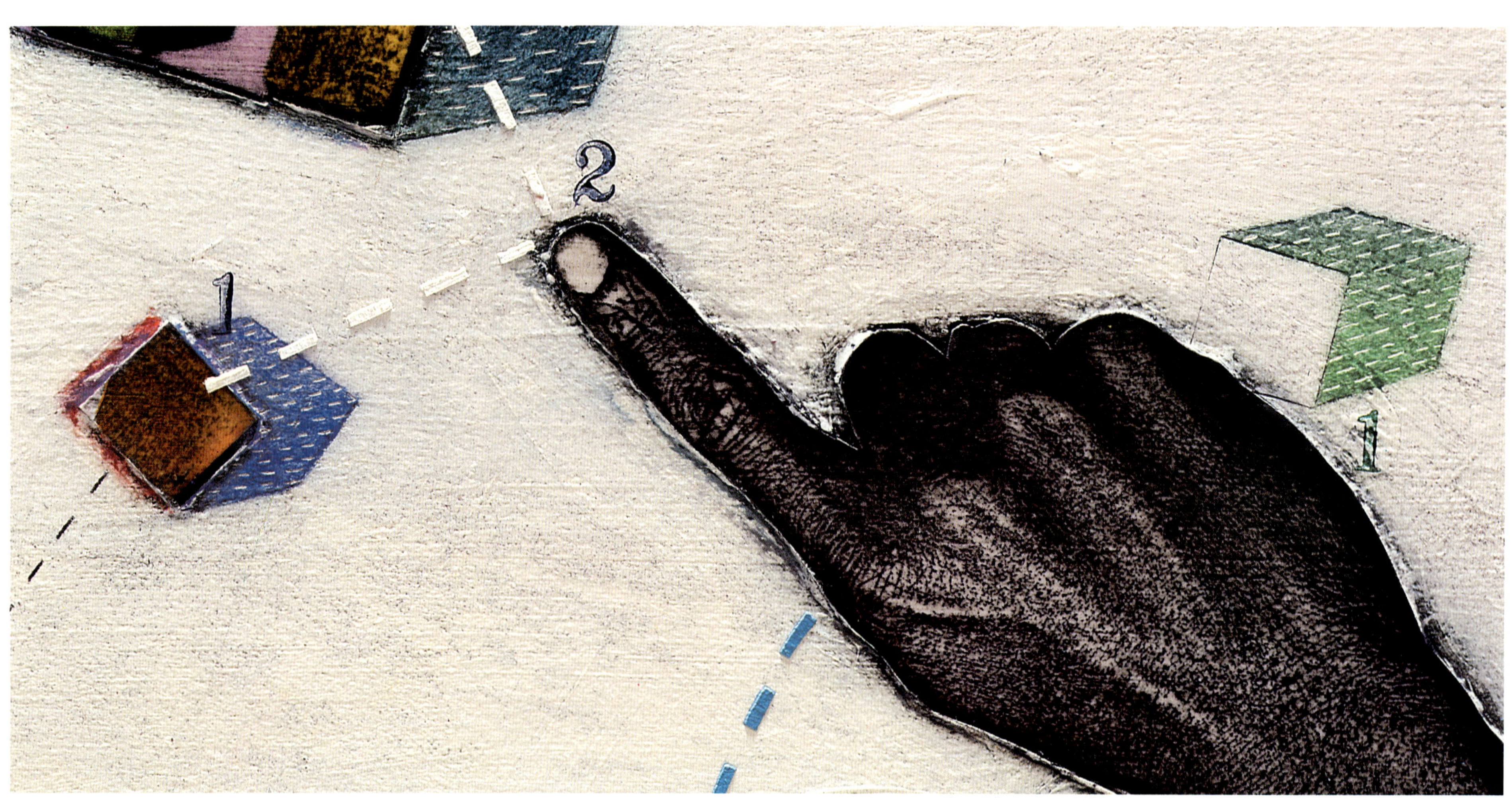

Access to health care services for people who cannot pay and for those needing scarce health care technologies should be improved.

care services to be provided to all of these groups is a critical issue, recommendations affecting the private and public sectors vis-a-vis access to needed health care are addressed in Chapter VI. In that chapter, the roles and responsibilities of federal, state, and local governments, and the need for a basic health insurance benefit package to ensure baseline coverage for all Americans, health care for the medically indigent and uninsurable, health insurance for children, and catastrophic and long-term care insurance are outlined.

Access to Scarce Health Care Technologies

Scarce health care refers to those items and services for which the demand exceeds the existing supply (such as liver, kidney, or heart transplants) and advanced technologies (such as magnetic resonance imaging). National criteria to ensure equity of access to these services do not exist. Currently, individuals or their families who are able to gain the attention and support of the local community and/or the nation are more likely to receive assistance in obtaining needed scarce health care. Therefore, some mechanism is needed to ensure that, insofar as possible, apportionment of care is carried out on a logical and fair basis.

Health care facilities should have or should establish review bodies (such as hospital ethics committees) to resolve conflicts over access to scarce health care technologies. In the event that a conflict over delivery of scarce health care technologies cannot be mediated satisfactorily, individuals should be able to seek redress through appropriate appeal mechanisms.

There are committees and agencies in existence that can aid individuals and health professionals in making decisions regarding the delivery and in determining the medical necessity of care. Examples of such bodies include hospital review committees, ethical boards, peer review organizations, and county, state or other health professional societies. These committees have been functioning satisfactorily at the facility level. Existing review mechanisms need to remain in effect, and facilities that do not currently have such a body need to implement a review system.

Using the private sector and groups currently involved in the allocation of scarce health care technologies, guidelines for determining who receives care and the financial responsibilities of third-party payors (including society as a whole) should be developed. The probability of success and the quality of life following receipt of care should be considered as key factors.

Facilities that are serving as a site of health care delivery should have an established mechanism to provide counseling to aid in making difficult treatment decisions, particularly decisions relating to scarce health care technologies. The review bodies should be multidisciplinary, incorporating physicians, additional health care professionals, consumers, ethicists and clergy, among others. In making decisions, the review body should consider fully the individual factors presented in each case, and the review process should use the precedents established for similar situations in similar settings.

One of the responsibilities of the review body should be to serve as the primary source of internal conflict resolution. Reasonable criteria should be applied to the conflict resolution, and the review process should take place as close to the site of conflict as possible. The review process also should include a local or regional system for appeal of facility treatment decisions for any party dissatisfied with a decision.

The Transfer of Technology

Health care technology consists of the pharmaceutical products, medical equipment, procedures, and techniques used in the delivery of health care. Pharmaceutical products are the drugs, both prescription and over-the-counter, that are regulated by the Food and Drug Administration. Medical equipment includes devices purchased by health care providers (for example, life support equipment and surgical instruments) and consumers (for example, eyeglasses and hearing aids). Medical procedures are those treatments, such as surgery, laboratory tests, and diagnostic and therapeutic radiology, performed to diagnose or alleviate particular health problems. Procedures may have multiple techniques. For example, suturing an incision is a procedure, but the choice of suture methods is a technique.

The transfer of health care technology is a process which begins with the generation of new knowledge and ends with the application of new technologies for the improvement of health care. The decision to use any type of technology involves a consideration of the delicate balance between meeting the needs of individuals, minimizing the risk of premature use, and satisfying the demands placed on the health care system by society. In making these kinds of decisions, safety, effectiveness, and cost must be primary considerations.

Technology transfer is influenced by many factors, including the nature of the technology, the level of research funding, the degree of government regulation, and third-party payor reimbursement. Additionally, it is influenced by the various groups— manufacturers, health care professionals, and consumers—involved in the availability, diffusion, and application of technology. Each group involved in the transfer of technology has specific responsibilities, and the responsibilities of the nine major groups are outlined below:

□ *Manufacturers* of health care technologies directly influence the transfer of technologies through decisions that determine whether products are developed and marketed. These decisions occur after consideration of the economic potential on the intended market, the state and federal regulatory environment, and reimbursement policies of both public and private third-party payors.

□ *The federal government* influences the transfer of technology by virtue of its power to regulate, through the FDA, the availability of new drugs and devices in the nation as a whole.

□ *State governments* similarly influence the transfer of technology through legal mechanisms, such as certificate-of-need regulations. These regulations require hospitals to show evidence of need (based on minimum utilization) before being allowed to buy equipment or to construct additional facilities costing more than a specified amount. Because the determinations are made at regional, state, or local levels, a particular technology may be more widely available in one part of the country than in another.

□ *Public third-party payors,* through programs such as Medicare and Medicaid, influence the transfer of technology through policies regarding coverage. For example, before the passage of the Social Security Amendments of 1972, end-stage renal dialysis was distributed to only a select group of patients. But once Medicare covered dialysis, all end-stage renal disease patients who would benefit from dialysis could receive it. The government acts as a fiscal intermediary, and therefore influences financial accessibility to technology.

□ *Private third-party payors* affect the transfer of technology by deciding what types of technology will be covered under their plans or contracts. Major payors can form coalitions to acquire greater influence and decision-making power over what they will pay for and therefore what technology will be made available. High-cost technology that private third-party payors will not finance will usually not be widely used.

□ *Health care facilities* influence the transfer of technology through decisions regarding the scope of practice within the facility, and through decisions concerning the purchase of medical equipment and/or drugs for use by the health professionals and the patients they serve.

□ *Professional and scientific associations* influence technology through their judgments as to the safety, efficacy, and clinical indications for use of different technologies, and by promulgating standards for use of such technologies.

□ *Individual health professionals* influence the transfer of technology through decisions as to the appropriateness of specific technologies for their patients, as well as through decisions to purchase specific medical equipment.

□ *Consumers* primarily influence the transfer of technology through exercising their preferences for specific drugs and equipment and, to a lesser degree, through expressing their preferences for specific procedures and techniques, either alone or in conjunction with a health professional.

New technologies are major resources that can in many cases enhance the quality of patient care and at the same time reduce the cost of producing a specific therapeutic outcome. An integral part of the technology transfer process is the use of new products and new applications of existing products; manufacturers have been, and continue to be, in the forefront of product innovation. However, despite the benefits that can accrue to individuals and society as a whole through product innovation, all potential risks cannot be known at the time of innovation, and there is an irreducible minimum risk for those individuals who use medical products. Solutions to the problems of product liability were extensively discussed by the Health Policy Agenda, but it was not possible to reach a consensus. Therefore, this issue is not addressed in the report.

All participants in the health care system—providers, payors, manufacturers, government, and consumers—have responsibilities in the technology transfer process. The roles of participants are delineated in the following recommendations.

Factors Affecting the Use of Health Care Technology

The particular role of each group in the transfer of any given technology depends in large measure on the characteristics of the technology in question. A pluralistic approach to influencing and determining the transfer of technology should be continued, but with a clear delineation of which groups should be involved and the nature of that involvement.

All providers, payors, manufacturers, health care facilities, governmental units, and consumers of health care have an obligation to contribute to an orderly process of technology diffusion. The nature of each group's involvement should be based on the characteristics of the technology, which include safety and effectiveness, potential for societal benefit, and cost. The groups involved in technology transfer should assess the need for and nature of their involvement in influencing the transfer of any given technology based on the following guidelines; these guidelines should be considered as a whole as they are interdependent.

□ *Effectiveness* is the degree to which a diagnostic, preventive, therapeutic or other action achieves the intended result under usual or normal circumstances. Thus, effectiveness requires a consideration of outcomes.

When a technology is *moderately to highly effective,* its transfer should be influenced by consumer preference, and by health professionals and professional associations through encouraging the use of the technology for appropriate patients.

However, when a technology's effectiveness is found to be *low or marginal,* its transfer should be influenced by both private and public payors, either through withholding coverage for the technology in general or by withholding coverage for specific, inappropriate applications of the technology. It should also be influenced by professional associations through consensus statements on ineffectiveness, and by health professionals through refusal to order or use the technology. Health facilities should influence its transfer through refusal to allow use of the technology within the facility. Its transfer can also be influenced through educational programs, such as the FDA's Health Fraud Program, which provides information to consumers on technologies lacking proven effectiveness.

□ *Safety* is the probability that use of a particular drug, device or medical procedure will not cause unintended or unanticipated hurt, disease, or injury. Safety is, in this context, a relative concept that must be balanced against the effectiveness of the drug or procedure in question. Drugs or procedures known to cause hurt, disease, or injury when used are not usually thought of as unsafe if the benefits they give exceed the damage.

The issue of safety is inextricably linked to the issue of risk. Even though a drug, device, or medical procedure does not result in unintended harm, and it is therefore deemed to be safe, there is always an element of risk involved in its use. This is why safety is defined in terms of probabilities. For example, aspirin is considered to be safe, but there are risks involved in its use, especially if one is allergic to it. There are other unintended consequences which may result from its use, so there is a risk involved even though it is safe.

When the safety of a technology is *high* (the risk from use is negligible) its transfer should be influenced by consumer preferences. When the use of a technology is *relatively safe* (there is some risk but it is still low), manufacturers and providers of the technology should provide accurate information on its benefits and risks to the individuals using it through labeling and package inserts.

However, when the safety of a technology is *moderate to low* (the risk involved in use is moderate to high), its transfer should be influenced through federal regulations governing the availability of new drugs and devices. Private and public payors should decide whether to provide coverage in general or for specific applications of the technology. Professional associations should make recommendations to members about safety, appropriate clinical indications, and qualifications of providers. Health facilities play a role in delineation of professional privileges within the facility. Finally, health professionals should make judgments as to appropriateness for individual patients.

□ *Benefit to Society.* There are instances in which the application of a particular technology will benefit only a very few individuals, and there are instances in which the application of a particular technology will benefit society as a whole. Immunization against infectious disease is an example of the latter case.

When a technology's potential benefit to society as a whole is *low,* its transfer should be influenced by consumer preference. However, when a technology's potential benefit to society is *high,* its transfer should be encouraged by public and private payors through offering coverage for its use, by state and federal governments through *requiring* its coverage by public and private payors, and by health professionals and professional associations through encouraging widespread use of the technology.

□ *Cost.* In this era of trying to control expenditures for health care, the issue of technology transfer and cost is very sensitive. The role of cost is addressed in the next recommendation.

The Role of Cost in the Use of Health Care Technologies

Basing treatment decisions on both health and monetary considerations is a difficult task, and the process itself can raise serious ethical questions. The data required to make decisions based on effectiveness, benefit, and cost may not be complete, available, or reliable. Furthermore, some medical choices are influenced by factors that cannot readily be quantified or assigned a dollar value. For example, how much is "pain relief" worth? How much is the reassurance provided by a negative test result worth?

Despite the difficulties inherent in making decisions of this kind, some parameters need to be defined and applied to assist in the process of deciding when and how technology transfer is to occur. Cost-effectiveness and cost-benefit analysis take into consideration both monetary and nonmonetary factors that need to be used to guide the decision-making process. As classically defined, cost-effectiveness analysis is the comparison of dollar costs to results or benefits that are expressed in nonmonetary terms, such as years of life saved or sickness/disability days prevented. Cost-benefit analysis is the comparison of dollar costs to results or benefits that are also expressed in monetary terms.

The availability and application of technology should never be limited in the health care sector because of cost alone, but continuing analysis of cost-effectiveness and cost-benefit should always be a major factor in the continued availability and utilization of a given technology. Furthermore, public and private payors should make coverage available for any costly technology that can be demonstrated to improve health or quality of life and that is cost-effective. Coverage decisions by payors should be based on clear criteria for clinical indications and contraindications. Costs for application of a technology should always be considered in the context of other technologies or interventions available, and the health outcomes and benefits derived from such use.

Cost-benefit assessments of a given technology in relation to expected benefits for an individual patient can best be done by the health professional. However, systematic attempts are needed to evaluate cumulative data on the cost-versus-health benefits of technologies for specific categories of patients, as well as the cost-effectiveness of specific technologies in relation to other available interventions or treatments for the same condition. Such evaluations can best be made by the type of public-private sector technology assessment consortium recommended in Chapter V in the section on the evaluation of health care technology. This technology assessment consortium would be funded by and composed of representatives from the health professions and providers, and from public and private payors, including self-insured groups, business, labor, government agencies, consumer groups and other organizations involved in or concerned with technology assessment activity. It would be charged with identifying, collecting, synthesizing,

Payment for health care technology should be related to its resource costs, i.e., the amount of time, skills, and training required to use the technology appropriately.

and disseminating data from public and private sector studies on the safety, efficacy, indications for use, cost-benefit, and cost-effectiveness of new and existing technology, with analysis of existing technology assessment methodology and development of improved methodologies where indicated.

The discussions and findings of this consortium with respect to safety, efficacy, clinical indications, and cost-effectiveness provide a foundation upon which individual private and public payors could base their coverage decisions.

Third-Party Payor Role in Diffusion and Regionalization of Technology

Experience with certificate-of-need laws has shown that government regulation alone is of mixed effectiveness in promoting cost-effective regionalization of health care technology. A potentially more effective strategy is for payors to encourage the regionalization of technology by reimbursing only certain providers. Third-party payors should support and promote limited diffusion of new technologies and regionalization of all technologies that are costly or resource-intensive. Third-party payors should accomplish this by limiting payment to those providers that demonstrate, according to professionally-developed standards, that they possess (1) a critical mass of potential patients for whom the technology is appropriate; (2) the resources to use the technology at a volume sufficient to achieve clinical proficiencies; and (3) an institutional commitment to maintain adequate standards of proficiency. An example of the kind of professional standards for utilization and proficiency that could be used by payors in establishing selective payment policies are those prepared by the American College of Obstetricians and Gynecologists for perinatal care units.

Third-Party Reimbursement for New Technologies

Payment for health care technology should be related to its resource costs, i.e., the amount of time, skills, and training required to use the technology appropriately. For new technologies, especially those for which there are few analogues, third-party payors have difficulty in establishing fair and reasonable reimbursement. Because of the uncertainties inherent in any new technology, professional associations must be included as participants in the development and revision of payment schedules. Therefore, third-party payors and professional associations should jointly determine, based on a technology's resource costs relative to other technologies, the payment level for a new technology. Additionally, because the resource costs of a new technology may decrease substantially once it is integrated into the health care delivery system, payors should frequently re-evaluate their payment levels for new technologies, using the same resource-cost approach.

Health Care Facilities and the Acquisition of Health Care Technology

Technology transfer decision-making in health care facilities is multifaceted in nature, and includes medical, legal, economic, and ethical considerations. Such decisions require input from a variety of sources, including medical researchers and practitioners, consumers, suppliers, and a range of disciplines within the facility itself.

The decision-making process concerning technology use should be incorporated and coordinated with the overall institutional planning process. Health care facilities should use processes that incorporate data regarding safety, effectiveness, cost, and conditions of use; and these factors should be balanced with the institution's mission, community need, delivery capacity, and financial feasibility in decisions regarding the acquisition of costly or resource-intensive technology. The analysis of community need should take into account other available resources in the community, and the opportunity for cooperation and coordinated use of resources. A technology assessment process based on these principles, supported by a financing system that allows for real growth to support efficacious advances, is the best guarantee of quality care at a reasonable cost.

Health care facilities should continue to develop and use internal management and planning processes for the acquisition of costly technology. The evaluation process should include the participation of staff from a number of disciplines, including physicians and other health care professionals knowledgeable about the technology and patient care needs; hospital planners; facility engineers; purchasing managers; and financial managers. Management should be responsible for conducting such planning and evaluation processes and must accept final accountability for decision-making.

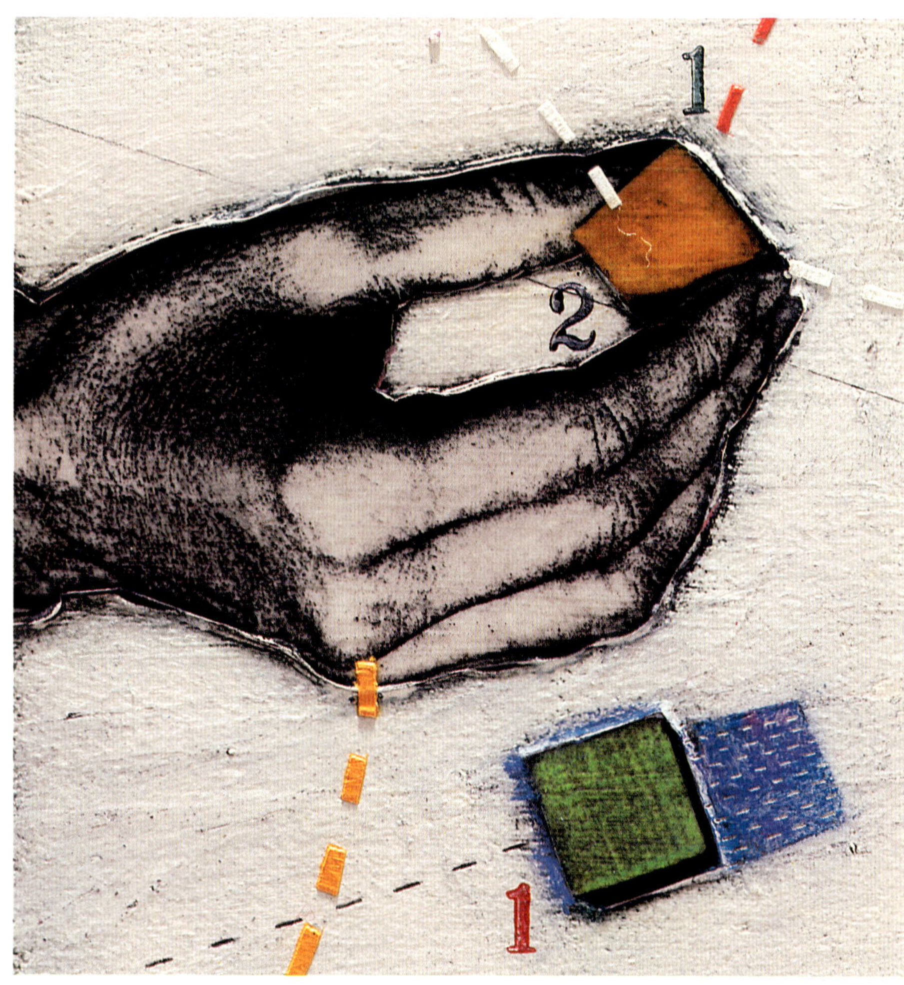

Manufacturers, government, third-party payors, health care professionals, and consumers must all assume a role in ensuring optimal use of technologies.

Third-Party Payor Support for Technological Innovations and Clinical Research
Payment systems have a major impact on the transfer of a technology—reimbursement decisions concerning the use of a new technology or reconsideration of the use of an existing technology markedly affects its availability. The potential impact of reimbursement decisions on technology transfer can be illustrated using the Medicare prospective payment system as an example. Because Medicare is the largest third-party payor, its actions often influence all other reimbursement decisions. Under the prospective payment system, the development and diffusion of costly but effective new technologies may be stifled. An adjustment factor has been incorporated into the payment system to provide funds for the acquisition of new technology; but, under current regulations, funds for the acquisition of new technology must come from the money saved as a result of hospital efficiency. This limitation makes it very difficult for facilities to acquire costly but effective technology.

Technological innovations are also impeded by the high costs of conducting clinical research, which serves as a basis for improvements and advances in medical therapy and is an integral component of the technology transfer process. Preliminary data support the view held by many clinical researchers that patients in a research study consume more health care resources than those patients with the same diagnosis that are not enrolled in a study. For example, the cost of patients receiving cancer therapy as part of a research protocol is estimated to be about 30% higher than for nonprotocol patients. However, by statute, Medicare cannot pay for research-related costs, leaving researchers in the position of trying to find supplemental funds to cover the extra costs of research. Clinical research in the area of mental illness also requires some consideration because the National Institute of Mental Health has no program to cover the costs of patient care in its research grants.

Many believe that prospective payment systems have the potential to seriously disrupt the technology transfer process. Academic medical centers are particularly concerned that clinical research activities will be disrupted and researchers forced to abandon their studies to maintain the solvency of the hospital or department. Third-party payors should contribute to the acquisition of technologies that may be expensive but that improve the quality of care; they should also contribute to clinical research for the development, refinement, and evaluation of new and established therapies.

The Health Care Financing Administration (HCFA) could provide the necessary adjustments in its payment system for the acquisition of effective but expensive technologies. These adjustments are necessary for fostering the continued development of new technologies in disease management. The level of payment needs to be recalibrated frequently to reflect the impact of more costly technology; delays in recalibration will negatively influence manufacturer decisions to commit the time and financial resources for research and development of new technologies that offer improved patient care at a higher cost.

With respect to clinical research, more data need to be gathered to determine the actual differences in health care costs incurred by research and nonresearch protocol patients. Using this information, a joint study of the problems of patient care costs in research could be conducted by major third-party payors and supporters of clinical research. This group should explore possible ways of covering the additional costs for patient care in clinical research; legislative amendments will be required to allow HCFA to cover an equitable share of these costs.

Communication of Research Findings

The accurate and timely flow of information from the biomedical research community to the practicing community is necessary for the development, application, and replication of new findings. Traditionally, biomedical information has been disseminated through publications, scientific meetings, and informal peer-to-peer contact. However, the need for editorial changes and peer review introduces delays in the communication of findings, and there is some concern that some types of medical information are disseminated too slowly to those who might benefit the most. Certainly, the validation of findings by peer review is necessary, but the communication of important medical news should not be impeded by the extensive delays that often result from the journal review process.

Health care professionals and their organizations should ensure that the results of biomedical research and of technology assessment are communicated in an accurate and timely manner to both the research and the practicing communities. Electronic technologies offer many opportunities to enhance the efficiency of journal review and to rapidly communicate published findings to the health care community. On-line computer databases, television, and radio are three forms of electronic communication that can be used.

The journal peer review process can be expedited by the use of computers in the submission of articles to journals, in manuscript changes, in transmitting notices of acceptance or rejection, and in sending manuscripts to the publisher for printing. Health care professionals should be familiar with computer-based information systems. Medical television and radio programs should be expanded, and consumer and insurance groups should be encouraged to contribute to electronic sources of information. However, the use of electronic media does not preclude the need for validation of findings through the peer review process.

Associations of health professionals and specialty societies sponsor many activities to transmit information on the use of new technologies to the practicing community. Their activities include the development of guidelines, recommendations, or consensus statements on the safety, efficacy, and clinical applications of new and existing technologies. They also sponsor continuing education programs, including formal self-assessment and voluntary recertification for their members.

Specialty societies, health care professional organizations, and local and state medical societies should intensify their efforts to disseminate information to their members on the effective use of technology. These groups should identify "opinion leaders"—those individuals who influence attitudes and behavior in a desired way—to communicate information on new technologies. Although journals, continuing education, and scientific meetings are important sources of information, the actual decision to use a new technology does not usually occur until a respected peer has validated its use by reporting favorable results. Opinion leaders can be very effective in establishing the use of new technologies in the practicing community.

The Use of Peer Review by Scientific Journals

The dissemination and validation of the results of biomedical research and technology assessment depend in large measure on the peer review that is conducted by scientific journals prior to publication of articles. The peer review system is designed to screen reports that are poorly conceived, designed, or executed, or otherwise suffer from severe shortcomings. Additionally, peer review can lead to improvements in the quality of manuscripts.

Although there is a consensus that the current system for peer review works reasonably well, the peer review system used by professional journals should be strengthened by health professionals and their organizations. A private or public sector study group should be created to analyze the policies and practices of the peer review system used by professional journals. The goal of this study would be to improve the ability of journals to promote scientific advancement and to enhance patient care. Potential areas for analysis include but are not limited to a study of the validity of peer review; a study of the time spent between receipt of a manuscript and final rejection or acceptance for publication; and a study of the fate of articles which are not accepted for publication. The entire scientific community, including journal editors, reviewers, authors, and professional societies and organizations, should lend its support to this effort.

Additionally, scientific journal editors should inform readers and authors of what happens to a manuscript after it is submitted for publication. Disclosure of a journal's method of review would be helpful in a critical assessment of different review processes.

Continuing Education and the Use of Health Care Technology

The primary goal of continuing education for health professionals is to ensure that skills do not become obsolete with the passage of time. The introduction of new technologies after a practitioner has completed formal training necessarily implies that health care professionals have a responsibility to engage in continuing education activities to improve patient care.

Health care professionals should employ a variety of methods, including formal continuing medical education and self-directed studies, to acquire the necessary knowledge to use technology appropriately. Continuing education can include formal courses and seminars, professional meetings, reading, and consultations with colleagues. The value of self-directed, individualized learning experiences, such as those made available by professional associations and specialty societies, should not be overlooked.

Consumer Use of Health Care Technologies

As previously stated, the nature of each group's involvement in the transfer of technology should be based on the characteristics—including the safety and effectiveness—of the technology. To enable them to use a health care technology, individual consumers have a right to receive sufficient information from suppliers of health care technology, providers of health care, and relevant governmental agencies. In turn, consumers have an obligation to comply with the instructions for the use of health care technologies. Health professionals have traditionally advised their patients on the effective use of drugs, devices, and procedures. This activity should be expanded to improve the patient-provider relationship, to promote patient compliance with treatment regimens, and to reduce the risk involved in the use of any technology.

Regarding the use of low-risk technologies—such as over-the-counter drugs, blood pressure measurement devices, diagnostic screening tests, and cardiopulmonary resuscitation—individual consumers are the most effective decision-makers. Providers should make available sufficient information to allow self-administration of low-risk technologies, and consumers should exercise their preferences for these technologies either independently or in conjunction with the appropriate health care professional.

A number of organizations—industry, professional, and consumer—prepare and disseminate patient education materials; these organizations should consider the joint development of informational packets on the most commonly used drugs, devices, and procedures. Health professional associations should encourage the distribution of these materials to patients.

The Role of Government in the Development of Health Care Technology
Certainly the public must be protected against dangerous and ineffective technology. The Food and Drug Administration currently assures the safety and efficacy of pharmaceutical products and medical devices entering the marketplace. Over the past 25 years, the FDA has been very cautious in allowing the availability and use of potentially useful drugs for consumers, even when alternative treatments are not available.

Although some time lag is necessary before a new technology should gain widespread use in medicine and surgery, long and unnecessary delays are undesirable and potentially damaging to innovation. The rate of new drug introductions has sharply declined, and the costs associated with introduction of new drugs have rapidly risen over the past quarter century. Although there have been no rigorous analyses of the impact of stricter regulations governing the introduction of new medical devices, it is expected that the end result of these regulations will be fewer new devices, decreased diversity of suppliers, reduced competition, and rising prices of medical devices.

In addition to assuring safety and efficacy, federal regulatory agencies should be given the additional charge of assessing the long-term effects of their activities on the development of new technologies. These agencies should be given the necessary resources to perform this activity. Legislation will be required to allow the FDA to assess the long-term impact of its regulatory activities on product development. Funds will need to be allocated to analyze the problem and to acquire the additional qualified personnel to conduct the research. Congress should consider making an additional change in FDA directives to allow increased input from industry-affiliated experts who may not otherwise be allowed to participate in this assignment. Collaboration between industry representatives and the FDA would inject additional expertise and manpower into this new activity and into the mandated drug and device reviews for safety and efficacy.

Development of Health Care Technologies for Rare Disorders
There are a number of rare disorders—such as Huntington's disease, Lou Gehrig's disease, and Tourette syndrome—that affect a relatively small number of individuals. Effective treatment of these disorders is stymied by limited understanding of the disease process and by the lack of financial incentives for manufacturers to invest in the development of new and potentially useful treatments. Because the commercial market is so limited, few manufacturers want to take the risk of investing time and money in these products of limited use, which are also known as "orphan" products. As a result, several federal governmental agencies have collaborated with industry to make some orphan drugs or devices available. One of the major obstacles for manufacturers was addressed in the Orphan Drug Act of 1983, which provides marketing exclusivity (for seven years) to unpatentable designated orphan drugs.

Manufacturers have performed an important public service in the past by providing products for rare disorders; but as the patents on many profitable drugs expire, some pharmaceutical firms may have to reevaluate this service in light of their financial positions. However, manufacturers and the government do have an obligation to provide technologies for rare disorders. Manufacturers of health care technologies and the Department of Health and Human Services and its branches should continue to cooperate in the research of rare disorders and in the development of technologies for rare disorders. Additionally, manufacturers should maintain the availability of currently utilized investigational and marketed products. The federal government should improve the interagency coordination of research efforts and product regulation.

Government-industry cooperative research in rare disorders is perhaps best illustrated using the National Cancer Institute (NCI) as an example. The NCI modified its agreements with industry to preserve trade secrets and patents, and its drug-screening program for anticancer agents soon became the largest of its kind. Allowances for trade secrets and patents can stimulate collaborative drug development programs, as can the provision for exclusive marketing provided by the Orphan Drug Act. Research and development of orphan products may be approached by more than one manufacturer through the use of joint ventures.

Additionally, clinical research involving orphan products that are supported by the National Institutes of Health should be conducted, when possible, with the dual purposes of expanding the understanding of the underlying disease process and drug mechanisms, and of satisfying the FDA's regulatory requirements of safety and efficacy. This approach may help reduce duplicative clinical trials needed to gain marketing approval.

FDA and Manufacturer Involvement in Postmarketing Surveillance
Safety and efficacy data compiled by manufacturers to support a New Drug or Device Application of the FDA are usually based on a limited population of 1,000 to 2,000 patients. Because of the relatively small number of patients exposed to the new product and the acute nature of exposure, there is no information on the potential subacute and chronic toxicity that may occur in a larger exposed population.

Significant information on adverse reactions—frequently from anecdotal reports of the product's effects—is determined after a drug or device is marketed to larger and more clinically diverse populations. Rare reactions may only be detected at 1:1000. Additionally, certain demographic groups, such as elderly and pediatric patients, may show a higher rate of adverse reactions. Special considerations exist for subpopulations that receive long-term therapy for a particular condition, such as epilepsy or diabetes.

The Food and Drug Administration and other appropriate government agencies should be allocated greater resources with which to strengthen postmarketing surveillance programs. With regard to the FDA, pharmaceutical and device manufacturers should modify their postmarketing surveillance activities to augment FDA activity. More complete information on the potential adverse reactions attributed to the use of a drug or device would allow the health care professional and consumer to make better informed decisions about utilization. A more comprehensive postmarketing surveillance system needs to be established for data collection and for the initiation of case control and cohort studies to provide quantitative measure of relative risk and rate of occurrence of adverse reactions.

The FDA has long-range plans to strengthen its postmarketing surveillance activity by upgrading its existing program and by working with health care professionals to promote prompt and more complete reporting of adverse drug reactions. The FDA should be given the resources to expand its registries and survey programs which provide information on trends and demographic distribution. Epidemiological capabilities could be enhanced to allow a greater number of case-control and cohort studies to be performed. Manufacturers should continue and increase the involvement of their sales representatives in soliciting reports from health care professionals and in conducting surveys.

Promotional and Marketing Strategies for Health Care Technologies
Advertisements, promotional literature, and detail personnel are primary sources of information on health care technologies. Because all three of these sources exert considerable influence on the use of such technologies, manufacturers and suppliers of health care technologies should ensure that promotional material and marketing strategies provide accurate and balanced information regarding the risks, benefits, and uses of products to be used in health care. Despite Food and Drug Administration regulations governing advertising and promotion, the FDA still finds that guidelines are not always followed. For example, only selected and highly favorable information may be used, or claims for usefulness may be made that extend beyond those approved by the FDA. Manufacturers often sponsor seminars on their products, and present various expert opinions that are useful sources of information. Because this information is used by health professionals, an accurate and balanced assessment of the particular technology should be made.

Although the moratorium on direct-to-consumer prescription drug advertising has been lifted, major drug companies have been reluctant to advertise these products. Should this type of advertising become commonplace, the FDA and the Federal Trade Commission (FTC) should monitor the content of advertising. Promotional and marketing strategies directed at the public should be patterned after those used for health care providers.

Summary

In this chapter, the need for planning at the community level was discussed; planning can ensure that the health care delivery system is responsive to changing needs, and that the health care needs of special populations are met. Specific issues concerning access to health care services—the role of the private and public sectors in ensuring access to care and access to scarce health care technologies—were discussed. Roles and responsibilities in the transfer of technology were also addressed to ensure the optimal use of the health care delivery system.

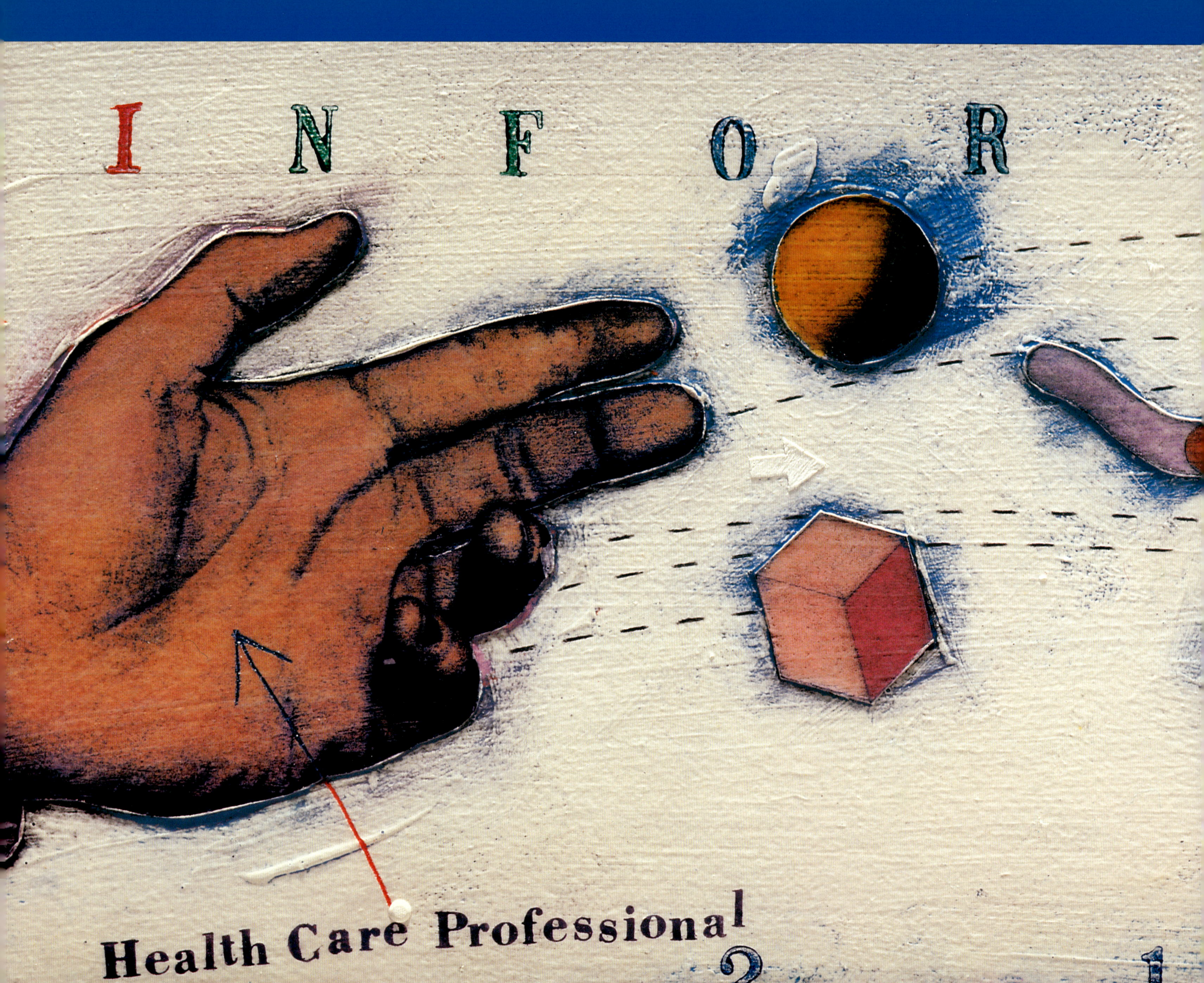

I N F O R
Health Care Professional
2
1

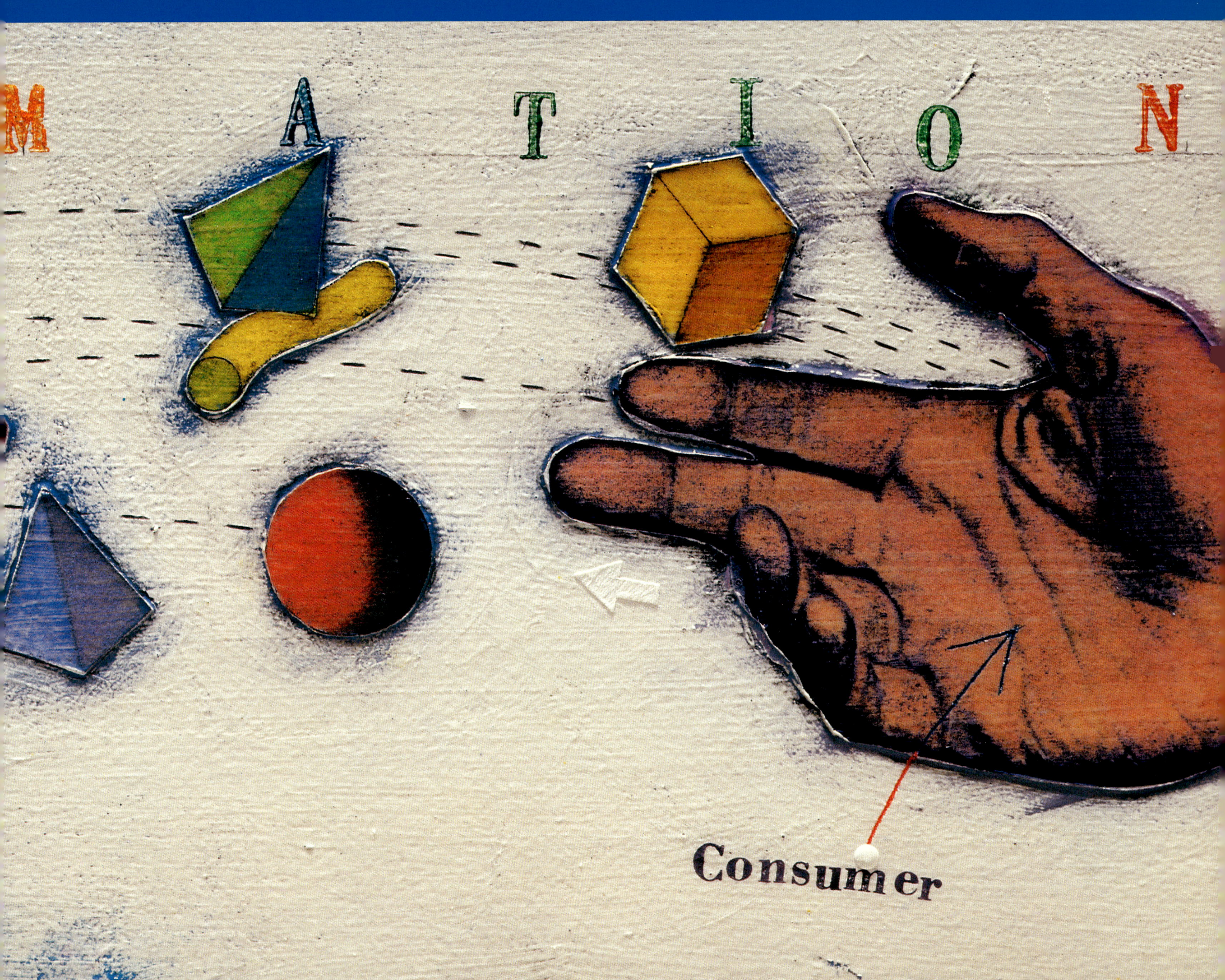
M A T I O N
Consumer

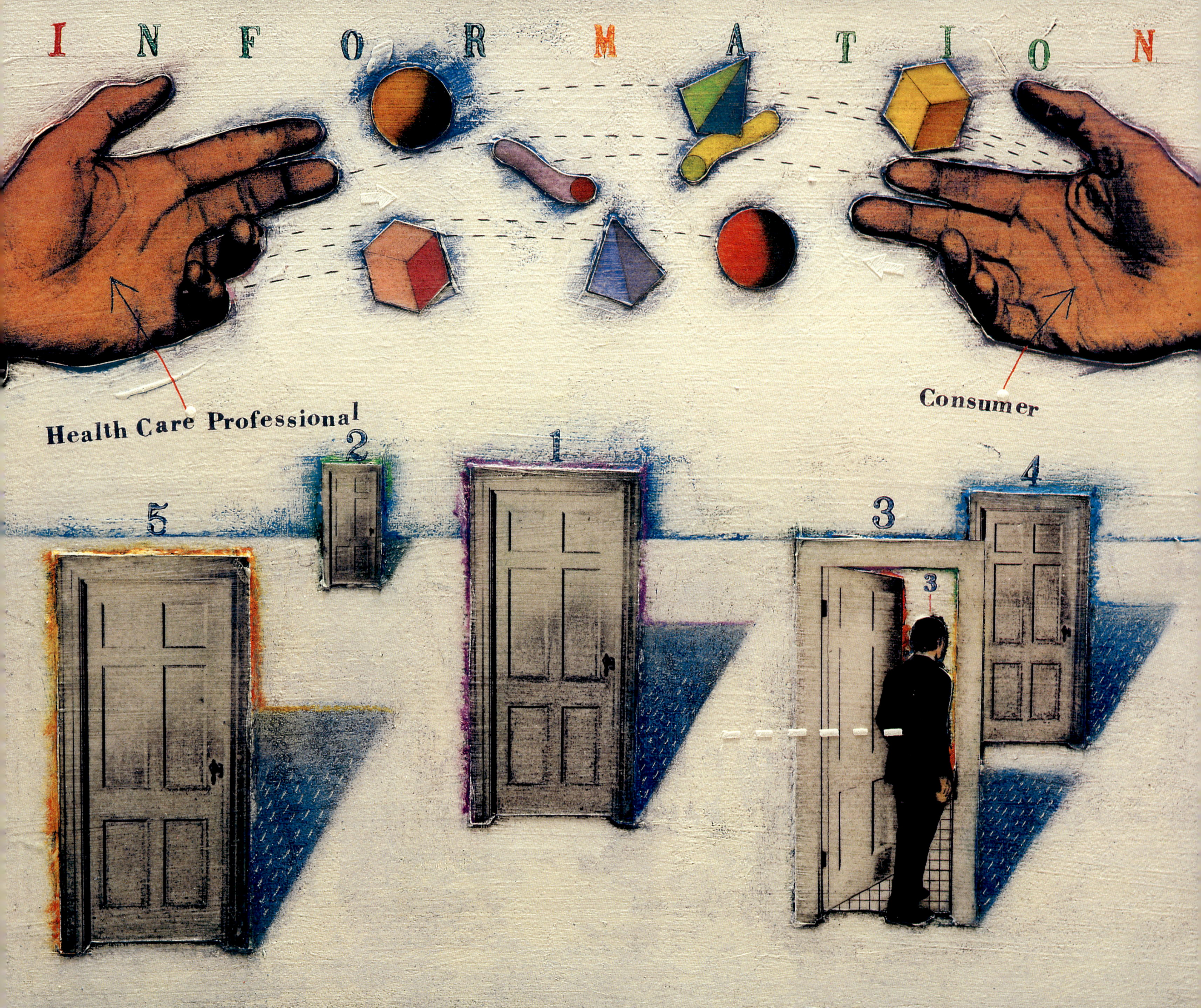

INFORMATION
Health Care Professional
Consumer
5
2
1
3
4
3

Ultimately, it is the individual who has the responsibility for his or her lifestyle and health. The collection of individual decisions to adopt healthy lifestyles and to be prudent users of the health care system will have a significant impact on the overall health status of the country.

To facilitate individual decision-making, it is necessary for the public to have a sound knowledge base of health care information. Much of the information that the public receives concerning health care comes from the mass media, and it takes a well-educated consumer to sort and sift through all of this information. And, of course, while individuals share a large part of the responsibility for their health care, the health care sector and society as a whole have certain responsibilities to protect and promote the health of the nation. Health care providers, employers, and governmental agencies all have specific responsibilities to ensure that information and education on health promotion, disease and injury prevention, and utilization of health care services is available and widely disseminated.

Open communication and shared decision-making between patients and their practitioners provide the foundation for optimal health care treatment. The goal of health care decision-making is to protect and foster the autonomy of the patient, and decisions concerning care are a shared responsibility between the patient and his or her health care professional. Patients have a responsibility to tell their health care professionals about their health status, and health care professionals have concomitant responsibilities both to protect the confidentiality of that information and to provide their patients with sufficient information to make informed decisions about their care. Protecting the confidentiality of information and fully informing patients of diagnoses and treatment alternatives will help to ensure that the trust between patients and their practitioners is maintained.

Finally, just as information and education programs can be used by the public to promote healthy lifestyles and effective utilization of health care services, public health care needs should be considered in the design of health professions education programs. Faculty and administrators of programs should be responsive to changing health care needs.

These issues—the need for health information and education to guide health promotion, injury and disease prevention, and effective use of the health care delivery system; informed consent and the need to protect the confidentiality of health care records and information; and the consideration of health care needs in the design of health professions educational programs—are discussed in this chapter.

Health Information and Education

Two activities that have positive effects on health and health care are an individual's adoption of a healthy lifestyle to reduce the risk of disease and injury, and an individual's ability to make knowledgeable decisions on the appropriate utilization of health care services. There is evidence that substantial progress needs to be made in both of these areas.

For example, preventable illness accounts for more than one-half of the total health care expenditures in the country. In a single year, preventable illness claims as many American lives as the grand total of all the deaths attributable to battle in all the wars fought by the United States from the Revolutionary War through Viet Nam. Smoking is a major contributing factor to cardiovascular disease and cancer, which are the two leading causes of death in the country. Alcohol abuse is a major factor in both accidents and disease; it accounts for one-half of all fatal vehicular accidents, and about one-half of all deaths from falls, drownings, burns, and suicides. Other lifestyle indiscretions, such as obesity, take significant years and comfort from the lives of many.

It is necessary, therefore, that health information and education activities continue. In addition to reducing the risk of injury and disease, health information and education can also increase the ability of the individual to make safe and effective choices in a changing and increasingly complex health care environment.

There are a large number of health education programs in a wide variety of settings. Health education can occur in the occupational, school, or health care setting. Community health programs, sponsored by hospitals, universities, professional and voluntary organizations, or local health departments, use many methods to achieve their goals, including screening, health fairs, and "hot line" services. About 70 national health and health-related organizations, such as the American Cancer Society, the American Heart Association, the American Lung Association, the March of Dimes, and the Red Cross, engage in broad public education within their respective areas of interest. Other national organizations, such as the Planned Parenthood Federation of America, the National Safety Council, and Alcoholics Anonymous, are not typically identified as health educators, but they do engage in important health education efforts.

Because of the enormous variety in health education programs, it is difficult to offer an assessment of their success. Some health education efforts are viewed as effective, but in general there has been an emphasis on the implementation of health education programs rather than on their evaluation. The lack of evaluation data poses a major obstacle for guiding health education program policy.

With the need to control health care costs, and because so many individuals actively contribute to their own injuries, diseases, and deaths, efforts to educate and inform the public are important. To be sure, many individuals have joined physical fitness centers, sports clubs, and exercise programs, and are paying more attention to nutrition. Nonetheless, there is a continuing need to inform and educate the American public on how to reduce the risk of disease and injury, and how to make knowledgeable decisions concerning the appropriate use of health care services.

Individual Responsibility for Health Promotion and Health Care Utilization

Individuals have the ultimate responsibility regarding their lifestyles and for making decisions to seek or not to seek treatment. The leading causes of death—cardiovascular disease, cancer, injury from accidents, pneumonia, cirrhosis of the liver, and emphysema— are all associated with risk factors which, if avoided, could prevent or reduce the incidence of disease and injury. Individuals should seek out and act upon information that promotes appropriate use of the health care system and that promotes a healthy lifestyle for themselves, their families, and others for whom they are responsible. They should seek information that will increase their awareness of risks associated with smoking, abusing alcohol or other substances, or practicing other unhealthy behaviors. To make informed choices about lifestyles, individuals should also seek information on the appropriate use of the health care system. This information will provide the knowledge to be an active participant in planning for health care, including an awareness of the treatments available in case of illness or injury.

Very few Americans use health care professionals as primary sources of health care information; in fact, four out of five Americans obtain most of their health information from newpapers, magazines, television, or radio. While the majority of information reported by the media is accurate, individuals should seek informed opinions from health care professionals regarding health information delivered by the mass media.

When appropriate, self-help and mutual aid groups, such as Alcoholics Anonymous, should be used to provide support to individuals and their families who share common life situations that affect health and well-being. Self-help and mutual aid groups are important components of health promotion/disease and injury prevention, and their development and maintenance should be promoted. These groups represent low-cost resources for those individuals who are coping with developmental disabilities, chronic conditions, and other afflictions. Self-help groups should make their presence known in a community through coalitions to develop and distribute directories of their services. The establishment of a self-help clearinghouse should be considered by self-help groups and their supporters as a means of integrating these efforts at the state level.

Employer and Employee Responsibilities for Health Promotion and Health Care Utilization Programs

The occupational setting is an important site for the delivery of health education. Most workers spend several years at the same company, which serves to enhance the effectiveness of education programs. A small but growing number of companies are providing health promotion programs for their employees. Some reasons for employer involvement are the potential to reduce health care costs and the opportunity to improve worker productivity and performance.

Since employers assume a large share of the costs of medical treatment for their employees, companies are also instituting programs for the appropriate use of the health care system. Employees who are educated about health care and health care costs have greater potential to be prudent users of health care benefit plans. In addition, many employees are now required to make decisions regarding a variety of benefit packages—HMOs, PPOs, cafeteria style benefits, and so forth. The rational exercise of choice requires adequate information and education on benefit options.

Employers should provide and employees should participate in programs on health awareness, safety, and the use of health care benefit packages. Where employee education programs do not exist, employer and employee groups should meet to identify specific needs and to develop strategies for program implementation, including strategies to encourage employee participation. When the costs of such programs cannot be absorbed by the employer or when technical assistance is needed, there are outside resources that can be used. For example, start-up grants might be obtained from state or federal public health agencies, and technical assistance may be offered by third-party payors or private and public health organizations. If companies belong to coalitions, they might want to share their resources in the development of programs. Health care professionals in the local community could also be contacted to determine if they might be interested in some type of cooperative agreement. To further promote employee health education, business coalitions, local planning bodies, and companies with established health education programs should engage in outreach efforts to assist employers in developing such programs.

Employer and Employee Responsibility for Worksite and Community Safety

Employers have a responsibility to their employees to provide as safe an environment as is possible consistent with the nature and inherent risks of employment activity. This includes a responsibility to inform employees, their representatives, and the appropriate governmental agencies of workplace hazards. While the Occupational Safety and Health Administration (OSHA) has legislative authority for monitoring workplace safety and engaging in employee education, the vastness of the workplace necessitates employer and employee participation in the maintenance of a safe environment.

The presence of various chemical substances in the workplace can pose health hazards to both employees and the community. Knowledge of hazardous substances is necessary to make informed decisions regarding job, place of residence, product handling, and waste disposal. A substance is defined as hazardous if it meets certain criteria established by a particular standard, such as containing a certain percentage of a known carcinogen. However, substances that are defined as hazardous vary among the states, and between states and OSHA. OSHA's Toxic and Hazardous Substance list names over 600 chemicals, while the substances covered in state statutes range from 300 to approximately 40,000.

In 1983, OSHA put into effect the Hazard Communication Standard, a federal requirement that certain employees be informed of chemical hazards in the workplace and by early 1985, workers right-to-know laws had been adopted by almost one-half of the states and a number of municipalities. However, the Hazard Communication Standard was challenged in court because it only covered employers in the manufacturing sector, and as a result OSHA officials have announced their intent to expand the standard to cover all employers. Rules governing this expansion have not yet been published.

Employers should provide a safe workplace and should contribute to a safe community environment. Further, they should promptly inform employees and the community when they know that hazardous substances are being used or produced at the worksite. Information concerning the use and/or production of hazardous substances should be provided to the appropriate community members, including medical professionals who may be able to use this information when making diagnoses, and emergency service personnel who may be able to use this information in preparing plans for workplace accidents. Employers should also identify and correct safety hazards. Employers can disseminate information using a variety of methods, including posters, newsletters, and education programs on safe worksite behavior.

Employers should be responsible for informing employees and the public about those substances that are known and have been proven to be hazardous. However, employers should not be responsible for informing employees and the public about every substance that is used in a given industry. Nor should employers be held accountable for failure to inform employees about those substances that are not known or suspected to be hazardous. Employees should be responsible for following safe work practices and safety rules and regulations.

Joint Employer and Government Responsibility for Health Promotion

Because of the public's interest regarding the safety and well-being of the worker at the worksite and because of business and industry concern with worker well-being, government, business, and industry should cooperatively develop effective worksite programs for health promotion and disease and injury prevention, with special emphasis on substance abuse. In the workplace, absenteeism alone costs American industry billions of dollars a year, not to mention the amounts spent for sick pay, health insurance, and time lost on the job that cannot be measured. Cooperative efforts would maximize the resources in the development of programs, closing gaps that presently exist and preventing duplicative efforts.

Representatives from government, business, and industry should meet to share information on existing health promotion programs and to designate committees to work on the development and implementation of programs where they currently do not exist.

Federal and State Support for Health Promotion

The federal and state governments have commitments to health promotion/disease prevention activities, including health education and information initiatives. At the federal level, a diverse group of programs in health, social services, education, transportation, safety, and environmental protection advance health promotion objectives. Within the Department of Health and Human Services, every agency contains programs with significant prevention components. Agencies that deal specifically with prevention efforts include the Office of Disease Prevention and Health Promotion, the Center for Health Promotion and Education, and the Office on Smoking and Health. The federal entity presently charged with coordinating activities at the federal level and between the federal and private sectors is the Office of Disease Prevention and Health Promotion in the

Department of Health and Human Services. The services of this office include the National Health Information Clearinghouse, which responds to requests for health information from the general public and health professionals.

State governments support health promotion/disease prevention activities through tax revenues and through the administration of federal block grants for health education. Presently, states are provided with federal block grants for four major categories of health promotion services: Alcohol, Drug Abuse, and Mental Health Services; Preventive Health and Health Services; Maternal and Child Health; and Primary Care. While the block grant program requires states to use specified portions of their grants for particular purposes, the federal government does not require detailed reporting of the specific programs conducted under the grants. Assumptions are made at the federal level that the total funding of the Preventive Health and Health Services grant, for instance, goes to prevention-related activities.

Federal and state governments are clearly committed to prevention and promotion programs, and they should continue to provide funds and allocate resources for health promotion and disease and injury prevention activities. Further efforts should be undertaken to increase coordination and public awareness of federal initiatives, to incorporate prevention services into government-funded health care programs, and to make states more accountable for expenditures related to prevention services.

Health-related organizations should lobby for adequate governmental funding to ensure the success of programs. Particular attention should be paid to strengthening the coordination of health promotion and disease prevention activities in the federal sector, and between the government and private sectors. Federal services and activities should be given greater visibility and accessibility. This can be accomplished through intensified media campaigns aimed at both health-related organizations and individual consumers.

Because of the importance of health promotion and disease and injury prevention services, government, as a major provider and payor of health care, should require that such services be an integral component of government-financed health care. Presently, health promotion services, such as routine eye or dental care in the Medicare program, are not given sufficient emphasis. Representatives of government-funded health programs (including Medicare, Medicaid, CHAMPUS, and state-administered grants such as Women, Infants, and Children programs) should meet with representatives of health professional organizations and consumer groups to reassess present coverage of promotion/prevention benefits and to incorporate appropriate additions to government-funded programs. When possible, studies of cost-benefit and cost-effectiveness should guide the selection of services to be covered, and these services should be gradually phased into health care programs.

To ensure that states allocate appropriate funding for preventive activities, states should be encouraged to allocate a certain percentage of their federal funds each year for the conduct of health promotion and disease and injury prevention activities. If necessary, the U. S. Congress should pass legislation to this effect. The private and public sectors should conduct research on health promotion and the prevention of disease and injury. States should utilize evaluation studies, when available, to assist them in choosing the most effective health promotion programs. State legislatures are currently required to conduct public hearings on how federal block grants are to be used for the following year. They should make this a more visible activity and seek input from organizations with health-related interests to identify significant health promotion and disease and injury prevention needs.

Fraudulent Health Care Treatments

It is estimated that consumers spend about $25 billion annually for remedies that are dangerous or are of no proven benefit to health. Health fraud is responsible not only for human suffering and a loss of dollars, but also represents a lost opportunity to use effective medical treatment. Victims of such fraud tend to be those suffering from chronic degenerative diseases for which there is no known cure, and the elderly comprise a population that is over-represented in the category of victims.

Public and private agencies should increase their efforts to identify and curtail false and misleading information on health and health care. Federal and state legislation should be reviewed to increase the penalties for health fraud. Federal regulations that classify various drugs as "food supplements"—which exempts them from Food and Drug Administration regulation as drugs—should be reviewed. Federal agencies entrusted with combating health fraud—for example, the FDA, the Federal Trade Commission, and the U. S. Post Office—should be supported in their surveillance activities. Business and health professional associations should be encouraged to alert the proper authorities of potential transgressions. Newspaper and magazine publishers should curtail misleading advertisements for fraudulent medical products by instituting more vigorous review of advertising copy. In health education programs, especially those in schools, an emphasis should be placed on the development and use of skills to better evaluate the credibility of health information.

Health Care Professionals' and Providers' Responsibilities for Health Promotion and Health Care Utilization

Health care professionals and providers are in a strategic position to have a positive effect on the promotion of both healthy lifestyles and cost-effective health care utilization. Patient education has traditionally occurred in hospitals, clinics, HMOs, and doctors' offices. A substantial amount of patient education is conducted informally in these settings, and recently there has been a significant increase in the number of formalized programs. A recent survey found that about 60% of community hospitals have one or more structured patient education programs.

While there has been an increase in patient education in health care settings, the potential is still unfulfilled. Health care professionals and providers should provide information on disease processes, healthy lifestyles, and the use of the health care delivery system to their patients and to the local community. Health care professionals should assume a lead role in preventive health care activities; efforts should include outreach activities, such as instruction of public officials, teachers, and individuals in private industry. Health care provider organizations should institute educational programs in health promotion and prevention, patient education, and cost-effective health care utilization.

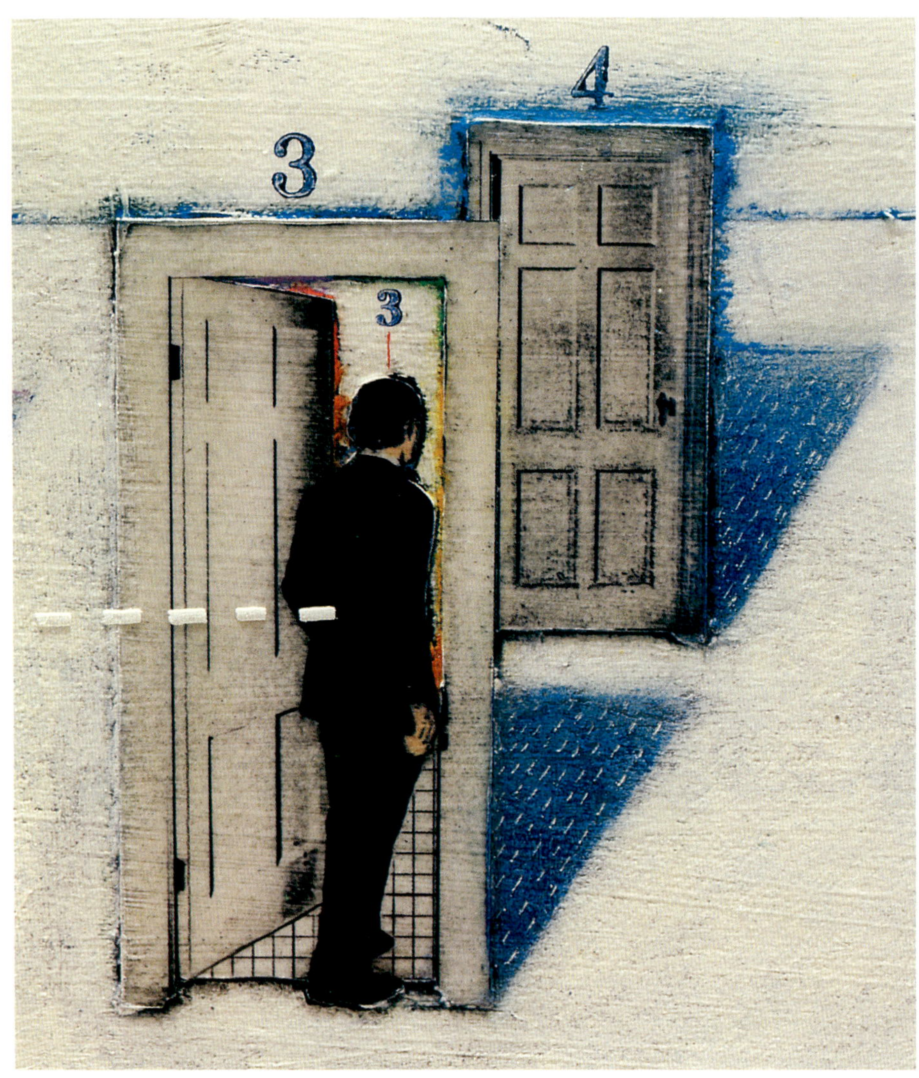

It is each individual's responsibility to adopt a healthy lifestyle to reduce the risk of disease and injury.

They should participate in the local planning process to increase the availability and accessibility of these services, and should advocate that health professions schools develop effective curricula for health promotion, disease prevention, and patient education.

"Truth in Advertising" and Health Care Providers

Advertising by health care providers and advertising of approved health care products are both legal activities, provided that such advertising is accurate and not misleading. In recent years, advertisement of health care services has increased dramatically, both in quantity and in intensity.

Advertisements for institutional delivery mechanisms are more aggressive than those of most health care professionals. This is so because advertising by health care professionals has always been an area of controversy. Recent Supreme Court decisions have removed barriers to advertising by health care professionals, but there is still a general negative attitude among some professionals toward such activity. While advertising may contribute to more competitive pricing, higher consumer awareness, better service, and decreased overall cost, there are concerns about the potential of advertising to mislead consumers, to lead to unrealistic expectations of outcomes, and to create a general mistrust of health care providers.

Information on health and health care should be presented in an accurate and objective manner. Health care providers who choose to advertise should make ethical considerations an integral component in the design of advertising strategies. Facilities, for instance, should designate an internal review board to develop standards for advertising. Professional associations should caution their members who advertise to apply the highest ethical standards in ensuring that their advertisements are accurate and not misleading.

Health Promotion and Patient Education in Health Professions Curricula

In the last decade, there has been increasing interest in health promotion and disease prevention strategies, including health education. Consumers want to understand their conditions and to participate more fully in therapy, and health education is an important factor in improving health outcomes, patient satisfaction, and adherence to therapeutic regimens. Still, there is concern that patient education courses are not receiving adequate prominence in many professional curricula.

Educational programs for health professionals at all levels should incorporate an appropriate emphasis on health promotion/disease and injury prevention and patient education in their curricula. Schools of health professions should evaluate the curriculum for adequate emphasis on health promotion, disease prevention, and patient education. National associations representing schools of health professions should take a lead role in encouraging their member institutions to incorporate such coursework in their curricula.

Third-Party Payors' Responsibilities for Health Promotion and Health Care Utilization

Third-party payors can play an instrumental role in informing consumers about the appropriate utilization of the health care services they cover. Third-party payors should provide options in benefit plans that enable employers and individuals to select plans that encourage healthy lifestyles and are most appropriate for their particular needs. They should also continue to develop and disseminate information on the appropriate utilization of health care services for the plans they market. Third-party payors and purchasers of health care benefits should engage in a thorough assessment of the health promotion and disease prevention needs of the population to be covered. Plan designs should not be bound by conventional coverage decisions, but should look to individual needs and the long-term cost savings of promotion and prevention services. Payors should also take the initiative in developing and implementing informational and educational programs on health care utilization.

State and Local Educational Agency Support for Health Education Programs

The school is an ideal setting for health promotion and disease prevention because it provides an opportunity to teach about and reinforce good health habits during the more formative years of an individual's life. While the overall health of the American child has improved dramatically, significant health concerns are manifest in many children. Both the suicide rate and pregnancy rate for teenagers are increasing. Other threats to the health of young people include smoking, sexually transmitted diseases, and accidents.

In spite of the need for health education, few school districts have well-developed programs, and only 28 states require a definite amount of health instruction prior to graduation. Comprehensive school health education (i.e., sequential instruction and curricula) is uncommon. In general, there is a tradition of low-priority, deficient content matter and ineffective educational methodologies. Funding is frequently inadequate, and teachers may not be as qualified to instruct students in this area as they could be.

State and local educational agencies should incorporate comprehensive health education programs into their curricula, with minimum standards for sex education, sexual responsibility, and substance abuse education. Teachers should be qualified and competent to instruct in health education programs. Responsibility for implementation of this recommendation resides at the state and local level since the administration of education occurs at the local level. Parent-teacher groups, health professional associations, civic associations, and voluntary health agencies should take lead roles in petitioning state departments of education and school districts to incorporate effective and comprehensive health education curricula where such curricula do not exist. Regarding subject matter, sex education and education on substance abuse are major needs of youth and should be a core component of comprehensive health education.

It is recognized that school districts may not have the resources to employ full-time health educators. However, through special instruction programs, teachers who are not exclusively trained as health educators can achieve greater competence in this area. A model for such instruction is the Summer Institute program conducted by the National Science Foundation for science teachers. Similar programs with a health education content should be developed by both the public and private sectors. In addition, all educational institutions granting degrees in primary and secondary education should make health education a component of the course curriculum.

Private Support of Health Promotion

The private sector is extensively involved in health education and information and has been responsible for the development of effective health education programs. Its continued involvement is important to ensure success of health promotion and disease and injury prevention efforts.

Private organizations should continue to support health promotion/disease and injury prevention activities by coordinating these activities, adequately funding them, and increasing public awareness of such services. A prime example of a private coordinating entity is the National Center for Health Education (NCHE). Created as a result of the President's Committee on Health Education in 1973, the NCHE serves as a coordinating body for health education through advocacy, technical assistance, research and evaluation, and information exchange. The NCHE works for the mutual collaboration of private and government organizations in national, state, and local settings. Such coordinating efforts in health education must be maintained.

Evaluation of Health Information and Education Efforts

As previously noted, the public receives most of its health care information from the mass media. Basic information is needed about those channels of communication used by the public to gather health information. Studies should be conducted on how well research news is disseminated by the media to the public. Researchers from the fields of journalism, biomedical science, social science, and health care should study the channels of communication used to publicize information on science and health. They should evaluate the strengths and limitations of these channels and offer suggestions to improve the dissemination of information. Funding should be made available to public and private organizations that have an interest in communications, science, and health.

In general, there has been more emphasis on the implementation of health education programs than on their evaluation. A major factor appears to be the high cost associated with performing rigorous evaluation. Moreover, valid research in this area is very complex. Many variables must be measured, including the behaviors that the program seeks to affect, the program setting, the populations served, and the time involved to assess the outcome. Yet, it is imperative that evaluation be undertaken so that

The goal of health care decision-making is to foster and protect the autonomy of the patient, and this is a shared responsibility between the patient and his or her health care professional.

the cost and relative benefit of different health education strategies can be assessed.

Evaluation should be undertaken to determine the effectiveness of health information and education efforts. When available, the results of evaluation studies should guide the selection of health education programs. Collaborative efforts should be undertaken to minimize the cost of evaluation and to provide for an exchange of methodologies. Pluralism in evaluation of programs should continue, such as that presently undertaken by the National Institutes of Health, the Centers for Disease Control, academic institutions, and private foundations. Clearinghouses—for example, the National Center for Health Services Research, the National Center for Health Education, and the American School Health Association—should be used to collect and disseminate evaluation outcomes and methodologies for the research that they fund.

Informed Consent and Decision-Making in Health Care

The goal of health care decision-making is to foster and protect the individual autonomy of the patient, and this is a shared responsibility between the patient and his or her health care professional. Patients have a responsibility to provide their health care professionals with necessary information, which can then be used to recommend a course of treatment. Health care professionals have a concomitant responsibility to provide their patients with sufficient information to make informed decisions about their health care. The ability of patients to make decisions about their own care is a function of the doctrine of informed consent.

The concept of informed consent is based on two fundamental principles. A person in whom another person has placed a special trust is required to act in good faith, and in the interest of the person placing the trust. This concept is called a fiduciary relationship. Because of the knowledge and training of health care practitioners and the variable awareness of the patient about his or her own condition, the practitioner has a responsibility to discuss the full range of treatment alternatives, including the alternative of no treatment. The second principle involves patient self-determination. Legally competent individuals have the right to make decisions about their care, and do not have to

accept treatment based on someone else's mandate. Thus, the doctrine of informed consent is based on respect for the individual's rights coupled with the freedom to make one's own decisions.

Shared decision-making in health care is a component of the patient-provider relationship that promotes partnership in care, and the ability of patients to make wise choices about their care hinges in part on the doctrine of informed consent. Informed consent plays an important role in promoting patient trust, improving therapeutic outcomes, and decreasing provider anxiety over legal liability.

The participants of the Health Policy Agenda believe that the responsibility of shared decision-making can best be met by fully informing patients of the diagnosis and treatment alternatives, except in rare situations in which such information would cause serious harm to the patient. Additionally, individuals should consider a wide range of advance directives, e.g., living wills, durable powers of attorney, and designation of surrogate decision-makers to act for them in the event of incapacity.

Responsibility of Health Care Professionals to Obtain Informed Consent

As previously noted, informed consent is an integral part of the communication and shared decision-making process between patient and provider. However, both parties seem somewhat unclear as to what constitutes informed consent. In a survey conducted in 1982 by the President's Commission for the Study of Ethical Problems in Medicine and Biomedical and Behavioral Research, both the public and practitioners were asked what informed consent meant to them. Both groups gave varying definitions, and only about 10% of the public and about 50% of the practitioners mentioned that patients should be informed of the risks of treatment alternatives. Health care professionals should inform patients or their surrogates of their clinical impression or diagnosis; alternative treatments and consequences of treatments, including the consequence of no treatment; and recommendations for treatment. Health care practitioners should communicate the known facts about the patient's illness, as well as the uncertainties involved in the diagnosis. The extent of the information to be discussed may vary and will depend on individual circumstances. However, communication must remain at a level at which patients understand their illness and their options for treatment.

Information must be disclosed in a sensitive manner. Attention to the choice of language, the framing of the information, the timing of the disclosure, and the discussion setting can enhance the communication between patient and practitioner. When the proposed treatment plan entails potential grave consequences, patients should be encouraged to discuss alternatives with their families and those close to them. Patients should also be encouraged to reflect on their own values and priorities in making treatment decisions. When a patient is not competent to give informed consent and no surrogate decision-maker has been named in advance, the treating health care professional should follow applicable law providing for substitute consent.

Risk management programs should serve to maintain standards of disclosure necessary for good patient care with full recognition that what is necessary and appropriate in one situation will not automatically be necessary and appropriate in another situation. Failure by practitioners to provide information that meets standards of care for disclosure would result in liability. Professional journals can include information that will serve to guide health care professionals in the communication and disclosure process. Health care professionals, lawyers, and counselors should be available to speak at consumer forums to answer questions about disclosure and decision-making in health care.

Designating and Using Surrogate Decision-Makers
Anyone may at any time become incapable of making health care decisions. This may occur on a temporary basis, e.g., as a result of medication or trauma, or it may be a permanent condition, e.g., irreversible coma. To receive health care that is consistent with their goals and values, individuals should designate surrogate decision-makers to act for them in the event of incapacity, and should provide instructions regarding their care. Discussions concerning the possibility of incapacity and the appointment of a surrogate

should occur, for example, when health care professionals take medical histories, when lawyers prepare wills, and when hospital employees admit patients. Organizations that serve these professionals are urged to educate their members on the importance of issues surrounding decisional incapacity. Social service agencies are encouraged to advise individuals of state requirements regarding preparation of living wills and the execution of powers of attorney for health care decision-making. Issues that should be addressed explicitly include designation of a surrogate, organ donation, and the types of life-sustaining treatments that are desired in the event of incapacity, including the administration of nutrition and hydration. Each state should distribute to the public its legal requirements and the procedures for naming a surrogate decision-maker.

The surrogate's primary responsibility is to make decisions consistent with the patient's own previously expressed or known desires, beliefs, attitudes, and values—even though the surrogate may believe that what the patient would have wanted would not be "in the patient's best interests." Only if there is no evidence of what the patient would have wanted is the surrogate permitted to use "substitute judgment" in order to decide what would be in the patient's best interests. When a patient is incapable of making health care decisions, such decisions should be made by a surrogate acting pursuant to the previously expressed wishes of the patient, and when such wishes are not known or feasible, the surrogate should act in the best interests of the patient. The surrogate should make decisions only when the patient cannot.

The circumstances under which patients may be declared incapable of rational decision-making may at times be unclear. The criteria to be used to declare certain categories of patients—for example, psychiatric patients or those suffering from Alzheimer's disease—incapable of making their own decisions are uncertain. Additionally, although older minors are perfectly capable of making decisions, the law is usually clear that an adult must give informed consent on behalf of a minor. The application of this general law can be complicated when an older minor requires emergency treatment and the parents are not available to provide consent.

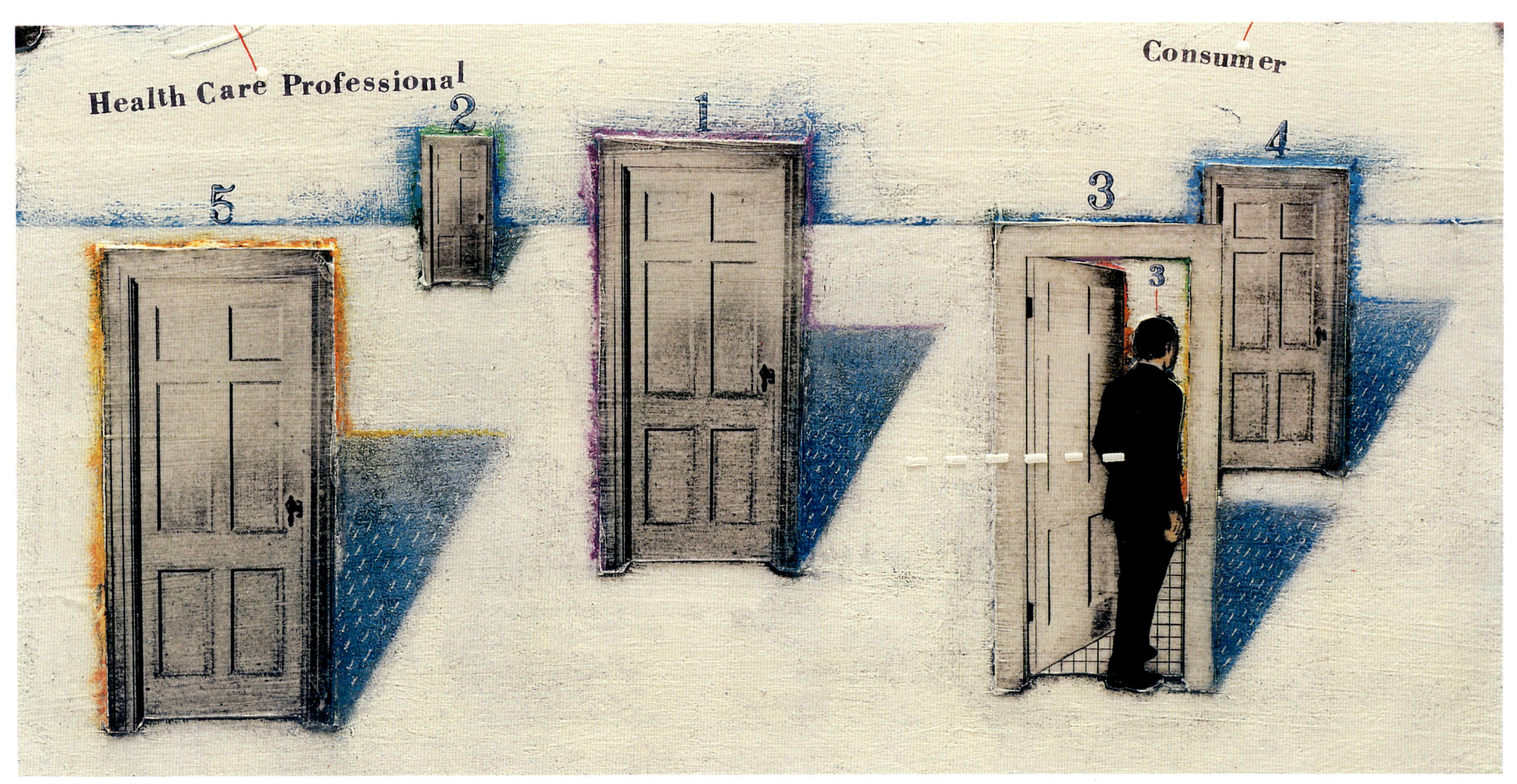

We must work toward a patient-provider relationship that promotes partnership in health care.

State bar associations should research their state laws to determine the legal requirements for a finding of incapacity, as well as the requirements for appointing a surrogate when none has been explicitly named by the patient. Health care professional associations, bar associations, and consumer groups should form committees to review the status of state laws and to recommend any needed modifications.

Confidentiality of Health Care Records and Information

Optimal health care treatment is highly dependent upon full and open communication between the practitioner and the patient. Disclosure by the patient and maintenance of confidentiality by the practitioner form the foundation of the trust in the patient-provider relationship. The responsibility of the practitioner to keep that information confidential is implicit in this exchange.

Many factors contribute to the concern about the confidentiality of health care records and information. For example, the technological sophistication of health care has increased the need for more patient information. Increasing specialization and the subsequent need for consultation has increased the number of practitioners who have access to health records. An increasing number of organizations and individuals—for example, peer review organizations (PROs) and self-insured employers—have access to health care records and information.

Patients are expressing concern about what information is being tabulated and used, the extent of its accuracy, the necessity to control its dissemination, and the extent to which they have have access to, and the opportunity to verify and correct, their personal health records. Patients need to be informed of the parameters that govern the confidentiality, disclosure, redisclosure, and access to their records. Confidentiality of this information protects patients against harm to reputation or personal relationships, threats against employment, or exploitation by public agencies or private interests.

The participants of the Health Policy Agenda believe that the patient's right to privacy should be preserved at all costs, except when serious health hazard or harm could come to the patient or another party if the information were not disclosed. Every effort should be made to use and enforce security measures to protect the confidentiality of health care records and disciplinary action should be taken when proper measures are not used. Additionally, the patient's health record should include information that is sufficient to enable another professional to provide treatment. Patients should have access to the information in their own health care records. In a small percentage of cases, access to records may be injurious to the patient or others; in those cases, access should be limited. Disclosure of information about a patient to a third party should be made only upon authorization by the patient or when the third party has a legal or predetermined right to such information.

The Contents of Health Care Records

A patient's health record should include sufficient information for another health care professional to assess previous treatment, to ensure continuity of care, and to avoid unnecessary or inappropriate tests or therapy. A health record includes the following information: professional observations by health care providers; patient observations; historical health events; ancillary studies obtained, such as x-rays, ultrasound, radioisotope studies, ECGs, or laboratory studies; tentative and final diagnoses; treatment advised or taken; medications advised or taken; consultation reports; and hospitalization summaries.

Information included in health records should be essential for patient care. Because the health record is used as the basis for care, specific patient care objectives will guide decisions about what information is included in the record. In the current health care environment, in which a patient will meet with a variety of health care providers, health records are a critical factor in the continuity of care. They are also of assistance in determining the need for additional or repetitive studies.

Health care professional associations should develop guidelines for their respective professions on health recordkeeping. Health care facilities should develop institution-specific guidelines and practices that are required of the health care professionals practicing in that setting. Additional input should be sought from governmental and voluntary accreditation agencies, along with review of federal and state requirements.

Confidentiality of Patient Health Care Records and Information

Confidentiality of patient information is an integral aspect of the patient-practitioner relationship. Assurance to patients that what they disclose to their practitioner will be kept confidential is of paramount importance. However, patients and practitioners alike must recognize that confidentiality cannot be absolute. There may be certain circumstances in which disclosure of confidential information is appropriate, such as to avoid direct and significant risk to public health. Accountability to third-party payors and to employers who may be the purchasers of insurance requires patient authorization to release confidential information. Conflicts between a patient's right to privacy and a third-party's need to know should be resolved in favor of patient privacy, except where that would result in serious health hazard or harm to the patient or others.

When there is an overriding need or legal requirement for a third party to have access to health care information, it is permissible for a practitioner to disclose the necessary information. Examples of legal requirements are the reporting of communicable diseases and gunshot wounds. Another example in which an unauthorized breach of patient confidentiality may be appropriate is the disclosure by a patient of the intent to inflict serious bodily harm to self or others.

Health care professional associations are encouraged to follow the example of the American Psychiatric Association, which has developed guidelines for patient confidentiality. When protection of others from specific harm justifies the breach of confidentiality, every effort should be made to be as discreet as possible.

Maintenance of Privacy of Health Care Records and Information

The owner of the health record is that health care facility or professional who has compiled the record. Those individuals or facilities that are patient-authorized to access health records are accountable for the protection of the record while it is in their possession. Furthermore, only those individuals who have a need to know what is in the records should have access to them. These individuals must understand the issues of patient-identifiable information and know how to protect patients' privacy.

Although protection of the confidentiality of health records is properly the responsibility of the health care provider, and although patient authorization is usually necessary prior to disclosure, the confidentiality of patient information is sometimes weakly guarded. A relatively new cause for concern derives from the growth of computer capabilities to collect and store vast amounts of patient-identifiable information. Computerized recordkeeping systems are subject to security risks just as manual systems are. Potential problems with the use of computers include inadvertent alterations, releases, or loss of information; and unauthorized use of information, including the transfer of information with malicious intent. The majority of Americans believe that privileged information between practitioner and patient is secure. Health care facilities and practitioners must ensure that public confidence in their security measures continues to be justified.

Holders of health record information should be held responsible for reasonable security measures through their respective licensing laws; it should be grounds for disciplinary action not to utilize proper security measures. Third parties that are granted access to patient health care information should be held responsible for reasonable security measures and should be subject to sanctions when confidentiality is breached. Facilities and practitioners can address security risks in computerized record systems by investigating information-intensive industries and industries dealing with sensitive information, and by implementing those models that most closely approximate their own. At minimum, legal, software, hardware, and medical record expertise should be included in developing and implementing record security systems. Breaches of security, either with manual or automated records, must be met with disciplinary action through licensing boards and other mechanisms. State consumer protection laws should specifically provide for protection of health record information in the possession of third parties.

Over the past several years, there has been a trend in legislation toward patient access to the information contained in health records. Germane to the idea of self-determination is the belief that the contents of a health record, which affect the patient to whom the record relates more than anyone else, should be available to the patient. A patient should have access to the information in his or her health record, except for that information which, in the opinion of the health care professional, would cause harm to the patient or to other people. For example, in the case of psychiatric records, access to the information may be available, except to those portions which in the opinion of the coordinating practitioner, will cause harm to the patient or another person. There may be other circumstances in which it would be harmful to another party to allow the patient to see the complete health record, and professional judgment needs to be exercised. Certainly, a patient's personal representative or duly authorized nominee, upon good cause shown by such a person, may be granted reasonable access to information contained within the patient's health record.

At present, state laws address the issues pertaining to patient access to information contained in health records. While these laws may be appropriate and necessary to delineate the respective rights of the parties, health care professionals and health care facilities should, on their own, be responsive to patients' interests in their own health records. Treating the patient as a partner in health care is an important function in furthering the patient-practitioner relationship.

Disclosure of Health Records and/or Information to Third Parties

To support self-determination, it is mandatory that patient authorization for disclosure of health information be secured in situations where there is a choice involved. Disclosures of health information about a patient to a third party may only be made upon consent by the patient or the patient's lawfully authorized nominee, except in those cases in which the third party has a legal or predetermined right to gain access to such information. Circumstances that may require disclosure without prior authorization include compli-

ance with laws and regulations, situations affecting public health and safety, and conduct of research projects. Examples of these include communicable diseases, wounds inflicted with weapons, child abuse, and occupational diseases. Additionally, employers may require prospective employees to take a physical examination as a condition of employment. When employment is contingent upon the results of the physical, the employer, if authorized by the patient, is entitled to the results of that examination. Although disclosure of nonconfidential information may be made under some circumstances without authorization, it is important that patients be notified when their health information is being released. It is an area of concern that patients are not informed that most insurance company release forms authorize the redistribution of health information to a central clearinghouse that makes the information available to a variety of insurance companies.

It is of paramount importance to keep health information confidential when employers are self-insured. Additionally, employers who administer their employees' health insurance must provide protection for the employee's confidentiality and not let an employee's medical or psychiatric condition interfere with employment status unless the employee's condition materially affects job performance or the safety of others. Such situations should be guided by federal and state requirements.

Valid court orders requiring disclosure of information must also be honored. State bar associations and state health care professional associations should form committees within their respective states to study and recommend procedures by which the confidentiality of patient records that are the subject of court orders can best be protected. In many circumstances, it is possible to uphold the tenets of the patient-practitioner relationship by informing the patient of the parties requesting his or her personal information and securing the patient's authorization.

Health care professionals and health care facilities should take it upon themselves to comply with this recommendation. Patients should be alerted if disclosures of health information are anticipated and prior authorization should be sought. Recipients of confidential information should find cost-effective means of notifying patients whose health records they are requesting or when they intend to disclose individually-identifiable information to other persons or organizations. General release of information should not be required as a condition of employment.

Additionally, when information from a health record is disclosed to a third party, only that information which is relevant to the needs of the requestor should be disclosed. Patients should have the opportunity to give authorization for specific information rather than blanket authorization. Blanket authorizations, such as those required by insurance companies, should be no broader than necessary to accomplish the specific purpose at hand. Blanket authorizations should include the names of each person, firm, corporation, or public body to which information or copies of records may be released by the custodian of the health care record so that the patient knows when a credit bureau or other party has been contacted to obtain health information; the specified time expiration date, if consistent with the purpose of the disclosure; and prohibition of proposed new use of information without additional consent by the patient or his/her nominee. Federal law and regulations should be amended as necessary to make it a violation of the Equal Employment Opportunity Commission Act for an employer to use improperly employee health information.

Meeting Public Health Care Needs through Health Professions Education

In addition to their primary responsibility for determining and implementing the curriculum for health professions programs, faculty and administrators must be responsive to changing public health care needs. Faculty must determine what those needs are and modify the curriculum in light of those needs. They should also participate in the education of the public regarding health matters and should serve on boards and other bodies to guide the development of public health care policy.

Health Professions Education and Public Health Care Needs

The content and administration of programs of education for the health professions are critically important in meeting the need for well-educated professionals. The inherent difficulty of identifying the elements of a good education has led to a general recognition that there are many ways to educate health professionals. There is also general recogni-

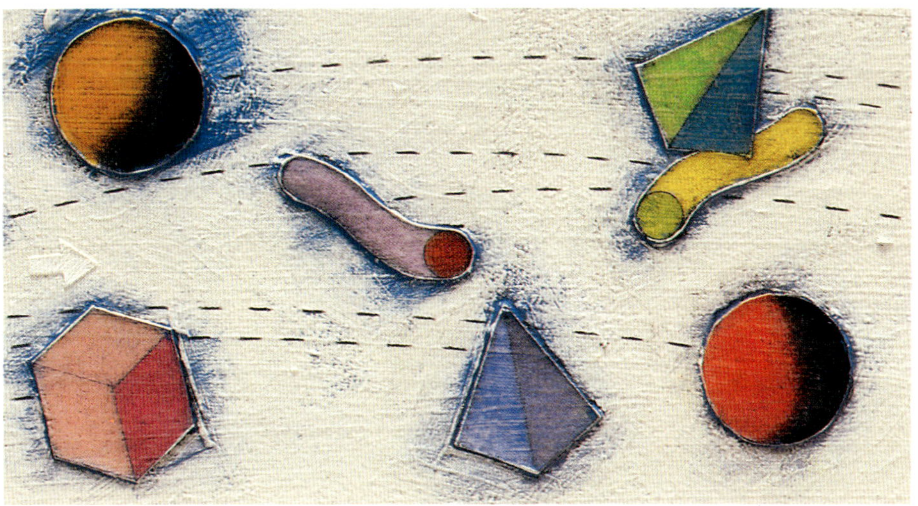

The responsibility of shared decision-making between patient and provider can best be met by fully informing each patient of the diagnosis and treatment alternatives.

tion that the public and many governmental and private organizations, as well as the health professions and their organizations, have legitimate interests in meeting the changing needs of society. Faculty members, students, and school administrators are involved in reviewing and revising curriculum, requirements for admission, and requirements for promotion and graduation. The general public is also concerned with health professions education, and has input into establishing the curriculum and educational content of programs. Faculties of programs of health professions education should be responsive to the expectations of the public in regard to the practice of health professions. Faculty and administrators, based on their intimate knowledge of an involvement in the educational process, must retain the major responsibility for determining the content of health professions education programs. In determining curriculum content, faculties should consider the variety of practice circumstances in which new professionals will practice. Faculties should add curriculum segments to ensure that graduates are cognizant of the services that various health care professionals and alternative delivery systems provide. Because of the dominant role of public bodies in setting the standards for practice, courses on health policy are appropriate for health professions education. At the same time, faculty must be willing to modify programs in response to public concerns. There are many ways to receive input from the public regarding educational programs. Information from legislatures, governmental and accrediting agencies, licensing boards, and professional organizations can be used as a basis for considering changing societal needs. Judgment should be used in deciding which comments represent genuine long-term public needs.

Additionally, governing boards of programs of education for the health professions, as well as the boards of the institutions in which these programs are frequently located, should ensure that programs respond to changing societal needs. Governing boards should ensure that programs have developed long-range plans that take public needs into account and are appropriate to the mission of the program. They should also ensure that programs are not diverted from their mission in efforts to provide services to the public not within the scope of the educational program.

The public receives a great deal of information about health care from the media, from practitioners, and from such informal sources as general conversations. Much of this information is accurate but some of it is not. For the most part, health professions educators have tended to concentrate on educating their students and have not taken a major role in programs directed at the public. There are some notable exceptions, and an increasing number of educators are involved in or affiliated with efforts to publish newsletters concerning health matters that are specifically directed toward the public. Health professions educators should be involved in the education of the public regarding health matters. The extensive knowledge of health professions educators and their experiences in education make them valuable resources for public education activities. Educators can undertake education activities through the public schools, universities, civic organizations, and the media.

Institutions with health professions educational programs have traditionally provided care to patients who are unable to pay. For both educational and social reasons, programs of health professions education should continue to provide care to patients regardless of the patient's ability to pay and they should continue to cooperate in programs designed to provide health practitioners in medically underserved areas.

Involvement of Faculty and Administrators in Determining Public Policy

Many educators are not experienced in policy development, public relations, or public debates, and are therefore reluctant to participate in public discussions of policies concerning health professions education or health care. However, educators should be involved in public policy discussions for two reasons. First, they will gain a better understanding of the public's views and, second, they can use this knowledge to implement any needed changes in their own educational programs or in policy development. Faculty and administrators of health professions education programs should participate in efforts to establish public policy in regard to health professions education. Educators who choose to participate in the debate of public policy should be thoroughly versed in educational issues and should learn to respond in an effective manner to the sometimes contentious discussion that can develop in public forums.

Educators are also involved in legislative activities, and it is common for them to represent a single health profession. To support common rather than individual goals, educators from the health professions should collaborate with health providers and practitioners in efforts to guide the development of public policy on health care and health professions education. Faculty members and administrators involved in representational activities should participate in multidisciplinary committees to enhance the representation of all health professions.

Summary

In this chapter, the need for information and education to guide health promotion, injury and disease prevention, and effective use of the health care delivery system were discussed. Informed consent, confidentiality of health care records and information, and the consideration of public health care needs in the design of health professions educational programs were also discussed.

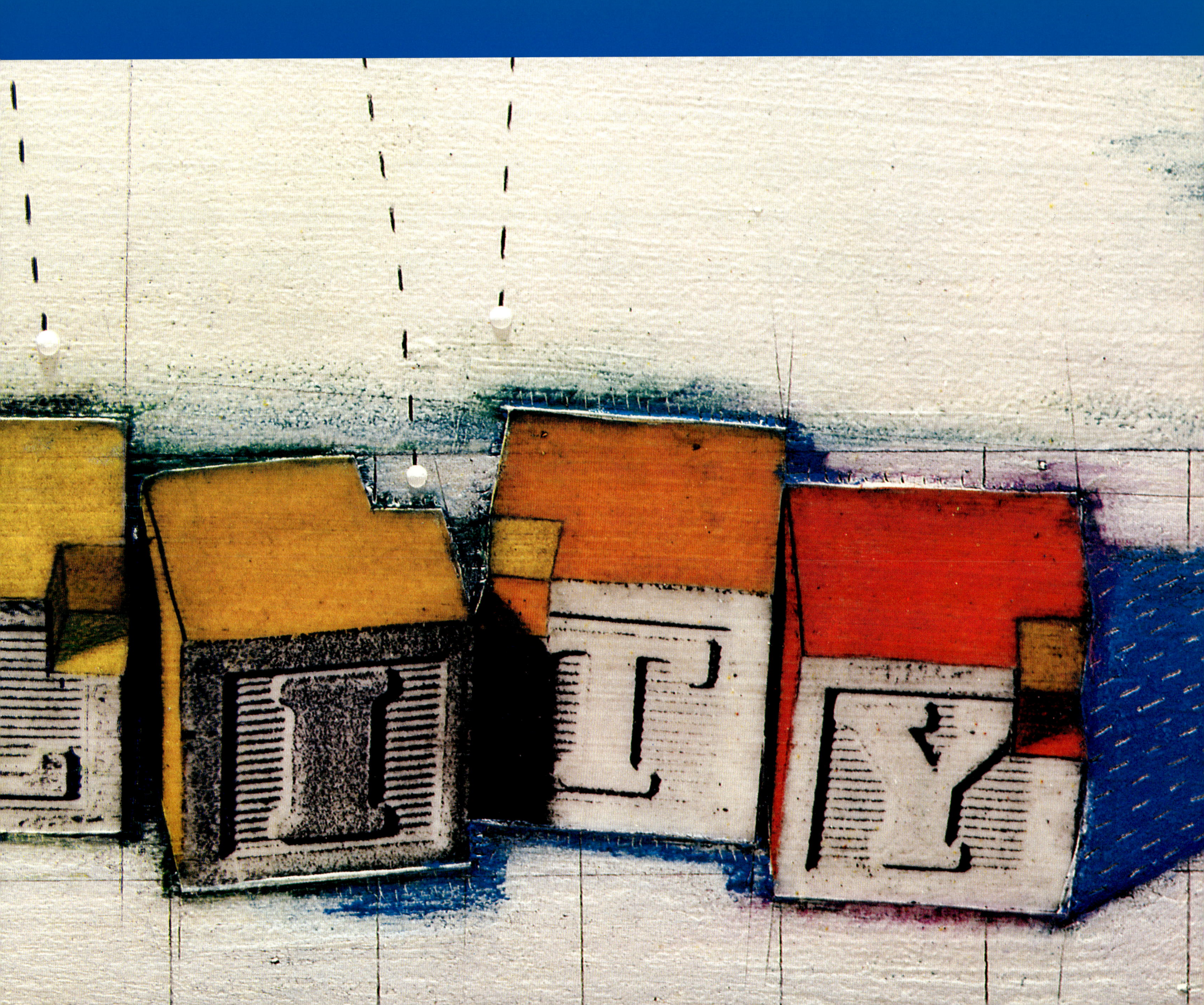

The fundamental goal of the health care delivery system is to provide quality health care services to the American public. However, providing "quality" health care services is no longer as simple as it once seemed to be. Only 10 years ago, there was little public debate about the quality of health care. Consumers expected to receive the "best" care in the world, providers seemed able to meet this expectation, and payors seemed willing to reimburse for the services provided. But, as the cost of health care rose, and kept on rising, it became evident that expectations had to be adjusted. Along with rising expenditures for health care, the nation also began to confront ethical dilemmas in the use of some health care technologies—technologies that potentially affect everyone from the unborn to the aged. The assurance of quality has evolved to the point where it is now one of the central policy issues in health care.

Through expanded quality assurance, we can integrate changes into the health care system while maintaining the high quality of care available in our society.

Despite changes in the health care environment, the fundamental goal of the health care system—to provide quality care—has remained unchanged. Quality health care is care that is appropriate, available, and accessible; it should be provided through a system that is affordable to society and accountable to consumers, providers, and payors alike. The delivery of quality health care is achieved through a high level of professional skill on the part of the provider, a compassionate concern for the patient, the effective and efficient use of the appropriate resources, continuity in patient care, and a consideration of the risk-benefit ratio in the selection of treatment approaches. The measurement of quality should encompass all of these factors. Additionally, patient satisfaction with health care services should be included in the measurement, since it influences compliance with treatment instructions and cooperation with providers; and, it may also affect use of health care services.

Two terms that will recur frequently in the discussion of quality—quality assessment and quality assurance—must be defined. Quality assessment involves the measurement of the level of quality at some point in time; it connotes no effort to change or improve that level of care. Quality assessment is the first step in quality assurance, which involves the measurement of the level of care provided and, when necessary, efforts to improve it.

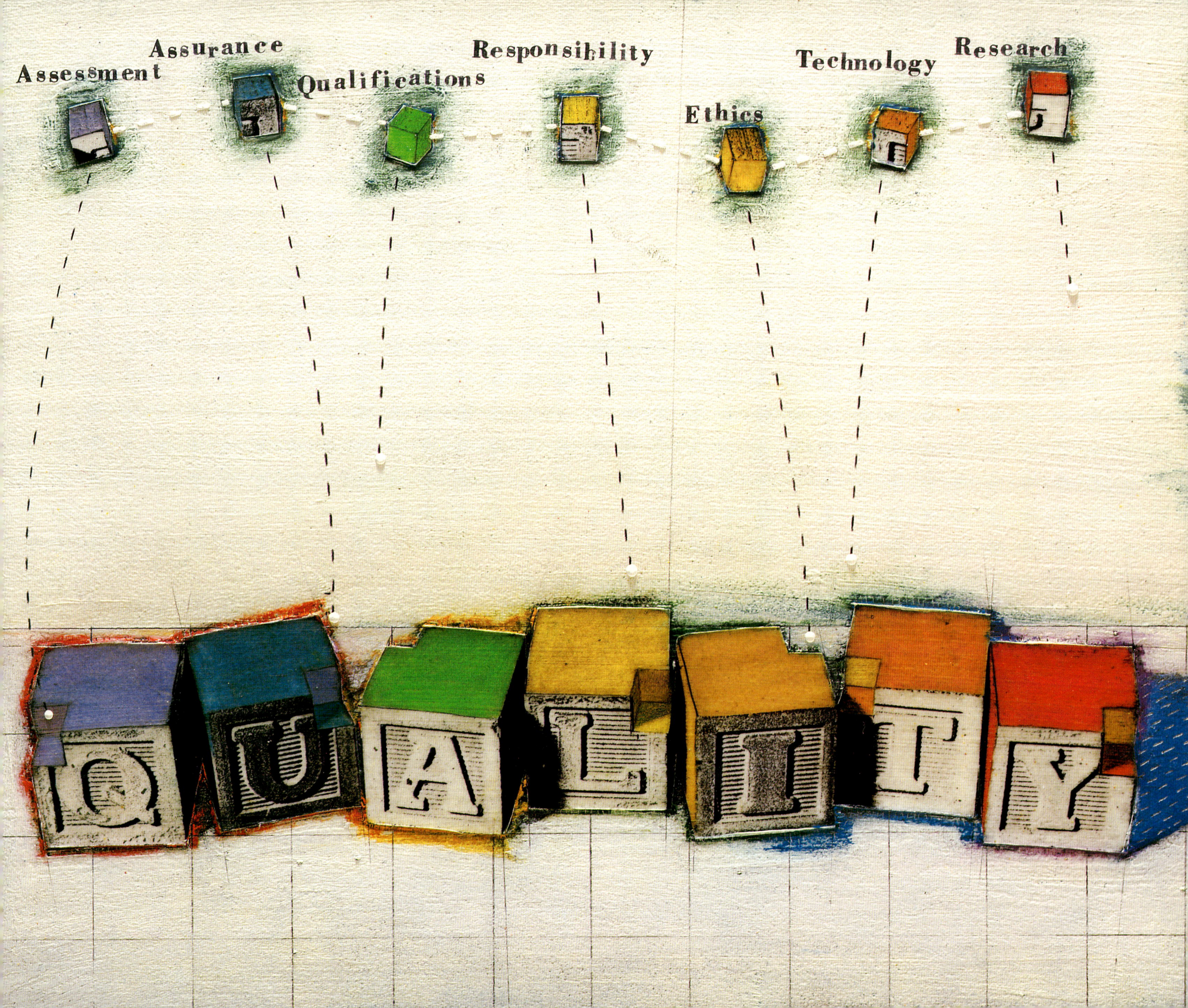

Assessment
Assurance
Qualifications
Responsibility
Ethics
Technology
Research
QUALITY

Quality assurance is a cyclical activity that usually involves the collection of two kinds of information: information on the qualifications of health care professionals and facilities, including licensure, certification, accreditation, equipment, space, safety, recordkeeping, organization, etc.; and information on what is actually done for patients and what the consequences are. This information can be gathered internally by providers themselves (e.g., by hospitals or other health care facilities) or externally (e.g., by insurance agencies, government bureaus, or government-mandated, quasi-public bodies, such as peer review organizations). In either case, the purpose of quality assurance is to correct identified deficiencies in the quality of health care services.

Many different mechanisms have been developed to ensure the quality of health care. Health care professionals are licensed and/or certified to ensure the health, safety, and welfare of the public. As the types of health care professionals seeking licensure continue to increase, state licensure laws and proposed legislation should be reviewed on a regular basis to determine which should be enacted, updated, revised, or repealed. Private certifying agencies are encouraged to continue their certification programs for all health care professionals. The importance of accreditation in ensuring the accountability of the health care delivery system has already been discussed, as has the need for continuing education (see, respectively, the section in Chapter II on the licensure of health care facilities and the section in Chapter I on maintaining competence of health professionals). These topics will not be addressed in detail in this chapter.

The continuing debate about professional liability has led to agreement that costs for obtaining liability insurance have escalated. The effectiveness of the tort system should be evaluated and a demonstration study of a new patient compensation system should be conducted. Additionally, more careful review of health professionals is needed.

As previously indicated, rapid advances in health care technology have made ethical considerations an increasingly important part of quality evaluation. Treatment decisions should be based on mutual understanding between health professionals and their patients, and emphasis should be placed on ethics in health professions educational programs and in the peer review process. Assessment of the safety and efficacy of health care technology should lead to increased use of effective technology, thereby improving the quality of care. A coordinated health services research and evaluation effort is needed to provide information for the development of a national health care policy.

All of these topics are addressed in detail in this chapter. Much attention is paid to quality assessment and quality assurance mechanisms—especially the measurement of quality—because failure to address these issues will result in inadequate national health care policy.

Assessment of the Quality of Health Care Services

Quality health care is care that consistently contributes to the maintenance or improvement of the quality and/or duration of life. This definition characterizes care that is consistently related to favorable patient outcomes. Implicit in this definition, then, is the need to develop more precise and meaningful criteria to measure "favorable" outcomes.

Quality assessment can be defined as the measurement of the level of quality of health care at some point in time, and it is essentially a two-stage process. In the first stage, the individual elements that, taken together, comprise quality in health care are identified. In the second stage, these elements are transformed into measures that can be used to evaluate the quality of patient care.

Although there are many different ways to measure the quality of care, perhaps the most useful approach is one that considers the structure, process, and outcome of health care. Under this approach, the assessment of structure involves the evaluation of the setting in which care was provided and a comparison of the available services and technologies with those that were actually used in the delivery of care. Two assumptions underlie the structural assessment of health care: the first is that better care is provided when qualified staff, adequate physical facilities, and effective administrative structures are present; the second is that it is possible to identify the characteristics of staff, technology, and administrative structure that actually contribute to quality.

The assessment of process is the evaluation of the activities of health care professionals and institutions in the management of patients, with the standard of measurement being the degree to which the management of patients complies with the models of care developed by health care professionals.

Patient outcome is viewed by many as the ultimate indicator of quality of care, and the increased attention to outcome evaluation represents a significant improvement in quality assessment methods. However, it is perhaps the most difficult of the three variables to measure because many factors other than health care—for example, the patient's age, sex, genetic individuality, prior injury or disease, and attitude—can influence the outcome. Nonetheless, gross measurements of patient outcome can be made using case fatality rates, disability rates, and levels of patient satisfaction with the services provided.

Quality health care requires both technical competence and appropriate concern for the patient's physical, psychological, and social needs. The participants of the Health Policy Agenda believe that quality assurance is the responsibility of the health care professionals, and that standards of care should be developed by their professional organizations for local use and interpretation. Standards should include a range of optimal treatments for a particular illness or condition, and should reflect scientific knowledge, the clinical expertise of the providers, and the availability of resources. Multidisciplinary research is needed to assess the quality of health care, and the findings of this research should be used to improve quality assurance programs. Finally, educational programs should be developed for the public so that it has a better understanding of how to obtain quality health care services.

Evaluation of Quality of Health Care by Health Professionals and Providers

Health care professionals have been and continue to be concerned with issues surrounding the evaluation of quality of care. Health care professionals and providers conducting quality of care evaluations should examine the process, structure, and outcome of health care services. Emphasis should be placed on the relationships between these three variables rather than on isolated examinations of each. Because it may be difficult to distinguish between the effects of care provided and other factors which can also influence patient outcome (e.g., the patient's age, past history and lifestyle, stage of disease, and attitude toward illness), outcome studies should be conducted on both a retrospective and prospective basis. As opposed to the "after-the-fact" outcome evaluation, the identification of an "expected" outcome on a pre-service basis with subsequent comparison to actual results can allow better identification of individual risk factors. The possibility of assessing intermediate rather than final outcomes should be considered, since the direct effects of care may be progressively obscured by time. Treatment outcomes should include a measurement of patient satisfaction. Finally, the assessment process itself should be subject to continued evaluation and modifications as needed. Using the results of research on quality assessment, quality assurance, treatment outcomes, and technology evaluation, health care professionals should develop criteria to evaluate patient care. These criteria should, in turn, be used to develop treatment models that include a range of optimal treatments for a particular illness or condition. Both the criteria and treatment models should reflect current scientific knowledge, the clinical experience of health care providers, and the varying availability of health care resources. As scientific knowledge expands, the criteria and treatment models should be reviewed for usefulness and updated when necessary.

Research on the Quality of Health Care

Multidisciplinary research to assess the quality of health care should be conducted. This research should concentrate on patient outcome relative to the structure and process of health care delivery, and should be broad enough in scope to be applicable to a multitude of health care settings. Research findings should be used to evaluate and improve quality assurance programs used by health care professionals and facilities. Research on quality of care should examine standards of care, relate these standards to outcome, study alternative ways of achieving favorable outcomes, and identify the most efficient and effective methods. To measure the process, structure, and outcome variables, considerable refinement of criteria for assessing overall quality of care is essential and needs to be, in itself, a major research goal. The measurement of outcome should include a measure of patient satisfaction when possible. If appropriate outcome measures are not available, process measures can be used to approximate the same results. In evaluating new services or techniques, in establishing review systems when none have previously existed, or in expanding review into settings not previously subject to review, the structure of delivery may be the only criteria that can be measured. Additionally, the varying definitions of quality health care services that providers, patients, and payors may want to use should be considered; there may be some difficulty in the development of measures of quality that simultaneously satisfy the concerns of each group.

Improved research methods will assist the public, health care providers, and payors to determine how successful quality assurance programs are in promoting quality health care. Improvements will also facilitate efforts to address resource allocation issues so that available resources are directed into treatment modalities that serve the best interests of all patients. Research directed toward quality assurance can also provide a framework to evaluate the relative benefits and costs, which are essential elements in improving both the efficiency of the health care sector and the quality of care.

Appropriate health care organizations should initiate discussions with major private foundations so that quality assurance research is given a high funding priority. It is the responsibility of health care professionals, providers, and public representatives to develop measures and to ensure that these measures are applied in the evaluation of care.

Educational Programs for the Public on Quality of Health Care

Educational programs that assist people in making informed choices about their personal health and about the appropriate uses of both self-care and professional care should be established. The content of these programs should include information about the costs and benefits associated with potential and alternative courses of treatment; the use of professional health care services that permit the early detection and treatment, or the prevention, of illnesses; lifestyle issues and personal responsibilities in preventing illnesses; and the effective use of the health care system.

Health care providers, through their professional and trade associations, should develop ongoing programs of public education on health issues, and should provide guidance to schools, community groups, and individual providers who wish to develop patient education programs. Health care providers should, as a normal component of their patient care activities, educate patients so that they can maintain their health or be restored to healthy lives.

Quality Assurance in Health Care

The primary goals of quality assurance are the improvement of care through identification and resolution of problems and to thereby render the health care system accountable to patients, health care professionals, and the public. Quality assurance activities and programs must include educational or other components intended to remedy identified deficiencies in quality, as well as the components (e.g., peer review, utilization review, tissue review, or mortality conferences) needed to identify such deficiencies and to assess the program's effectiveness. In general, two distinct but interrelated activities—peer review and utilization review—are included under the rubric of quality assurance.

Peer review is the evaluation by practicing professionals of the effectiveness, appropriateness, and efficiency of services ordered or performed by other practicing professionals in the same profession or specialty. Effective peer review depends on the existence of explicit screening criteria acceptable to the local health care community. Cases at variance with these criteria are reviewed on a case-by-case basis. A case may not fall within the local community standards for a number of reasons; it may have been an unusually complex or protracted illness that was appropriately managed; it may represent substandard care in one way or another; or it may represent an improvement in established methods of patient care. Peer review can be sponsored or conducted by professional societies or associations, hospital medical staffs, payors, foundations, corporate review programs, or federal agencies, and it can be either voluntary or mandatory. Under voluntary peer review, there usually is no coordinating body, except when the health care facility has requested coordination. Under mandatory programs, peer review activities are coordinated by a centralized body. In either case, peer review also serves as a continuing education activity.

Utilization review is a multidisciplinary evaluation of the necessity, appropriateness, and efficiency of the use of professional services, procedures, and facilities in comparison with preestablished standards and criteria. In a hospital, this includes the review of the appropriateness of admissions, services ordered and provided, length-of-stay, and discharge practices on either a preadmission, concurrent, or retrospective basis. Utilization review may be performed by an in-house utilization review committee, a peer review organization, public agencies (such as a state Medicaid agency), or by third-party payors (such as insurers or employers).

Thus, quality assurance provides an objective, problem-oriented approach for reviewing and evaluating the safety, efficacy, and quality of patient care in health care facilities. Paradoxically, the emphasis on cost containment has led to a proliferation in the number of formal quality assurance and risk management programs, some of which are expensive to operate. Furthermore, mechanisms to ensure quality of care in facilities— licensure, accreditation, and institutional quality assurance and risk management programs—may at times have overlapping requirements and therefore result in a duplication of effort. Pressures to contain health care costs demand that duplication be kept at a minimum.

To meet their responsibilities for ensuring the quality of care, health care facilities must comply with existing federal, state, and local regulations; additionally, some seek voluntary accreditation and/or formulate their own standards. The participants of the Health Policy Agenda believe that quality assurance activities should be extended to all health care facilities and settings, and that there should be both internal and external review procedures to evaluate the quality of care at health care facilities. Voluntary accreditation programs with standards that exceed those of state licensure and that focus on quality of care issues should be offered to all health care facilities. Third-party payors should limit their reimbursement for services provided in health care facilities to those that meet standards of acceptable quality. Educational programs on quality assurance issues should be expanded for both health care professionals and the public. Recently identified variations in practice and utilization patterns should continue to be analyzed, and research on the effects of peer review programs and payment mechanisms on quality of health care is also needed. Finally, there is a need for a data base that can be used to analyze and improve quality assurance activities.

Quality Assurance in All Health Care Facilities and Settings

Most health care is not provided in the hospital and is therefore not subject to the quality assurance mechanisms that operate in institutional settings. Cost-containment efforts, changing reimbursement mechanisms, and increasing competition among health care providers are likely to lead to further shifts in the amount of care provided in ambulatory settings. Diverse entities that have been established for the delivery of health care include health maintenance organizations, independent practice associations, preferred provider organizations, freestanding emergency centers, and ambulatory surgery centers. In addition, the increasing number of elderly patients has led to the development of facilities which specialize in long-term care.

With the development of nontraditional health care settings and new practice configurations, providers and patients alike would be well-served by the expansion of quality assurance mechanisms to all health care delivery settings whenever such expansion is feasible and cost-effective. Accountability through quality assurance mechanisms should be part of every system of health care delivery. Quality assurance activities must be expanded into nontraditional settings, new practice configurations, and specifically into the areas of chronic illness and long-term and ambulatory care. This effort must be a unified interdisciplinary approach with consumer participation where appropriate. The cost of quality assurance programs and activities should be considered a legitimate element in the cost of care.

As a first step, quality assurance review in nonhospital settings should be voluntarily conducted by groups of health professionals on a peer-to-peer basis. Findings regarding identified problem areas may be communicated to hospital professional staffs. Ambulatory review should also be conducted locally and on a voluntary basis, and at least in part under the aegis of hospital medical staffs, whose efforts would be monitored for validity and comparability by peer review organizations and the Joint Commission on Accreditation of Hospitals.

In addition, local health professional societies should undertake voluntary performance review with special emphasis on office care. The dental profession and the American Board of Family Practice have developed models of office review, and these mechanisms could operate in conjunction with or independently of the hospital medical staff.

Risk Management Programs at Health Care Facilities

Risk management programs, like quality assurance programs, may be required by licensing agencies, accreditation organizations, or health care facilities themselves. While quality assurance programs generally focus on the clinical aspects of health care, most risk management programs are designed to identify and correct potential problems in the quality of care and to minimize the risks of liability. For example, risk management programs may include activities as diverse as changing the salting procedures on the icy steps at the entrance of a hospital and instituting new procedures to prevent errors in the coding of blood samples.

Currently, risk management programs are primarily found in hospitals, but there are other settings in which they could be useful. All health care facilities should be required to undertake or continue risk management programs. While the problems in other health care settings may differ from those of hospitals, risk management programs may be useful for identifying, analyzing, and correcting problems that could result in harm to patients. For example, nursing homes, ambulatory care facilities, and office-based practices could all benefit from risk management programs. Enhancing the relationship between the professional and the patient, especially through clear and empathic explanations of treatment alternatives, is one important risk management activity that is applicable in any setting. Health care professionals should be encouraged to become involved in these programs, to enroll in courses that address the identification of potential risks, and to support insurers' requirements for risk management activities.

Internal and External Procedures to Evaluate Quality of Care at Health Care Facilities

To maximize the quality of health care services, all health care facilities should have both external and internal review processes. External review processes include all participants in the health care delivery system, while internal review processes include those individu-als who are most directly involved in providing patient care services. Thus, participants in external review processes should include the public, and participants in internal review processes should primarily include health care professionals.

The external review process will be discussed first. To fulfill its fundamental responsibility to maximize the quality of services, each health care facility should establish, through its governing body, a formal structure and process to evaluate and enhance the quality of its health care services. This should be accomplished by participation of the professional staff, management, patients, and the general public. The external process for the review of quality of health care services should include consideration of accreditation standards and government regulations through professional associations, payors, business and industry, community members, court rulings, and liability insurers.

Internal quality assurance activities occur at various levels in health care facilities; therefore, to ensure quality care at all levels for all patients, these activities should be coordinated by a central body within each health care facility. Every health care facility licensed or certified to provide any kind of health care should be required by its licensing or accrediting body to establish a formal committee to coordinate all quality assurance activities that occur among the various health care professions within the facility. Each of these committees should have at least one representative who is not an active member of that facility's health care staff, such as a representative from the Board of Directors. At a minimum, the internal process should include the review, assessment, and evaluation of personnel (including professional staff) and patient care (including patient feedback). There should be an informal exchange of information among these quality assurance committees at the community level as well.

Voluntary Accreditation of Health Care Facilities

Health care facility accreditation is voluntary; however, the influence of accreditation programs should not be underestimated because of their voluntary, nongovernmental nature. In fact, in many jurisdictions, facility accreditation may be linked to state licensure. A number of benefits accrue to facilities as a result of accreditation. In addition to being a visible sign of quality to patients, providers, and third-party payors, accreditation offers tangible financial rewards, such as reduced liability premiums and eligibility for third-party reimbursement.

The Joint Commission on Accreditation of Hospitals (JCAH) is the most well-established and influential accrediting agency. The JCAH accredits about 75% of the nation's community hospitals, and over 95% of those hospitals with more than 200 beds. In addition to accrediting hospitals, the JCAH also accredits psychiatric and substance abuse facilities, long-term care facilities, nonhospital ambulatory care facilities, and hospice programs.

In recent years, with the rapid rise in the number of nonhospital facilities—such as freestanding emergency centers, ambulatory surgery centers, and birthing centers—several smaller and more specialized accrediting bodies have been founded. These organizations, like the JCAH, are voluntary and nongovernmental. They include the Accreditation Association for Ambulatory Health Care, the College of American Pathologists' Laboratory Accreditation Program, the American Association for Accreditation of Ambulatory Plastic Surgery, the American College of Radiology's Committee on Accreditation, the American Association of Blood Banks' Inspection and Accreditation Program, the National League for Nursing's Accreditation Program for Home Care and Community Health, and the Commission on Accreditation of Rehabilitation Facilities.

Licensure of health care facilities ensures that minimum standards have been met, but most voluntary accreditation standards are higher than those required for licensure. Voluntary accreditation programs with standards that exceed those of state licensure and that focus on quality of care issues should be offered to all health care facilities. Existing accreditation agencies, through a review of the types of facilities and their programs, and when appropriate through the implementation of new programs that are consistent with their goals and expertise, should be encouraged to expand their activities. Accreditation agencies should also include in their activities studies on the effect of accreditation standards on the quality of care.

However, accreditation programs should not be expanded to the extent that they result in increased costs, duplication of effort, and competition among accreditation agencies. Various agencies that accredit health care facilities should develop a formal interagency structure to coordinate their activities and to resolve any interorganizational problems that may arise. These agencies should work together toward the common goal of ensuring quality health care without expensive duplication of effort.

Third-Party Payors and the Quality of Care in Health Care Facilities
The costs of developing and implementing a structure and process for maintaining quality health care services in health care facilities are—like the costs for utilities and personnel—necessary costs, and should be included in the price of health care services. Furthermore, third-party payors, like individual users, should encourage improvements in the quality of services. Public and private payment programs should limit their coverage for services provided in health care facilities to those that meet standards of acceptable quality, should structure their reimbursement to support the improvement of quality, and should provide information on quality for the benefit of their subscribers. Neither individuals nor other payors should pay for substandard care. Payors should develop criteria to measure the quality of care in various types of facilities. Hospitals accredited by the JCAH are deemed to have met standards that qualify those institutions to receive Medicare reimbursement. Subscribers should be informed as to what these criteria are, how to determine if a particular facility meets them, and how to select a quality facility.

Educational Programs on Quality Assurance for Health Care Professionals
Health care professionals have a responsibility to participate in quality assurance programs throughout their careers; unfortunately, this is not happening to the extent that it should be. Educational programs on quality assurance issues for health care professionals should be expanded through the inclusion of such material in health professions education programs, in preceptorships, in clinical graduate training, and in continuing education programs. Academic institutions should participate in the research and evaluation of programs to improve the quality of care. Additionally, they can offer course work on the development of criteria to assess outcomes of care, the identification of geographic

variations in the delivery of health care services, and joint clinical administrative monitoring programs in the hospital. Many such programs already exist and could be replicated at other institutions.

Public Information on Quality of Care in Health Care Facilities
Inadequate information concerning all aspects of health care has been identified as a major source of patient dissatisfaction with the health care system. Most of the public knows little, if anything, about the quality assurance activities that occur within the various professions or in health care facilities. Because educational programs are an integral component in the provision of quality health care, they should be developed to inform the public about the various aspects of quality assurance. Many hospitals and other delivery systems have developed "patient awareness" and "patient education" programs; these have been used primarily to acquaint patients with the inpatient environment and to explain the procedures and processes that will be encountered during their stay. Activities of this kind should be expanded by professional associations and hospitals. A multidisciplinary approach should be taken to develop educational programs and activities for the public. For example, health care professionals from nursing and medicine might jointly sponsor public service announcements for use on radio or television. The content of these announcements could vary from message to message, with some focusing on quality assurance activities within particular facilities, locales, or professions, and with others focusing on the future of American health care. The public should also be informed that peer review and other quality assurance mechanisms represent the application of standards to local and individual cases by professional peers to assure both quality and the appropriate use of resources.

Additionally, health care facilities and national and local health care organizations should make information available to the public about the factors that determine the quality of care provided by health care facilities, and about the extent to which individual health care facilities meet acceptable standards of quality. A facility might make information relating to its licensure and/or accreditation status, the qualifications of its professional staff, and internal quality assurance and risk management activities

available to current and potential users. A nationally-agreed-upon list of quality measures could be developed, and each facility could be required to disseminate information on its position regarding the criteria to anyone requesting such information. As an alternative, health care facilities could work with national and local health care organizations to develop information suitable for distribution. For example, a brochure could outline what consumers should look for in selecting a health care facility. It could also be accompanied by a listing of currently accepted measurements of quality and sources of specific information on individual facilities.

Variations in Practice Patterns
Evidence that there are wide geographic variations in practice patterns of health care professionals in the United States has been emerging over the past decade. Variations in practice patterns are not limited to any particular area of the country, health care delivery system, or specialty. These variations have been well-documented, but researchers have not reached definitive conclusions as to why they exist. Potential explanations include differing patient needs, differentials in health care practice style, and inappropriate utilization. Variations often arise from a lack of well-established data on the effectiveness of alternative treatment programs.

Certainly, inappropriate utilization adversely affects the quality of health care. But it is just as true that standardization to the point where there is no allowable deviation from the norm can also adversely affect the quality of care. The analysis of utilization patterns should take economics into consideration but not at the expense of delivering quality health care services. Government and private sector peer review groups should evaluate variations in the utilization of health services and should provide information about the characteristics of health care practices within the hospital staff, the local community, and the geographic region to health care professional groups and the public. The prospective payment system under Medicare, the quantitative utilization objectives of peer review organizations, and much of the selective contracting within the private sector are all indicators of the growing pressures to reduce variations in utilization. As the focus of cost containment efforts turns toward standardization in the provision of care, third-party payors are regarding geographic variations per se as indicators of inappropriate care and are using them as a means of identifying potential cost savings. If utilization patterns are changed solely on the basis of economic considerations, quality of care may be lessened, future health care innovation may be seriously endangered, and the scope of professional judgment may be severely circumscribed.

Research on the Effects of Peer Review Programs and Payment Mechanisms on the Quality of Care

While specific quality assurance methods have changed over time, the basic goal of ensuring the provision of quality care has not changed. Recent pressures on the health care system and health care professionals, however, have led to changes in the way quality assurance programs are conducted. Two major pressures are the consideration of efficiency as a criterion in the evaluation of health care, and the need to stem the persistent increases in health care costs. These pressures have led to an increasing tendency, particularly on the part of those who are paying for health care, to emphasize the cost-effectiveness of quality assurance.

The Utilization and Quality Control Peer Review Organization (PRO) Program, the peer review conducted by practicing professionals, and various payment mechanisms— for example, the prospective payment system under Medicare—can all have direct effects on the quality of care received by patients. Research should be undertaken to assess the effects of peer review programs and payment mechanisms on the overall quality of health care. Some research on the effects of these programs has already been initiated. The Prospective Payment Assessment Commission is currently conducting a number of studies on the effect of the prospective payment system on quality of care. Utilization review programs are viewed by some as a primary vehicle for reducing inappropriate variations in health care, and research is being conducted in this area as well. Results of these studies should be carefully evaluated to ensure that there are no adverse effects on the quality of care.

The U.S. Department of Health and Human Services, in consultation with affected health care professionals, should conduct evaluations of the effects of PROs on quality of care. The research should focus on outcomes of patient care, costs of patient care, and administrative costs to patients and providers. An assessment of patients' perceptions will be an important element of this research. Indemnification of peer reviewers to protect them against liability and restraint of trade charges should be addressed.

Quality Assurance and Data Collection

Consistent and coordinated data collection and analyses are extremely important to the effective evaluation of health care services, including quality assurance activities. Health care data are currently collected and analyzed in a very fragmented fashion and at great expense. In addition, there is no consistency in the data collected. There should be a coordinated and cost-effective system for data collection, analyses, and dissemination on a national level to improve quality assurance activities on the local level. The establishment of a unified data system requires the participation of payors, providers, patients, and employers so that the data needs of all parties can be met by the system. Representatives of these groups, as well as other interested parties, should formulate a specific plan for defining what data should be collected, and to coordinate the analyses and dissemination of the data. An initial step in this effort might be the assessment of the various statewide data collection systems that have been established. Policies relating to the confidentiality of data should be defined to protect the individual rights of patients and providers, and decisions should be made concerning procedures for access to the data.

Qualifications of Health Professionals

The quality of health care received by the public is highly dependent upon the qualifications, including the education and experience, of health care professionals delivering these services. Licensure and certification have been developed to assist in the determination of qualifications of health care professionals, and both are important elements in protecting the health, safety, and welfare of the public.

Licensure is the process by which an agency of government grants permission to an individual to engage in a given profession or occupation upon finding that the

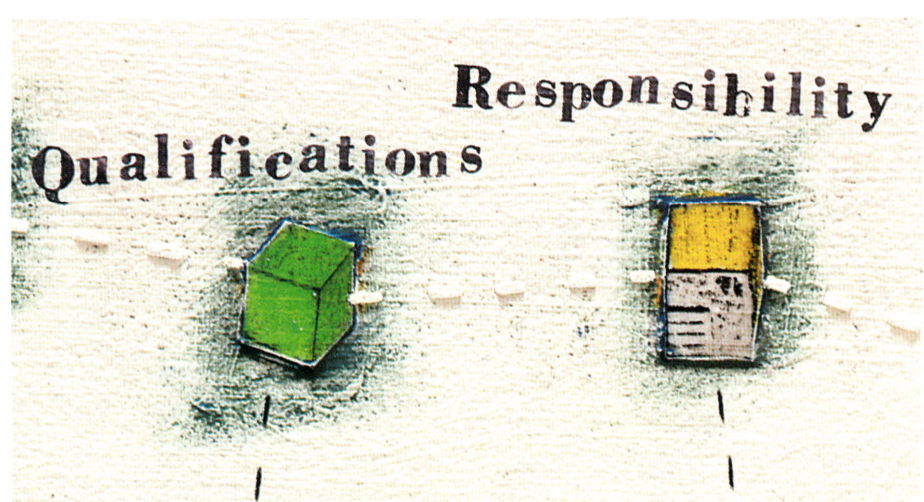

Quality health care requires both technical competence and appropriate concern for the patient's physical, psychological, and social needs.

applicant has met acceptable qualification standards. Since the law establishing a licensed profession or occupation usually sets forth the "scope of practice," licensing laws are often referred to as "practice acts." Requirements for initial licensure typically include criteria relating to personal integrity, education, training or experience, and successful completion of an examination. All 50 states and the District of Columbia require that licenses be obtained to engage in the practice of dentistry, medicine, nursing, optometry, osteopathy, pharmacy, and podiatry. In addition to the authority for granting licenses, states also have the authority to revoke or otherwise restrict an individual's license to practice; for those professions which require licensure, practicing without a license is a violation of state law. Maintaining a license usually requires periodic payment of licensure fees and avoidance of disciplinary actions (such as suspension or revocation of the license). Completion of continuing education courses may also be required.

Certification is the process by which a governmental or nongovernmental agency or association grants authority to use a specified title to an individual who has met predetermined qualifications. Certification can be either public or private. Public certification is a governmental recognition of an individual's having met certain requirements; for purposes of this discussion, both governmental authorization to practice a health profession or occupation and public certification will be referred to as licensure. Private certification is the formal recognition of the qualifications of an individual in a profession or occupation by an established group of professional peers. It is voluntary and is a function of the private sector.

Licensure and private certification are two distinct processes. While state governments may require licensure for the practice of a particular profession, private certification is a nongovernmental process to which individuals may subject themselves in order to be recognized by the certifying agency. For example, while physicians must obtain a license to practice medicine, they may or may not choose to subject themselves and their credentials to examination by a medical specialty board to become "board certified" in that particular specialty. However, over time, medical specialty certification has become a quasi-requirement of many hospital medical staffs for the granting of hospital privileges and, in many cases, acts as a classification system for varying levels of reimbursement under public and private insurance plans. As a result of public concern, some of the specialty boards have adopted in principle the need to recertify physicians periodically as evidence of their professional commitment to quality health care.

The growth in the number of health occupations comprised of individuals whose training ranges from vocational to scientific and who are classified as "allied health professionals" has increased the demand for private certification. Allied health professional certification requires graduation from an accredited training program, successful completion of written or clinical examinations, and usually some work experience.

Increasing competition for health care dollars, increasing specialization in health care delivery, and projected surpluses in some health care specialties will affect licensing and certification processes to some degree. As changes occur, however, it should be remembered that the ultimate purpose of licensure and certification is to ensure the health, safety, and welfare of the public. The participants of the Health Policy Agenda believe that state licensing laws should be reviewed on a regular basis to determine which laws should be enacted, updated, revised, or repealed. Continued certification for the health care professions is encouraged. Additionally, licensing and certifying bodies, as well as the health professions themselves, should be encouraged to identify deficient health care professionals.

Review of State Licensure Laws

Advances in technology leading to new specialties in both medicine and allied health continue to increase the numbers and types of health care professionals; consequently, the number of health professionals seeking initial licensure is increasing. Currently, at least 145 health occupations are listed by the U.S. Bureau of Health Manpower, and 44 are regulated by at least one state. It is not unreasonable to assume that many of the remaining occupations will seek licensure at some time in the future. Furthermore, some health care professionals are seeking changes in scope of practice legislation.

Given these circumstances, state legislatures should develop a mechanism to consider the need for new health professional licensure laws; additionally, they should review existing health professional licensure laws to determine which should be strengthened to protect the public and which should be repealed because they are no longer necessary. The assessment of the need for new and continued licensure laws should be politically nonpartisan. Mechanisms for assessment may include sunset reviews and impact reports that forecast the effect of licensure on the cost of and access to health care services.

Certification of Health Care Professionals

An increasing number of health care facilities and agencies in the private sector are requiring that physicians be certified as specialists in order to receive certain appointments and benefits. Currently, over 80% of all graduates of American medical programs achieve certified status. It is estimated that by 1990 about 90% of U.S. medical school graduates will achieve board certification in some field, and this figure is expected to rise to 100% by 2010. Additionally, the federal government now lists close to 30 nongovernmental associations, boards, or other groups that certify various categories of allied health professionals.

Private certifying organizations should be encouraged to continue certification programs for all health professionals and to communicate to the public the qualifications and standards they require for certification. Decisions concerning recertification should be made by the certifying organizations. Private certifying organizations should adopt policies for the improvement of quality and for the enhancement of the professions. Informational materials explaining the qualifications and standards for certification should be available to the public through certificate holders, public health departments, and issuing organizations.

Identification of "Deficient" Health Care Professionals

There is some controversy surrounding the perceived effectiveness of licensing and disciplinary boards in identifying or taking appropriate action against "deficient" health professionals (those lacking in skills or ability to perform at an acceptable level). Furthermore, there is a public perception that health care professionals are sometimes aware of deficiencies in the practices of colleagues, but that only rarely is any action taken to correct these situations. This matter needs to be addressed by health care professionals and their associations, licensing and disciplinary boards, and the public.

Each health care profession (as well as professional associations for health care facilities and nursing homes) needs to take an active role, within the scope of the law, to correct substandard behavior by a practitioner or a facility. Working with state licensing and certifying boards, health care professions should use the results of quality assurance activities to ensure that substandard practitioner behavior is dealt with in a professional and timely manner. Licensure and disciplinary boards, in cooperation with their respective professional and occupational associations, should be encouraged to work to identify "deficient" health care professionals. Health care professional associations should create advisory committees to develop plans under which deficient practitioners can be identified without abridging patient or practitioner rights. When necessary, licensure and disciplinary boards should consult with these advisory committees on the competence and qualifications of practitioners. Finally, the public should be encouraged to report their concerns about specific health care professionals to either the advisory committees, or to licensure or disciplinary boards. Information concerning these activities should be made available to the public. For more extensive discussion of this topic, see the next section in this chapter.

Professional and Societal Responsibilities Regarding Patient Injury

The issues of patient injury, compensation for injury, and professional liability are very complex and subject to various interpretations. However, there is general agreement that some injured patients are not compensated fairly or expeditiously, that some patient injury could be averted by more aggressive discipline of health care professionals and, finally, that costs for obtaining liability insurance have escalated considerably.

In recent years, there has been growing public debate about the number of lawsuits brought against all kinds of businesses, professions, and governmental agencies. Health care professionals have been particularly troubled by escalating professional liability premiums. Although there is disagreement about the causes of escalating premiums, there is agreement that premium increases have resulted in changes in practice patterns and in the availability of needed care in some cases. Despite rising premiums and increases in the size of awards, it is estimated that an insufficient proportion of the premium award is actually received by patients judged to be injured as a result of negligence. A substantial proportion is received by attorneys handling the cases. There appears to be inequity in the awards received by patients who have had equally bad outcomes, and some injured patients may receive nothing at all. Also, many patients are injured not because of fault but because of imperfect reactions by unpredictable biological systems or because of degenerative changes inherent in human life. Some of these people have no replacement source of income and no health insurance.

Professional liability problems arise when the patient believes that the health care provider has been negligent in the provision of care. The tort system is the patient's recourse against poor quality care. However, the problem is complicated by a perception that juries are increasingly willing to compensate patients for "maloccurrences," i.e., nonnegligent injuries that the tort system was not intended to address. The difference between a maloccurrence and negligence is as follows: negligence occurs when a health care provider fails to perform at the standard of care for which he or she is responsible; a maloccurrence is a poor outcome, but not as a result of provider negligence. Practically speaking, it may be difficult to differentiate between the causes of an injury in the litigation process, but the tort system should not be used as a vehicle to obtain compensation for maloccurrences. Negligence is always a quality of care issue, but professional liability is only one method of dealing with such concerns; others include quality assurance programs, licensure, and continuing education.

National attention was first focused on the issue of professional liability in the mid-1970s, and many states implemented one or more of a variety of measures to reduce the extent of a professional's legal exposure to malpractice claims. For example, some states shortened the statute of limitations, and some implemented a periodic payment system under which award payments were to be made over the actual lifetime of the plaintiff or for the actual period of disability. Others imposed an upper limit—a "cap"—on the amount of damages which could be recovered in malpractice judgments. However some consumer groups opposed caps on awards, and in some states, statutes attempting to limit the amount of damages were found to be in violation of either the U.S. or state constitutions. Still other states opted for the creation of pretrial screening panels to provide the parties to a malpractice dispute with an impartial, nonbinding assessment of the validity of the plaintiffs' claims; the purpose of this was to encourage settlement of claims before they reached the courts. However, in many states, the screening panels were and still are easily by-passed. To avoid granting awards beyond the damage suffered, some states modified their collateral source rules to allow for the introduction of evidence of compensation or payments received from some or all collateral sources. In addition, legislation was enacted in some states to allow regulation of attorneys' fees in liability cases; one approach was to use a sliding scale for establishing attorneys' fees as a percentage of the awards, another was to provide for court review of the proposed fees, with subsequent approval for what the court considered a "reasonable" fee to be. Finally, some states established compensation funds to underwrite large awards.

Although these changes seemed to ease the situation somewhat, they evidently did not address the underlying factors that originally caused it, for in the 1980s, public attention was once again directed toward the issue of professional liability. The number of patient claims continued to increase, and the frequency and the average size of awards and judgments continued to grow, in part because of general and medical inflation, population growth, and real wage increases. The number of physicians involved in malpractice suits continued to increase, and, as in the mid-1970s, several insurance companies stopped offering malpractice insurance.

As a result of these developments, many health care professionals have changed their practice patterns; they spend more time with patients, keep more detailed records, and increasingly refer difficult cases to more specialized colleagues. While some of these changes may have improved the quality of care, other changes are clearly not beneficial. Some specialties and procedures have been identified as "high liability risk,"

and as a result, some practitioners and institutions have restricted their scope of practice or service to reduce liability insurance premiums. Other health care professionals have decided to "go bare" (i.e., to carry no insurance), while others are underinsured. These actions have led to a number of unfortunate but predictable consequences. First, the number of health care professionals paying professional liability premiums has declined, and insurance company reserves, from which liability awards are paid, have declined. Second, those health care professionals who do not restrict their scope of practice are required to bear the costs of premiums necessary to fund the liabilities incurred in high risk areas. Third, talented and skilled physicians are not providing certain health care services, which leads to a loss to society as a whole. Fourth, a health professional who is either not insured or underinsured creates a risk for a patient injured by that professional's negligence.

The advent of prospective payment systems and other cost containment efforts that encourage providers to limit the services provided to patients may also lead to increasing exposure to liability risks. To cope with this and other pressures, many health professionals are engaging in the practice of "defensive medicine," which is essentially the management of a patient's care with one eye focused on the patient's welfare and one eye focused on preemptively fashioning an unassailable record in anticipation of possible future litigation. Thus, the fear of malpractice suits provides an incentive to order unnecessary services, such as an increased number of tests or confirming opinions. This adds to total health care costs—costs which are ultimately passed on to patients and insurers. Additionally, the threat of a liability suit creates distrust between the health care provider and the patient; to the extent that this distrust represents an obstacle to good communication, the quality of patient care is adversely affected. Society as a whole and patients in particular must deal with the limited availability of some needed health care services, the risks of seeing uninsured or underinsured health care professionals, paying for the costs of unneeded tests and services, and the atmosphere of distrust between patient and health care professional.

It must be acknowledged that despite the generally high quality of health care, some professionals are impaired or are incompetent to practice for other reasons. This is true for any professional group, but because those involved in health care provide services affecting personal health and well-being, they carry a special responsibility to "do no harm." Licensing boards generally have the responsibility to check on the qualifications of applicants and to test them to ensure that only those who meet certain standards are licensed. While licensing boards have been quite zealous about screening applicants for initial licensure, they have not been quite as aggressive in checking on those already licensed. In defense of licensing boards, however, it should be noted that in some cases their hands are tied because of inadequate resources, a limited range of disciplinary options, or weak laws that make it difficult to obtain administrative orders. Many individuals argue that there is inadequate use of disciplinary actions against those who engage in substandard practices or who are incompetent. There are many problems surrounding self-regulation in the health professions. (Most licensing boards are composed of members of the regulated profession, so the system is essentially one of self-regulation under the aegis of the state.) Health care professionals may have neither the opportunity to obtain the detailed information required to evaluate particular problems, nor the knowledge necessary to evaluate the various subspecialties of their professions. And, health professionals, out of concern for due process, tend to keep complaints about colleagues to themselves. Although professional organizations may deprive a practitioner of membership (or take even lesser actions) and hospitals may curtail or revoke privileges, both of these types of disciplinary measures are subject to challenge as being anticompetitive or discriminatory. Some problem professionals, after being disciplined, continue to practice outside the bounds of observability and influence. Some state licensing or disciplinary boards are so inadequately funded and staffed that they cannot respond in a timely manner to complaints referred to them.

The participants of the Health Policy Agenda believe that providers, patients, payors, and legislators must consider ways to improve the system to safeguard the quality of health care delivery, to compensate injured patients, and to control the costs of professional liability insurance. Ultimately, injured patients should have adequate funds to cover medical and living expenses; patients injured as a result of negligence should be expeditiously, fairly, and reasonably compensated; instances of incompetence should be dealt with promptly and aggressively; and costs associated with the liability system should match the benefits provided by this system. To accomplish these goals, the effectiveness of the tort system itself should be evaluated and a demonstration study of a new patient compensation system should be undertaken. A variety of investigative and disciplinary actions should be implemented to address the problem of substandard practitioners. The authority of state licensure/disciplinary boards should be expanded to aid in the identification and disciplining of substandard practitioners. Health care professionals and their professional associations, as well as health care facilities, should be required to report actions against or evidence relating to substandard practitioners to state licensure/disciplinary boards; and these boards should be required to review professional liability judgments and settlements against health care professionals. Informational systems should be expanded to ensure prompt interjurisdictional transfer of licensure and disciplinary information about health care professionals. Allied health professions should communicate information on malpractice decisions and disciplinary actions to a central clearinghouse, where this information will be available to health care facilities and the public. Licensure and disciplinary boards should be adequately funded to support the many activities for which they are responsible.

Modifications in the Tort System

The issue of professional liability arises when a patient believes that a health care provider has been negligent in the provision of care. The purpose of the tort system is to provide appropriate compensation to patients if such negligence has in fact occurred. The tort system, then, provides an avenue of recourse to address the problem of poor quality care.

Over 300 reforms in the tort system have been enacted by states since 1975. However, there is uncertainty about the legality of some of these reforms and about whether certain provisions limit plaintiffs' rights to recover for injuries. Even if the reforms

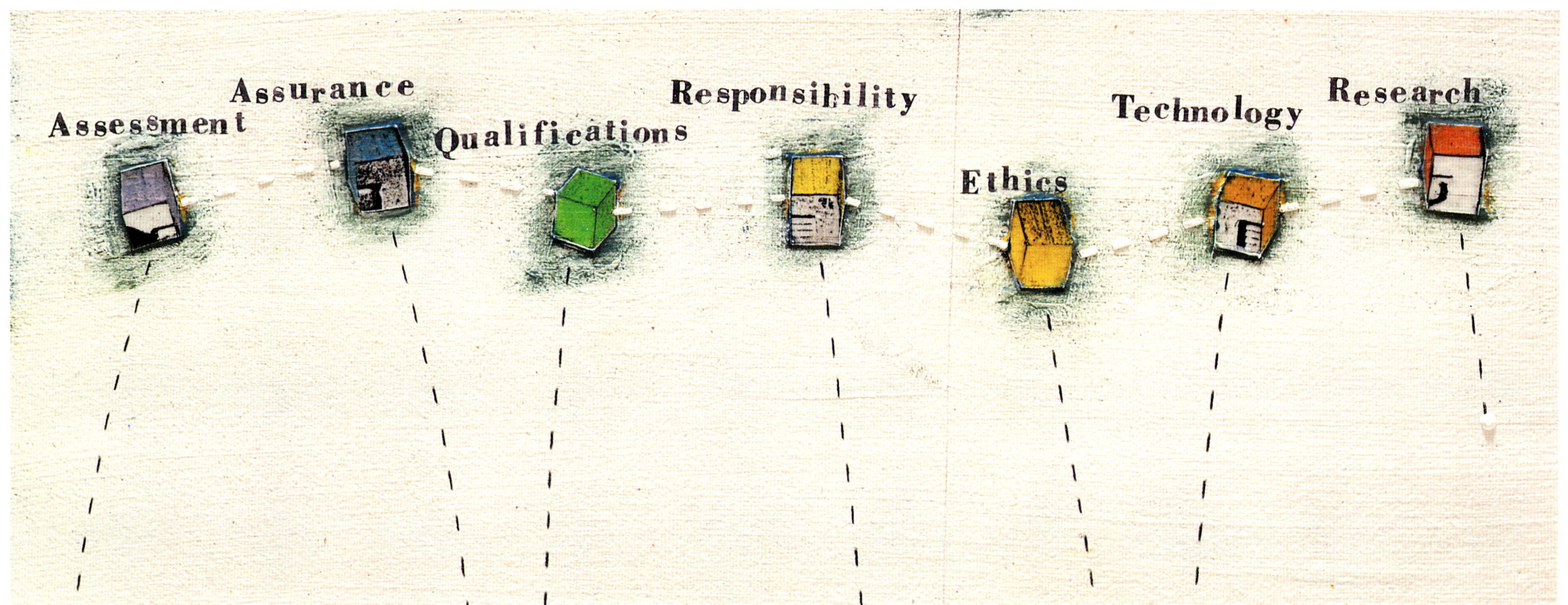

The delivery of quality health care encompasses the use of professional skills, compassionate concern for patients, effective utilization of resources, continuity in patient care, and consideration of the risks and benefits of treatment options.

are upheld in the courts, the effect of these reforms and modifications should be analyzed. Tort system modifications should be evaluated to determine the extent to which they provide expeditious, fair, and reasonable compensation in a cost-effective manner for injuries that occur as a result of negligence. Each state should report information about settlements and awards for economic losses, pain and suffering, and punitive damages. States should follow uniform reporting requirements established by the National Governors Association, which should compile the data and make it available to interested parties. Through careful evaluation, information will be available to examine the effect of modifications on the cost of liability insurance, on the level of patient compensation, and on the costs of "defensive medicine." The effect of the modifications should be evaluated against both the current tort system and predetermined desirable standards.

Demonstration Study of a New Patient Injury Compensation System

The states have traditionally had jurisdiction over the tort system. A demonstration study should be conducted to gather experience and information before changes are recommended. To determine if improvements can be made in the system for patient injury compensation, a demonstration study of a patient compensation fund, which would replace the tort system as the initial entry point into the system, should be undertaken by a state or group of states. In this demonstration study, a broadly representative panel should make expeditious determinations about compensation for injuries arising from medically related events. Payments should be made according to a predetermined schedule based on the severity of the injury and/or should include limitations on the compensation for pain and suffering. The patient compensation fund should be jointly financed by the public and private sectors; the initial portion of awards should be paid by the public sector, subject to a cap per case and reduced by the value of collateral sources. In the event that the injured or the defending party is not satisfied with the determination made by the panel, then that party should have the option to reject the panel's decision and to sue under state law, subject to more stringent standards established to parallel the compensation system (i.e., when a plaintiff rejects the panel's award, tougher tort law standards would be triggered, and when a defendant rejects the panel's award, current tort law standards would govern the case). A substantial monetary penalty should be imposed when the result of a lawsuit is less favorable to the party that rejected the panel's decision. If both parties accept the determination of the panel, then access to the tort system would be waived. A report, which includes a study of the costs, the number and types of cases, any cost-shifting, and the degree of satisfaction of those involved in the system, should be prepared as the basis for future decisions.

This demonstration study should be designed to balance the concerns of both patients and health care providers; injured parties would have an opportunity to receive swift compensation for their injuries, subject to a limitation on recovery for pain and suffering; the government would finance a limited portion of compensation, after all collateral benefits are deducted; and only the parties that have strong cases—whether plaintiff or defendant—could benefit by rejecting a decision of the compensation panel. Interested parties, working in conjunction with the appropriate state level organizations, the National Governors Association, and the National Conference of State Legislatures, should strongly encourage one representative state or group of states to become the demonstration site. Funding for the reports on the demonstration study should be secured through foundations that have an interest in making a social contribution through the alleviation of the problem of compensation for medically related injuries. Study results should be subject to the analyses of the interested parties and should be widely disseminated. If it is found that the costs of this system are predictable and reasonable, that negligence is deterred, that relationships between patients and providers are improved, and that compensation is fair, expeditious, and reasonable, then this system should be adopted on a wide scale at the state level.

Authority of State Licensure/Disciplinary Boards

Historically, licensure and disciplinary boards have only had the authority to either suspend or to revoke licenses upon finding a violation of practice acts. To increase flexibility and to allow sanctions commensurate with the nature of the violation, a number of state legislatures recently have expanded the types of disciplinary actions available to boards. In addition to the traditional authority to suspend or revoke licenses, some boards can now impose probation, fines, supervision, and practice restrictions. State licensure/ disciplinary boards should be given full and extensive disciplinary powers within constitutional limits. Licensure and disciplinary boards should have statutory authority to use broad disciplinary procedures, and members of these boards must be able to perform their responsibilities without fear of liability. Members of state licensure/disciplinary boards should be granted immunity for actions performed in good faith, and they should be indemnified at state expense against any legal actions brought under either state or federal law when they are acting in good faith in performance of their duties. Good faith does not include reckless, willful, or deliberate behavior that would restrain trade or discriminate against individuals who are subject to disciplinary action. These boards should have the authority to suspend licenses summarily in emergency situations, but they should ensure that individuals so affected have the opportunity for a prompt hearing. Disciplinary actions taken by boards should, by statute, be given force and effect pending any court appeal by the disciplined licensee in instances of clear danger to the public. Health professional organizations and other interested groups should encourage the amendment of state laws and practice acts to include the broad disciplinary powers enumerated above.

Reporting of Disciplinary Actions to State Licensure/Disciplinary Boards

Most health care professional associations are organized along county, state, and national lines. They urge the public to send in complaints against members, and promise to investigate and to take disciplinary action against a member when circumstances warrant. However, the strongest action they can take is to expel the member from the society; they have no way to prevent an expelled member from continuing to practice. Hospitals are supposed to check credentials and past performance before allowing admitting privileges, but the thoroughness with which screening is done varies from hospital to hospital. Professionals deprived of privileges in one hospital or who are having disciplinary actions taken against them may have little difficulty in arranging new affiliations.

However, professional associations and health care facilities are often privy to special knowledge about their members. Because health care professionals can cause serious harm to the public, health care professional associations and health care facilities should be required to notify state licensing/disciplinary boards when disciplinary action is taken against a health care professional. National and state professional associations and facilities located in the state should collaborate to amend state laws to codify these reporting obligations.

Professional associations should report to the state board any termination, revocation, or suspension of membership. Professional associations should be required to report any complaint which might be grounds for discipline under state laws and the reasons for the association not taking action. Health care facilities should report any actions to revoke, suspend, restrict, or condition a professional's privilege to practice or to treat patients in the institution. Institutional reporting of resignations prior to the conclusion of any disciplinary proceeding, or prior to the commencement of formal charges but after the professional had knowledge that formal charges were in preparation, will assist in the protection of the public.

Reporting of Potential Grounds for Disciplinary Action to State Licensure/ Disciplinary Boards

By reporting conduct which may indicate that a health care professional is incompetent or is medically or physically unable to engage safely in the practice of his or her profession, all health care professionals can ensure the safety of patients as well as maintain the integrity of their professions. Health care professionals should report personal knowledge of any conduct that they reasonably believe constitutes grounds for disciplinary action to the state licensing/disciplinary board. This recommendation formalizes the special responsibility incumbent upon each health care professional to act on behalf of patients, even when disciplinary action has not yet been contemplated. Model state legislation should be drafted by the National Conference of State Legislatures or by the National

Conference of Commissioners on Uniform State Laws for distribution to state health associations for use in amending state laws or practice acts.

Review of Professional Liability Judgments and Settlements by State Licensure/
Disciplinary Boards
A professional found to be negligent may not be incompetent. Only through vigilant follow-up can incompetent practitioners be identified, adequately disciplined and, when appropriate, have their licenses revoked. State licensing/disciplinary boards should be required to review judgments and settlements against health care professionals who have been judged negligent by the courts or who have settled claims which exceed a predetermined amount. Health care professional organizations and other interested groups should work to amend state laws to enable insurers and courts to report the names and addresses of professionals against whom settlements or awards were made; allegations contained in the claim or complaint which led to the settlements or awards; the dollar amount of each settlement or award; and any information which tends to substantiate a charge that a professional may have engaged in behavior prohibited by law. Courts and insurers should promptly report this information to the appropriate state licensure/ disciplinary board, which should review these cases.

Interjurisdictional Transfer of Licensure and Disciplinary Information about
Health Care Professionals
In some cases, health care professionals whose licenses have been suspended or revoked may attempt to practice in another location. All 50 states have reciprocity provisions or endorsements for physicians, for example, which facilitate the establishment of a practice in another state. The sharing of licensing and disciplinary information among jurisdictions (usually states) would enable licensing officials to flag applications of practitioners whose licenses have been suspended or revoked by another state, or who have voluntarily surrendered their licenses after an admission of wrongdoing. Having such information may decrease the likelihood that undesirable applicants will be licensed inadvertently.

Information systems should be expanded to allow prompt transfer among jurisdictions of pertinent licensure and disciplinary information about health care professionals.

Computer networks should be expanded and standardized among states, if possible, so that disciplined professionals cannot continue substandard practice in another jurisdiction. An example of such a system is that used by the Federation of State Medical Boards and the American Medical Association to transmit reports of official disciplinary actions taken against physicians to all states and jurisdictions. New systems, such as those being developed by nurses and dentists, should be developed as needed. Information should also be given to hospitals and other health care facilities for their use when making decisions about employment or privileges.

Reporting Obligations for the Allied Health Professions
Many allied health professionals make decisions and perform procedures that affect patient well-being as well as the liability of the attending physician and the health care facility. Just as there are some incompetent physicians and nurses, there are some incompetent allied health professionals. However, few of the allied health professional associations have the ability to deny them the right to practice by revoking a license. Also, health care facilities have no central contact point to use when screening prospective employees. In the case of allied health professions, malpractice decisions and disciplinary actions of licensing boards and certification agencies should be communicated to a central clearinghouse. Health care facilities should have access to the resources of the clearinghouse to screen prospective employees, and the public should be able to use the clearinghouse to gather data to make informed health care decisions. The Clearinghouse for Licensure, Enforcement and Regulation of the Council of State Governments currently acts as the repository of this type of information in 22 states; other states should be encouraged to use this same clearinghouse and this information should be widely disseminated to ensure that those who are unfit will have a difficult time securing or maintaining employment.

Funding for State Licensure/Disciplinary Boards

When a state determines that a health profession or occupation should be licensed, it has an obligation to ensure that the licensure law is adequately administered. However, it is generally acknowledged that the resources available to most, if not all, state boards are totally inadequate when compared to the requirements of the task. These boards cannot perform their legislated functions without staff, equipment, and other financial support. State licensure/disciplinary boards should be adequately funded to allow for appropriate investigation and disposition of complaints regarding quality of care and/or the competence of health professionals. Currently, funding of these state functions usually depends on the budget and appropriations in each state and the adequacy of funding varies from state to state.

Health professional organizations and other interested groups should aggressively pursue improved funding of licensure/disciplinary boards. At a minimum, revenue generated from licensure fees and disciplinary fines should be dedicated for use by the respective licensure/disciplinary boards or agencies. The use of licensure fees for unrelated state purposes is not recommended.

Ethical Considerations in Health Care

Debates about the role of ethics in health care are taking place at every level of society. To a large extent, these debates are being fueled by technological advances—for almost every life-threatening condition there is some intervention capable of delaying death. Artificial life-support systems provide a second chance to critically injured persons, and allow irreversibly comatose patients to stay "alive" indefinitely. Neonatal intensive care can provide a normal life for many three- and four-pound premature babies who would have died just a few years ago. Many decisions that were previously in the realm of fate are now in human hands.

Society has yet to develop an effective method of dealing with these issues. The President's Commission for the Study of Ethical Problems in Medicine and Biomedi-

cal and Behavioral Research enunciated three ethical principles that should be adhered to in the provision of health care services: that the well-being of people be promoted, that people's values and choices be respected, and that people be treated equitably. The government, through reports of this nature, through congressional investigations and hearings, and more recently through court decisions, is extensively involved in the discussion of ethical issues. Society seems increasingly inclined to rely on the courts for resolution of ethical dilemmas. In some cases, however, the ethical questions that need to be addressed from the perspective of the patient may not necessarily be the same questions that need to be posed from a societal perspective. Additionally, decisions that are made in one case are rarely directly applicable to other cases.

Many medical decisions now have an inescapable public dimension. No one individual can have the entire responsibility for making decisions regarding genetic engineering and screening, organ transplants, life-sustaining treatment, artificial insemination, and other ethical issues. Making decisions of this kind necessitates the realization that an inherent part of the process is the sharing of ethical responsibilities among individual patients, families, health care providers, and society as a whole.

The ultimate reason for considering ethical issues is the patient's and the public's need to be assured that health care professionals, institutions, and delivery systems will hold the patient's best interests as the highest priority in providing care. There seems to be a consensus that neither family members, institutions, nor health care professionals can act alone in making decisions concerning the provision or withdrawal of treatment. A new coordinated approach is emerging in which patients, families, health care professionals and institutions all have specifically defined roles. The participants of the Health Policy Agenda believe that the patient's interests are best served when ethical decisions concerning treatment are made on an individual basis between patients, or their authorized representatives, and their health care professionals. Ethical guidance on treatment decisions should be sought, when needed, from ethics committees. Health care

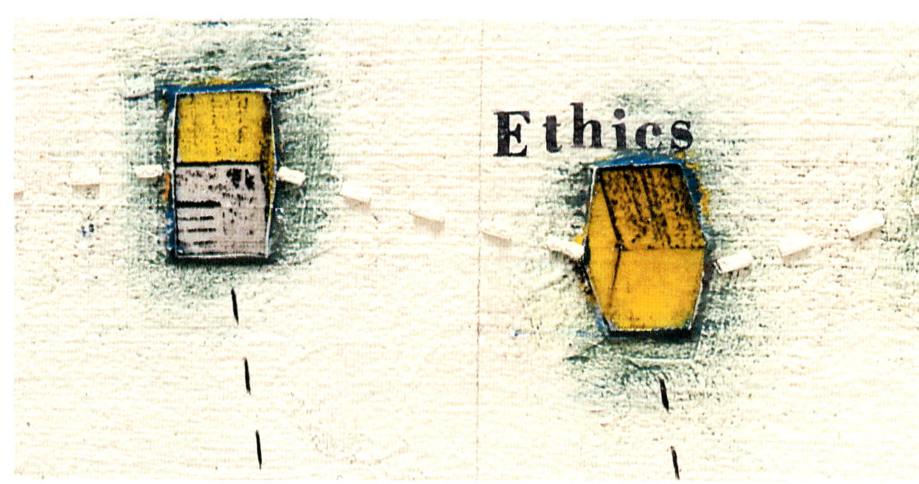

Health care professionals, institutions, and delivery systems should hold the patient's interests as the highest priority.

professionals and the public at large should be educated to better understand the moral and philosophical questions inherent in making ethical treatment decisions.

Decision-Making in Treatment Decisions Involving Ethical Considerations
Mutual participation and shared decision-making between health care professionals and their patients about ethical issues in treatment represent a high ideal. For the most part, patients depend on health care professionals for information regarding diagnosis, treatment alternatives, and treatment plans. In situations involving ethical choices between equally unsatisfactory alternatives, the patient may rely even more heavily on the health care professional for information and guidance. Patients and health care professionals must be able to communicate on such matters. In this exchange, it should be remembered that both health care professionals and patients are very susceptible to misunderstanding each other because of their own fears and anxieties.

When making treatment decisions that involve ethical choices, health care professionals and patients (or their authorized representatives) should strive for a high level of mutual understanding and shared decision-making. Considerations for patient dignity, trust, and integrity should be paramount in any discussion between patients and health care professionals. With improved communication, ethical dilemmas that may require guidance from ethics committees can be identified early in the decision-making process. Patients should have an opportunity to communicate their wishes and preferences in the event that they become incompetent to make their own decisions. In situations in which patients are incapable of making decisions for themselves, designated representatives and/or family members become very important elements in the shared decision-making process.

Many patients often do not understand enough about their own medical situation to know how or when to initiate appropriate communication. For this reason, the primary responsibility for initiating shared decision-making and helping patients to understand the decisions rests with health care professionals. However, this is does not preclude patient-initiated efforts or absolve patients of the responsibility for making their own decisions.

Emphasis should be placed on the education of both health care professionals and patients in fostering mutual participation and shared decision-making. Educational programs should address the gap between patients' expectations of health care and professional practice realities. Health care professionals should be instructed on how to educate patients, with an emphasis on the professional-patient relationship and the socio-cultural aspects of communication. Social phenomena that affect communication and influence health, behavior, habits, and treatment decisions should also be understood. Patients and the public should be instructed on the kinds of questions to ask, the appropriate timing of those questions, and methods to facilitate communication with health care professionals.

Local health professional societies, community hospitals, and local health planning agencies should cooperate in providing educational experiences for both health care professionals and the public. Local professional societies should provide seminars and workshops for local providers. Hospital outreach and social service departments should be responsible for holding general public workshops and for providing an orientation for all patients admitted to the hospital. The responsibility for coordinating these efforts on a community basis should rest with local planning agencies or, where no such agencies exist, with a voluntary body composed of representatives from the local professional societies and local health care facilities.

Establishment of Ethics Committees at Health Care Facilities

Ethics committees are often used to assist in the resolution of treatment decisions, but many facilities do not yet have such committees. Those facilities which do have ethics committees tend to be predominantly large urban teaching hospitals and tertiary care centers.

Ethics committees at health care facilities can serve several purposes. First, they can aid health care professionals and patients who are faced with difficult ethical decisions by facilitating communication and helping to resolve any disagreements. They can provide support to staff and families through confirmation of the ethical complexity of the issues and, in some cases, they can provide any needed reassurance of the social acceptability of their treatment decisions. Second, these committees can serve an educational purpose; they can educate health care professionals regarding the ethical issues involved in clinical care, and they can conduct retrospective reviews of previous decisions to guide future deliberations. Finally, they can serve as a catalyst for discussion of ethical issues both within the institution and in the larger community. They can thus be viewed as an attempt to further integrate ethical analyses into the comprehensive delivery of quality health care.

The establishment of ethics committees at health care facilities to provide ethical guidance to protect patients' rights and responsibilities should be encouraged. As noted above, most large health care facilities have ethics committees, and it may be impracticable to form ethics committees at some smaller facilities. Smaller hospitals often do not have the resources to establish a multidisciplinary ethics committee; some do not even have a sufficient number of health care professionals on staff to establish a credible committee. Many nursing homes, freestanding emergency centers, health maintenance organizations, and other types of facilities may also have limited resources. These facilities should investigate the possibility of establishing a community-wide committee to be shared and staffed by all health care facilities within a reasonable geographic area. In addition, these facilities may be able to use the resources of a referral hospital or a teaching institution in setting up a community forum.

The ethics committees should be composed of representatives from medicine, nursing, administration, clergy, social workers, and lay people from the community. These committees would not make decisions, but would assist those who are most involved in the care of the patient. Standards for committee membership and policy guidelines should be established at the local level. The issue of confidentiality of deliberations should be addressed, and there may be a need for state-level legislation to protect members of such committees from civil and criminal liability.

Health Professions Education Programs, the Peer Review Process, and Ethical Considerations in Health Care

An emphasis on ethical concerns in educational programs and the extension of these concerns into clinical training programs can serve several purposes. Discussions of ethical issues between ethicists and health care professionals can convey to trainees the moral and philosophical questions inherent in health care delivery, and can expose students to the decision-making processes that are used to resolve conflicts. Additionally, by providing educational programs on ethical considerations in health care, the professions will underscore their awareness of these serious issues.

Continued emphasis on ethics through traditional peer review activities permits the exchange of perspectives on an institutional level, and can help to ensure that community standards for ethical decision-making are adhered to in the delivery of health care.

The inclusion of ethics in the curricula of health professions education programs and emphasis on ethical concerns in the traditional peer review process should be encouraged. All health professions education programs are urged to formally incorporate discussions of ethical issues into their curricula and to consider requiring students to take these courses as part of their professional training. This curriculum development should be an element for consideration in accrediting health professions education programs of all kinds. In addition, health care professionals should work with local quality assurance programs to ensure that ethical considerations are incorporated into the peer review process.

Assessment of Health Care Technology

The proliferation of increasingly sophisticated health care technology and the concomitant cost implications of using this technology have been major forces in stimulating concern about technology assessment. Other factors that contribute to the heightened interest in health care technology assessment include the impact of technology on the quality of care, the implementation of the prospective payment system under Medicare, and the occasional use of ineffective treatments. Many forces—including the practice of "defensive medicine," promotion and advertising by manufacturers, and insurance coverage of high technology procedures—contribute to the accelerated use of technology. It is generally agreed that there is a need for an expanded and more coordinated effort in the assessment of health care technology.

The federal government has had a long-standing interest in the assessment of pharmaceuticals and medical devices for safety and efficacy before they are used on a widespread basis. And the government's interest in technology assessment was heightened to a considerable degree when it became a major payor of health care costs under the legislation that established the Medicare program. In 1972 Congress established the Professional Standards Review Organization (PSRO), a physician-sponsored organization charged with comprehensive and ongoing review of services provided under Medicare and Medicaid. The purpose of the PSRO review was to determine, for purposes of reimbursement under these programs, whether the services were medically necessary; provided in accordance with professional criteria, norms, and standards; and, in the case of institutional services, rendered in an appropriate setting. The National Center for Health Care Technology (NCHCT) sponsored evaluations of the safety, efficacy, and economic and ethical impact of health care technology; this information was, in turn, used by the Health Care Financing Administration and third-party payors to make reimbursement decisions.

In 1981, the majority of the responsibilities of the NCHCT were assumed by the Office of Health Technology Assessment, and in 1982, PSROs were replaced by Utilization and Quality Control Peer Review Organizations (PROs). Hospitals are mandated to contract with these organizations for review of quality of care and appropriateness of admissions and readmissions under Medicare's prospective payment system. The prospective payment system has influenced technology assessment and in some senses it acts as an implicit kind of technology assessment. Payment to health care providers on a per case basis has forced them to explicitly consider the cost-benefit ratio of additional services. Providers can no longer acquire expensive technology without regard to cost, and as a result there may be more standardization in the availability of health care technologies.

In addition to the Office of Health Technology Assessment and PROs, there are other federal agencies involved in technology assessment. These include the Office of Technology Assessment of the Congress, which synthesizes research on cost and effectiveness of technology; the Prospective Payment Assessment Commission, an independent governmental agency responsible for changes and adjustments in payments for hospital inpatient discharges; and the Office for Medical Applications of Research in the National Institutes of Health, which uses a consensus approach to identify and analyze clinical applications of research findings.

In the private sector, many associations, professional organizations, and medical specialty societies conduct technology assessment in areas that are of interest to them. Representative organizations conducting technology assessment include the American Medical Association, the American Hospital Association, the Blue Cross and Blue Shield Association, the American Academy of Neurology, the American Psychiatric Association, the American Dental Association, the American College of Physicians, the American College of Cardiology, the American College of Radiology, and the American College of Obstetricians and Gynecologists.

Many technology assessment activities are being "driven" by the need to contain health care costs. Estimates of the effect of health care technology on increased per diem hospital costs range from 33% to 75%, with 50% being the average figure. The contribution of health care technology to overall health care costs has led to some debate about the use of expensive technologies, such as computerized axial tomography (CAT) scanners. However, current analyses indicate that while CAT scanners are expensive, they actually provide a net cost saving to the health care system as a whole. In fact, it may be the cumulative expense of the thousands of small tests and procedures that is most responsible for the annual growth in medical expenditures. These small tests and procedures are commonly used by those practicing defensive medicine—about 40% prescribe additional diagnostic tests, 27% provide additional treatments, and 45% refer patients for further consultation—due, in large measure, to liability considerations.

Certainly the use of health care technology contributes to the cost of health care services. However, the task at hand is not to curb the growth of technology but to establish a national assessment program to ensure that information on the appropriate use of technology is available to improve the quality of care. At least 45 different organizations, both public and private, are involved in technology assessment activities of one kind or another. However, despite the extent of these activities, there is little or no exchange of information among the groups and, for the most part, assessment activities are modest in scope.

Technology assessment should ensure the appropriate distribution and use of health care technology to improve the quality of care. Health care technology assessment should lead to increased use of effective but underutilized technology, an enhanced capacity to make risk-benefit judgments for individual patients, and discontinuation of the use of ineffective and unsafe technology. Effective technology assessment mechanisms, with adequate funding to support them, are needed.

Objectives of Technology Assessment

Without an improved system for the assessment of health care technology, concern about the exposure of the public to unproven and possibly ineffective technology will persist and efforts to contain health care costs will be hindered. The primary goal of the assessment process should be the evaluation of the safety, efficacy, and conditions of use of existing and new health care technologies. Evaluations of the cost-effectiveness of such technologies should also be conducted, but as a separate process so as not to affect the evaluation of safety and efficacy. The assessment process must constitute an exercise distinct from decisions for coverage; coverage decisions are the ultimate responsibility of individual payors. Readily determinable and practical outcome measures of the impact of health care technology on the individual and on society as a whole also need to be developed.

The technology assessment process should not end simply because a given technology is in general use. Professional uncertainty regarding the superiority of new technologies may exist at the time of introduction; additionally, the initial resource costs of a new technology may drop substantially once it is used on a widespread basis. Health care technology should be evaluated on a continuing basis after its introduction, particularly if it is expensive or has potential for inappropriate applications in health care. The applications of the technology and the relationship between benefits and costs, both in general and with respect to specific patients, should be assessed through professionally-developed standards of utilization and peer review. To minimize unnecessary variations in the use of technologies, evaluation findings should be widely disseminated.

Technology Assessment Mechanisms
An expanded and more organized system should be established for the assessment of health care technology. Individual organizations should continue to pursue assessment activities that further their organizational and societal goals. Additionally, a public and private technology consortium should be established to evaluate, synthesize, and disseminate assessment data and to administer an independent Council for Research in Health Care Technology Assessment. This organizational structure would permit a centralized effort in health care technology assessment.

The first component of the system involves the individual voluntary activities of those organizations and individuals currently involved in health care technology assessment. These organizations and individuals should continue to pursue health care technology assessment activities that further their organizational or societal goals.

The second component is a public and private sector consortium of the various groups and members referred to in the first component. This consortium should be based in the private sector, and its activities should complement existing health care technology assessment activities. The consortium would serve primarily as a clearinghouse, tracking the activities and findings of various health care technology assessment bodies and communicating such information to practicing professionals, to policy-making bodies, and to the public. It should identify, collect, synthesize, and disseminate the results of technology assessment to facilitate both informed individual decisions in patient care and policy decision-making about the distribution and use of health care technologies. Additionally, this consortium should identify and prioritize existing and new technologies that need to be assessed. This consortium should in no way pre-empt the legislated responsibilities of the Food and Drug Administration (FDA) nor any other legally-mandated body; the marketing approval process for drugs and medical devices and the evaluative mechanism under which this approval process takes place at the FDA represent necessary functions of the federal government. The consortium should also set the agenda and provide funding for the third component of the system, the proposed Council for Research in Health Care Technology Assessment.

The Council for Research in Health Care Technology Assessment should be a nonbinding, nongovernmental advisory body charged specifically with developing and evaluating criteria and methodologies for health care technology assessment. This Council should also assess the applicability, utility, reliability, and validity of available methods. Studies should focus on ways to improve the clinical and economic evaluation of health care technologies, and the Council should conduct assessments of individual technologies only to the extent necessary to evaluate methodological competence.

This technology assessment system is intended to allow for the gathering, synthesizing, and dissemination of knowledge. A flexible organizational structure would permit the systematic identification and prioritization of health care technology assessment issues for a national agenda, the establishment of a comprehensive and uniform data base, the evaluation of existing methods for technology assessment and the development of new methodologies, and the dissemination of information to all interested parties.

Funding for Technology Assessment
Adequate funding for the administrative and organizational expenses of the public and private consortium and the Council for Research in Health Care Technology Assessment should be borne equitably by all voting members. A target annual budget should be established, and this budget should be increased incrementally as results are produced.

Health Services Research and Evaluation

Health services research is the study and analysis of all health care delivery components, including the operation, organization, costs, financing, and outcomes of health care delivery. Its focus is the overall efficiency and effectiveness of preventive, diagnostic, and treatment services, and it seeks to ensure the continuous evaluation of the quality, availability, and cost-effectiveness of health care delivery mechanisms. Research responsibilities include the evaluation of treatments, providers, and technologies used in the health care delivery system. Health services research should be distinguished from technology assessment, which addresses the safety and efficacy of individual treatment modalities.

The findings of health services research are used by both public and private decision-makers in the health care delivery system. Information is frequently needed and used by policy-makers at the federal, state, and local levels, and by health care providers and consumers. On the national level, there are a number of government-sponsored health services research activities. Examples include empirical analyses of the Medicare population conducted by the Health Care Financing Administration; surveys conducted by the federal government to collect data on health status, and the cost and use of services; and activities conducted by the National Heart, Lung, and Blood Institute, the Office of Smoking and Health, the National Institute on Alcohol Abuse and Alcoholism, and the National Institute of Diabetes and Digestive and Kidney Diseases. Additionally, health services research is conducted by the National Center for Health Services Research and Health Care Technology Assessment at the Department of Health and Human Services, and by the Veterans Administration. And, finally, national and regional research, financed by the public and private sectors, is conducted by private sector organizations, such as foundations and universities.

There are some concerns, however, with the relevance of the research, as well as concerns relating to the funding for research and the availability of research findings. Inadequate information for use in health care decision-making is often cited as a signifi-cant problem by those in policy positions in government and private industry. Another perceived shortcoming is the inability to collate, verify, and disseminate research results to relevant parties. Currently, no single entity is responsible for collecting and disseminating results from all public and private health services research initiatives.

The goal of health services research and evaluation should be to develop a rational and effective method to identify research needs, fund research projects, and disseminate research findings. The participants of the Health Policy Agenda believe that the reliability, validity, and timeliness of health services research should be regularly evaluated so that findings can be used in the development of national health policy. Priorities for health services research activities should be coordinated by a single entity, and funding for the various groups involved in research should be adequate to support their activities.

Health Services Research and Its Use in National Health Policy Development
One of the purposes of health services research is to facilitate decision-making by policy-makers, health care providers, and consumers. It is of the utmost importance, then, to ensure that such research is valid, reliable, and current before health care policies are implemented. However, all too often, health policies are developed and implemented prior to completion and verification of research studies. Research findings frequently are not supported by adequate research methods and designs, resulting in findings that are neither reliable nor valid. It is irresponsible for policy-makers to formulate health policies using preliminary research findings and in the absence of comparative and comprehensive analyses.

Health services research should be regularly evaluated for reliability, validity, and timeliness, and health services research findings should be used in the development of national health policy. Health services research should focus on the overall efficiency and effectiveness of the various delivery mechanisms and preventive, diagnostic, and treatment services. Research activities should include the analysis of the impact of new technology and delivery mechanisms on health manpower, the outcomes and costs of treatment, the overall quality of care, and ethical, moral, and legal issues in the delivery of care. National health policies should be based on health services research that includes the use of demonstration projects to ascertain whether policy objectives can be expected to be fulfilled on a nationwide basis.

Priorities for Health Services Research

As previously indicated, no single entity directs health services research investigations in a broad context, or identifies and assigns priorities to health policy issues to best meet public needs. The National Center for Health Services Research and Health Care Technology Assessment (NCHSR-HCTA), in conjunction with an Advisory Board, should be responsible for identifying informational needs and for determining the types of information to be collected to meet those needs. When appropriate, uniform standards for data collection to guide health services research activities should be established. Additionally, the work of the NCHSR-HCTA should be coordinated with all public sector research activities, including liaison with the National Center for Health Statistics, the National Committee on Vital and Health Statistics, and state health agencies. Finally, the Secretary of the Department of Health and Human Services should be responsible for assessing the validity and reliability of research activities and for correlating and disseminating health services research findings.

A National Advisory Council for the NCHSR-HCTA was recently created, but the sole function of this council is technology assessment. The responsibilities of the National Advisory Council should be expanded by legislation to include the generation of research activities in areas in which there are serious deficiencies. The involvement of the research and health communities, as well as the public, should be ensured. The Advisory Board should issue news releases on a regular basis, and reports should be made available to the research community and the public, as well as published in periodicals and the *Federal Register.*

Funding for Health Services Research

Just as there is no single entity to direct health services research, there is no integrated system for funding this research. Screening of research projects for funding often relies on a close relationship between the sponsoring organizations and the agencies that conduct the research. Funding is needed to support the activities of agencies and organizations involved in health services research. The National Center for Health Services Research and Health Care Technology Assessment (NCHSR-HCTA) should be adequately funded to support an appropriate number of research projects, educational programs in academic institutions, and graduate-level education. This funding will enable the NCHSR-HCTA to fulfill its primary responsibility for stimulating, organizing, and influencing the direction, expansion, and improvement of health services research activities. Funding should provide for ongoing research projects, institutional support to enhance faculty and equipment requirements, and graduate student assistance. The NCHSR-HCTA should supervise the distribution of funds to ensure the availability of career opportunities in health services research.

The National Center for Health Statistics (NCHS) should be funded to ensure the continuity and maintenance of its databases and survey activities. State health data systems should be funded at levels commensurate with their responsibilities to collect mortality and morbidity statistics that comply with national objectives and unite public health activities. The databases compiled, maintained, and analyzed by the NCHS provide valuable information that can be applied to identifying trends in health and health care, addressing critical research and educational needs, and allocating health care resources. Sustained support of state health data systems is necessary to provide information for decisions that may be necessary for resource allocation and public health measures. The support for both of these activities must be at a level to provide trend information that will allow continuity in health planning.

The private sector also has a role to play in funding health services research activities. All constituents of the health care industry should continue their investment in basic and applied health services research, and philanthropic foundations and organizations should continue their support of research and training in health services.

The funding of health services research, including funding for the Advisory

Board of the NCHSR-HCTA, should be derived from both private and public sources, and should be at a level that is commensurate with the priorities identified by the Advisory Board.

Dissemination of Health Services Research Data and Information

As previously indicated, there is inadequate synthesis and dissemination of health services research findings to policy-makers, health care providers, and consumers. Currently, over 40 clearinghouses disseminate information on health issues, but there is little or no linkage of these reference sources. A central body should be designated to act as a clearinghouse for the linkage, indexing, storage, and dissemination of health services research data and information. Data and information should protect the confidentiality of consumers, health care professionals, and health care facilities. Either the Library of Medicine or the National Technical Information Service might be able to serve as a central clearinghouse to organize, process, and disseminate reports of health services research activities in a format that would be useful to policy-makers and the public. Funding should be at a level to ensure the translation of scientific papers and research studies into useful documents. All information collected, analyzed, and indexed must protect confidentiality in accordance with Section 308(d) of the Public Health Service Act.

Summary

In this chapter, improvements that should be made in the mechanisms to ensure the quality of health care services were discussed. Both quality assessment and quality assurance activities were highlighted, as were the licensure and certification processes for health care professionals. Both health care professionals and society have a continuing responsibility regarding patient injuries, and emphasis was placed on the evaluation of the tort system as well as on increased efforts to identify substandard practitioners. The quality of health care can also be improved through the definition and promotion of ethical practices. Finally, the assessment of health care technology and health services research are important in ensuring the provision of quality health care services.

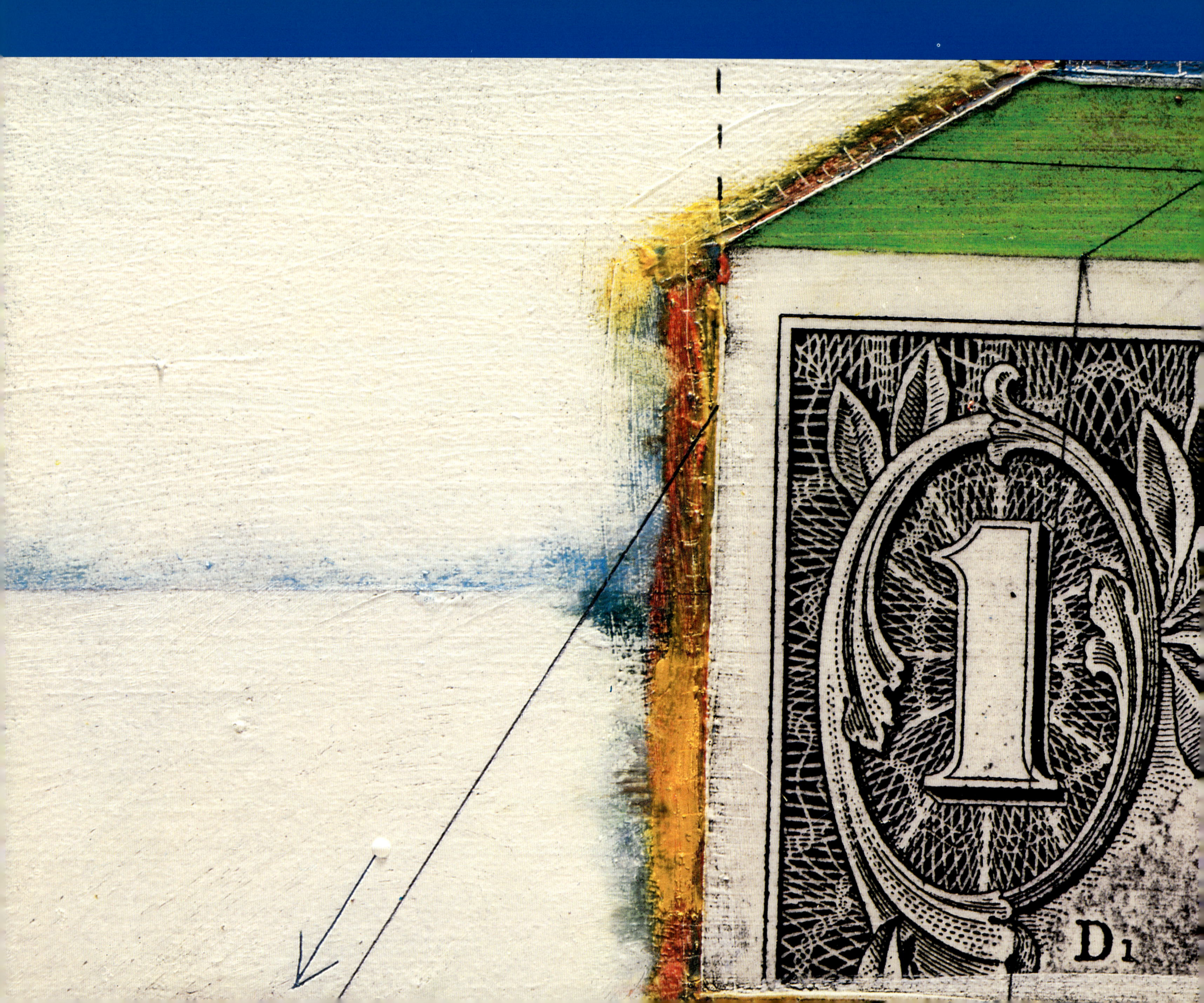

1
D1

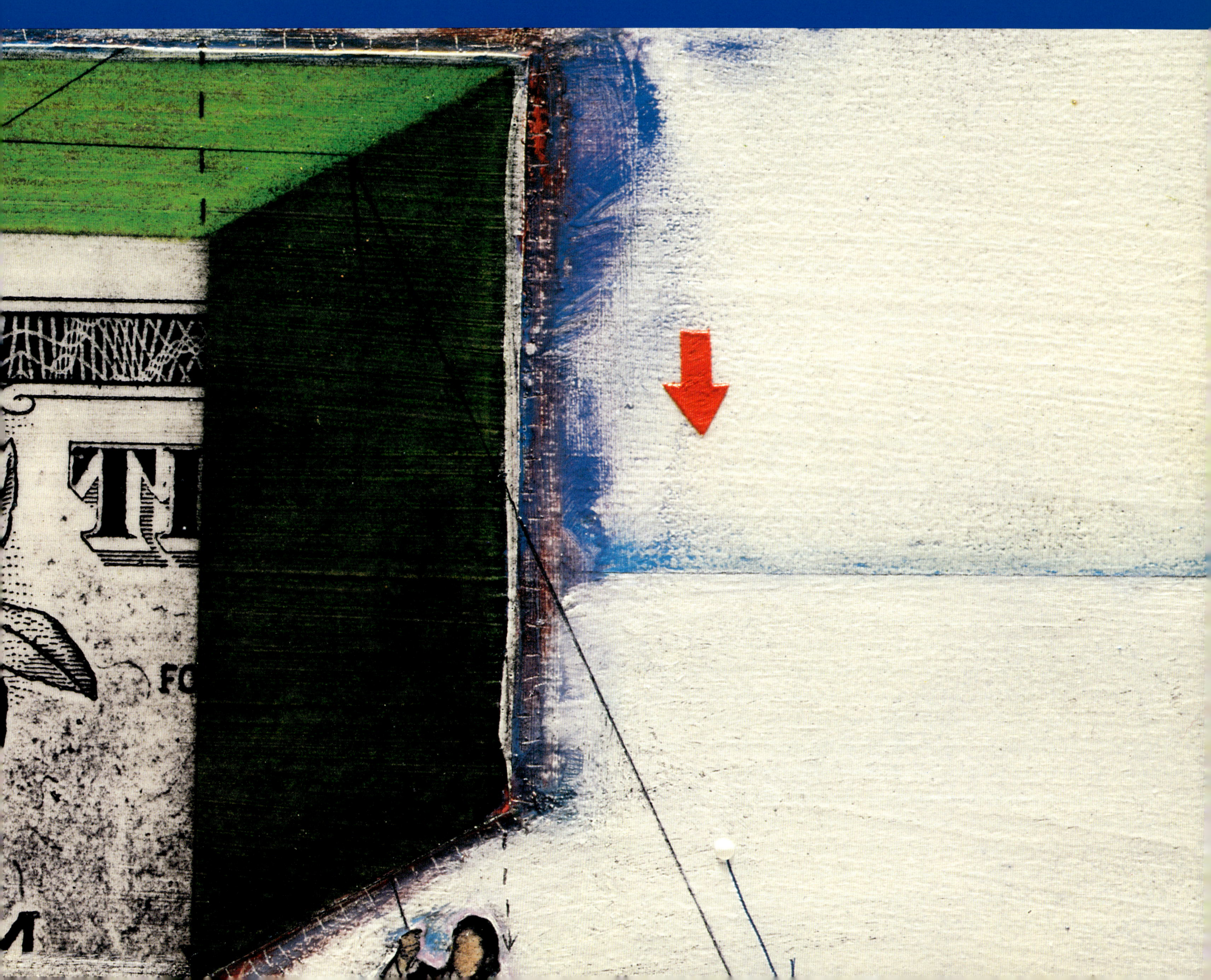

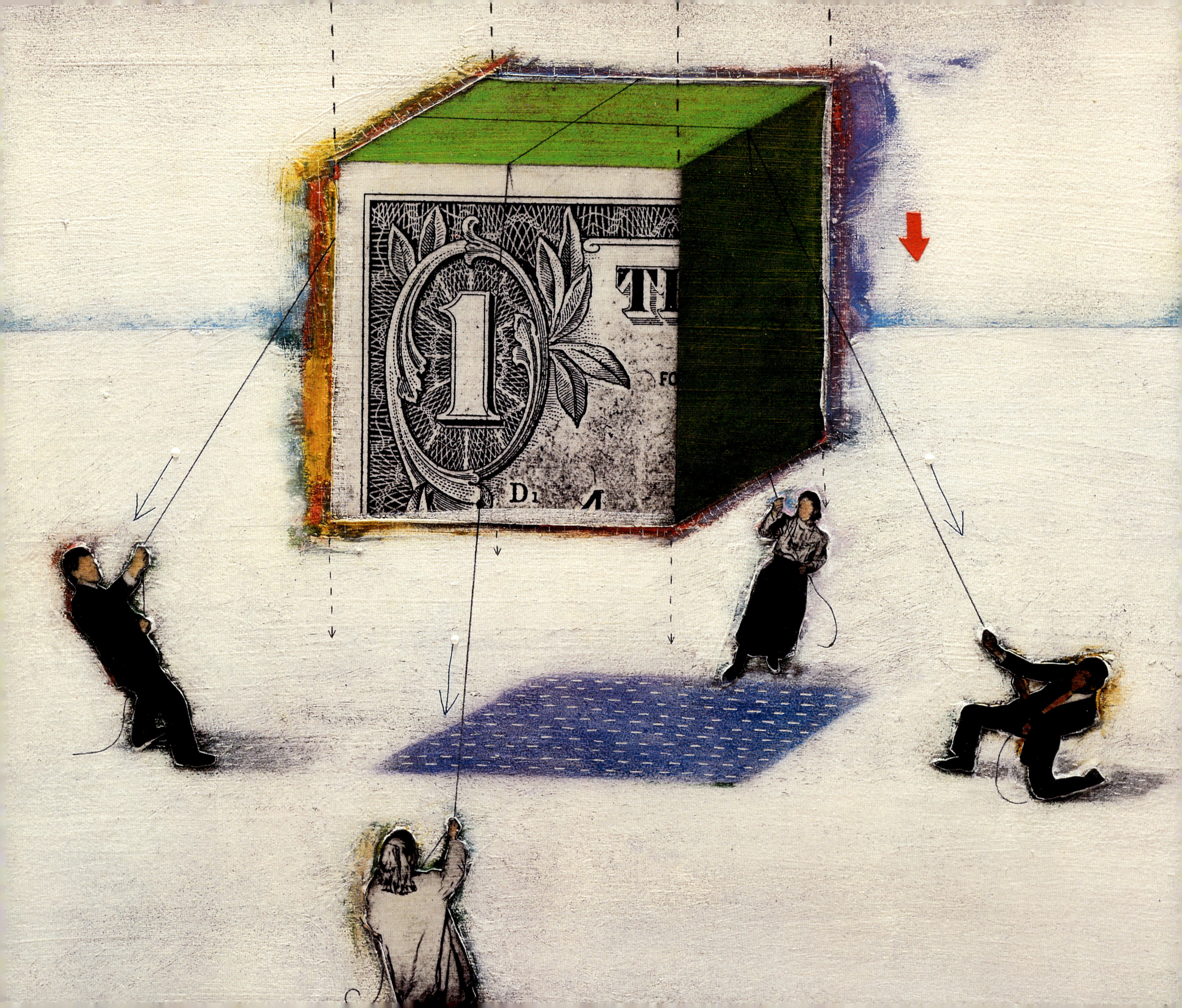

1
T
FO
D

About 88% of the $387.4 billion expenditure for health in 1984 was devoted to personal health care. For every dollar spent on personal health care, 46 cents went for hospital care, 22 cents for physicians' services, 9 cents for nursing home care, 8 cents for drugs and medical sundries, 7 cents for dentists' services, and 8 cents for other personal and professional services and supplies. About 59 cents of every dollar spent on health care came from the private sector; 41 cents came from the public sector—29 cents from the federal government and 12 cents from state and local governments.

From 1950 through 1965, the percentage of public funds devoted to national health care expenditures remained fairly constant at about 25%. By 1970, this percentage had increased to 37%, and by 1975 it had increased to about 42%. In 1966, federal, state, and local governments increased their commitments to providing health care coverage for the poor, the elderly, the disabled, and other select groups, and the establishment of programs such as Medicare and Medicaid contributed to the absolute increases in overall health care expenditures as well as to the significant increases in the percentage of money from the public sector used to finance health care. Over the past ten years (from 1975 to 1984) health care expenditures have continued to climb, but the percentage of public funding has remained fairly steady at about 42%. Analyses of the growth in spending reveal that four factors have made significant contributions to increasing health care expenditures in this period: general inflation alone accounts for about 55% in increased spending, growth in the intensity of health care services accounts for about 22%, medical care price increases in excess of general inflation account for about 16%, and aggregate population growth accounts for about 8% of increased spending.

Certainly the government, through the establishment of special programs to provide needed health care services, has contributed to the improved health status of many Americans. Life expectancy at birth has increased by nearly 12 years for males and by nearly 16 years for females since 1930, and most older Americans will enjoy 15 to 20 years of relatively healthy retirement. In the last two decades alone, the 65-and-over population has grown by 54%, compared with a growth rate of 24% in the under-65 population. If present trends continue, one in five persons will be 65 years of age or over by 2050, compared with about one in ten in 1980. The level of government involvement as payor and provider of health care services is evidenced in a few statistics: over 30 million individuals are enrolled in Medicare, Medicaid has about 21 million recipients, about 28 million veterans are eligible for care under the Veterans Administration (VA), the Department of Defense (DOD) provides care for more than two million active duty military personnel and their dependents, and about one million American Indians and Alaskan natives are eligible for care through the Indian Health Service (IHS).

The unabated increase in health care expenditures necessitates a reexamination and reformulation of the existing health care system. The role and magnitude of government involvement in health care must be evaluated, as well as the current reimbursement system, which generally provides coverage for health care services without incentives to contain costs. In redefining the role of government and in designing a cost-effective payment system, it must be remembered that public safety, access to health care, cost containment, and fair competition can be ensured only by maintaining an appropriate balance between the public and private sectors.

Designing a Cost-Effective Payment System

The increases in health care expenditures necessitate a reexamination and reformulation of the existing health care payment system. The health care payment system, which to one degree or another insulates providers, third-party payors, and individual health care recipients from the economic consequences of their decisions, is the focus of this section of the Health Policy Agenda. The methods used to pay providers, the kinds of services covered, and the role of health care recipients in delivery and payment mechansisms are all critical factors that influence the cost-effectiveness of the health care system.

Designing a cost-effective payment system requires an understanding of the term "cost-effective." For purposes of this discussion, a cost-effective payment system is one in which the least cost produces a desired effect or one in which the greatest effect results at a given level of cost. Payment programs that either improve health outcome and save money or deliver a health benefit at an acceptable cost will be considered cost-effective.

Health insurance provides a means of spreading the risk of unpredictable high-cost expenditures. Third-party coverage for health care costs began about 50 years ago. Earlier, people were largely responsible for paying for their own care. However, during the Depression of the 1930s many individuals were unable to pay for their health care, particularly hospitalization costs. The need for health insurance, coupled with the financial difficulties of hospitals, led to hospital prepayment, which ultimately became the Blue Cross system. Hospital coverage was followed by coverage of surgery and later by coverage of nonsurgical physicians' services. A significant factor in the rise of third-party payments was the 1949 Supreme Court decision on Inland Steel, which upheld the 1948 National Labor Relations Board ruling that companies must consider health benefits when negotiating with employees. This was followed by the passage of Medicare—now the largest third-party payment program—and Medicaid—now the second largest third-party payment program. The impact of providing insurance is evidenced by a few statistics: in 1940, less than 10% of the population had coverage for inpatient care, and very few had coverage for other types of care. Today, about 85% of the population has health insurance coverage. In monetary terms, for every dollar spent on health care in 1950, consumers directly contributed about 65 cents; today consumers contribute about 28 cents.

In general, then, the majority—about 85%—of Americans are covered under one kind or another of health insurance policy. However, 15% of the population—about 30 million individuals—is either uninsured or underinsured at any given time and may therefore be deprived of adequate health care. Recent attempts to define the population at risk show that almost one-third of the uninsured are children under age 18. More than one-half of those without adequate insurance work all or part of the year, and most unemployed people have no insurance at all. The lack of health insurance coverage for some unemployed individuals was partially addressed by the Consolidated Omnibus Budget Reconciliation Act of 1986. This act requires employers sponsoring health plans to employees and their families to offer "continuation coverage" at group rates in certain instances (e.g., death of the employee, termination of employment, or reduction in hours of employment) where coverage under the plan would otherwise end. However, this act does not address the health insurance needs of children, or of individuals who are not employed on a full-time basis, who are employed but without health insurance benefits, who are self-employed, or who are "uninsurable."

Access to health care services is intricately linked to the ability to pay for these services. Demographic trends and projections indicate that there are also growing numbers of individuals who require major health care services, such as catastrophic, long-term, and terminal health care. A cost-effective payment system needs to consider the needs of these individuals as well.

While ready access to health services is an essential component of quality health care, improper use of services can negatively affect the delivery of health care for all Americans. With the escalation of health care costs, a number of initiatives to contain costs have been undertaken. These include educational programs, financial incentives, health care coalitions, second opinions, case management, capitation, and prospective payment systems. To gain a better understanding of the role of cost in health care decision-making, educational programs have been used with both health care providers and consumers. Financial incentives have been used with consumers to increase their financial involvement in health care decision-making; these incentives seem to affect short-term cost and use decisions, but over the long-term cost sharing may discourage use of needed health care services and therefore result in poorer health and higher expenditures. Health care coalitions have had some success in containing costs, but for the most part their impact is limited to the communities in which they are located. The net effect of second opinions on cost-effectiveness and quality of care is subject to debate. Under the case management approach, a primary care physician is responsible for coordinating all aspects of care for a recipient; it appears that control over specialist care, stringent utilization review, and financial incentives are needed for this approach to be effective. Capitation, or per capita prospective payment, allocates a fixed-dollar amount to providers on behalf of each beneficiary, with the provider at risk for costs above the capitated level. Capitation appears to be most effective when there are limits

placed on the financial liability of providers. The impact of the prospective payment system under Medicare is still being evaluated; prospective payment may create cost-shifting problems and financial difficulties for providers serving large numbers of elderly and poor individuals.

There is little evidence to suggest that concern over health care costs will subside in the near future. However, emphasis on cost alone—without equal regard for access and quality of services—is short-sighted. A cost-effective payment system will ultimately shape the structure of the entire delivery system, and the competing objectives of containing cost, ensuring access, and providing quality health care must be balanced. This can be accomplished by defining the services that should be covered by third-party payors, by enhancing the decision-making capability and financial accountability of health care recipients, by placing providers at greater financial risk regarding resource utilization, and by clarifying the roles and responsibilities of all of the participants in the health care system.

The participants of the Health Policy Agenda believe that more information concerning the professions, licensure, treatment outcomes, and prices for services should be available for consumers, and that initial prices for services should be set by providers and subject to negotiation with health care recipients and third-party payors. A basic benefit package, with provisions for catastrophic and long-term care coverage should be designed. Health care recipients, providers, and third-party payors should all play a role in this payment system.

Information on Professions, Licensure, Treatment Outcomes, and Prices

For market forces to function, consumers must have sufficient information to make knowledgeable and cost-effective decisions regarding the use of available health care services. Many different types of health care providers offer similar or identical services. Given the complexity and diversity of the health care system, health care recipients need to know who can provide certain services, where those services are performed, the training and background of different providers, the success of particular providers in providing health care services, and the relative costs of providers. Information lacking in any of these areas can result in less than optimal selection of health care providers.

Health care recipients should have free choice of health care providers from among available resources. The following information should be made available through appropriate channels to the public:

□ each professional specialty group's standards of education and training, standards of practice, scope of practice, and initial and continuing standards of competence;

□ licensure standards, scope of practice permitted by the license, and licensed practitioners;

□ the treatment outcomes of health care providers, as well as the varied classifications of health care providers; and

□ the prices of health care services offered by different health providers.

Professional organizations, certifying and accrediting agencies, health care facilities and licensing agencies should prepare and make available to the public publications on education and training, standards and scope of practice, initial and continuing standards of competence, licensure standards, and licensed practitioners.

The dissemination of potentially misleading data about treatment outcomes is a major problem that needs to be resolved. A prerequisite for the dissemination of information about treatment outcomes is a more precise definition of what constitutes a "favorable" result or patient outcome. Quality assessment methodologies that clearly differentiate between the many factors that contribute to a favorable outcome are needed. Health professionals, health care facilities, and the research community should give priority to these needs. Representatives of the health professions, facilities, payors, business and labor, and the public should then jointly develop systems for providing such information to the public. This could be done on a local or regional basis by health care coalitions.

The dissemination of price information is also an area that needs to be addressed. For example, information on prices without regard to the quality of services could be misleading to consumers. Health professionals should be encouraged by their professional associations to provide information on their charges for typical or frequently performed services through patient information materials, community directories, or other channels. The professional associations themselves should provide general information to the public as to the typical range of charges for commonly performed procedures. Health care facilities should make available to health professionals and their patients the facility's charges both on a routine (per diem) basis and for specific, commonly ordered services.

Determination of Prices by Providers

For the most part, health care providers have been able to set their own prices. Providers are in the best position to determine—after considering their expenses, their practice style, and objectives in the marketplace—what their prices should be. With the exception of those professionals subject to mandatory price freezes and those providers located in states with mandatory rate-setting programs, individual providers should be able to determine what their prices will be for services offered. Furthermore, it should be noted that the actual payment received by the provider may differ from the list price because of a contractual agreement either between a provider and a third-party payor or between a provider and the recipient of health care services. Statutes that do not allow providers to determine their prices should be reviewed; where barriers exist, appropriate organizations should be charged with petitioning the government to change these laws.

Negotiation of Health Care Prices between Health Care Recipients and Providers

For a variety of reasons, many consumers do not engage in extensive "comparison shopping" when choosing a health care provider. In some cases, contracts with health maintenance organizations (HMOs) or preferred provider organizations (PPOs) preclude comparison shopping. In other cases, individuals may be acutely ill and more concerned about their immediate health than about the price of needed services. However, not all health care involves the treatment of acute illnesses, and in noncritical situations consumers can function as prudent purchasers of health care services. Health care recipients, individually and collectively, have the right and the responsibility to negotiate health care prices with providers when possible. Health care recipients can and should communicate with providers regarding the financial implications of pricing decisions.

Process for Determining Reimbursement from Third-Party Payors

Almost 75% of personal health care expenditures are paid for through third-party payors, and in some local markets several large third-party payors may account for over 70% of the payments for health care services. Contracting for services promotes pluralism in delivery and payment mechanisms, and contracting mechanisms should require neither excessive regulation nor excessive litigation. Individual providers and third-party payors should have the right to enter into contracts with each other. They should be allowed to designate their own bargaining agents in the negotiation process, and bargaining should take place at the national, regional, state, and/or local level as appropriate to the third-party payors involved. Providers and third-party payors should have the right to negotiate both the level of reimbursement and the payment mechanism.

At present, legal barriers may preclude implementation of these recommendations. Therefore, as a first step a council, composed of representatives from the business community, consumers, provider organizations, labor, private and public third-party payors, and government, should be established. This council should review existing laws and regulations to determine the changes needed. Second, the council should explore options regarding the structure of the negotiation process. The council, which should be jointly financed by private and public funds, should report its findings within two years.

Provider Consideration of Financial Circumstances of Individual Recipients in Determining Fees

At any given time there are several million Americans who are either unemployed, who have no health insurance, who are entirely dependent on government programs for payment of health care bills, or who have large out-of-pocket expenditures for health care. These persons are entitled to adequate health care even if they cannot pay the entire fee for the services at the time they are delivered. Health care providers should consider the financial circumstances of health care recipients and should accept reduced fees when warranted.

Peer Review of Professional Fees

Because they can provide professional judgment as to whether specific fees for services rendered are unreasonable, health care professions should have a role in the review of exorbitant fees that may be charged by their respective practitioners. The Federal Trade Commission (FTC) has publicly endorsed the concept of professional peer review of fees, but only if the particular program in question does not violate antitrust laws. According to the FTC, peer review of fees violates the law if it unreasonably restrains competition by threatening independent pricing by other professionals or dampens cost-control efforts by third-party payors.

Health care professional associations should explore the feasibility of establishing peer review panels to assist patients in the resolution of fee-related disputes as well as to aid cost-containment efforts of third-party payors. Programs for peer review of fees should be established with due consideration of legal risks, that is, they should involve themselves only in specific fee disputes and not in generalized discussions of fees, usual and customary charges, or fee schedules. Additionally, they should only be advisory and voluntary in nature. Decisions of these peer review panels should not be disseminated beyond the patient, the professional, and the third-party involved in the case.

Establishment of a Basic Benefit Package

A basic benefit package for all Americans should be defined to serve as the basis for private health insurance plans and for public programs that finance health care. A basic benefit package would ensure that beneficiaries are covered for important health care services, would facilitate "comparison shopping" by consumers, and would protect the public by identifying "basic benefits" that should be available. A basic package would be competitive in the marketplace, and insurers could continue to market plans with additional benefits and with variations in coverage and cost-sharing requirements.

A basic benefit package should focus on the health care services needed for diagnosis and treatment of illness and injury, and should not discriminate against any specific category of physical or mental illness. A provision for child health services and preventive services should be carefully considered to avert more costly treatments in later life. Additionally, coverage of hospice care should be considered for inclusion not only because it provides a cost-effective alternative to health care but because it can also improve the quality of life for the terminally ill.

To address these and other technical details, an ad hoc committee, composed of representatives from the health care professions, public and private third-party payors, employers, unions, and the public, should be established. This ad hoc committee should define the health care services to be included in the basic benefit package; prepare actuarial cost estimates for alternative benefit structures; evaluate the impact of alternative benefit structures on total expenditures for health care; analyze alternative risk-pooling structures that would minimize cost-shifting and ensure the availability of the basic benefit package to nongroup and high-risk purchasers; and develop a timetable for adoption, including the possible adoption of this package by Medicare, Medicaid, the Civilian Health and Medical Program of the Uniformed Services (CHAMPUS), and self-insured entities. Where the private marketplace for health care coverage cannot ensure provision of basic benefits, public programs should fill in the gaps. To the extent that current public funding is inadequate to ensure basic benefit coverage for those whose needs cannot be met in the private market, the ad hoc committee should develop a proposal to augment public funding. Potential problems of adverse selection should be given careful consideration as the basic benefit package is designed. Further responsibilities of the ad hoc committee for development of catastrophic and long-term coverage and consideration of cost-sharing requirements in the basic benefit package are outlined below.

Provision for Catastrophic Coverage in the Basic Benefit Package
Lack of catastrophic coverage can deplete the average household's resources as well as create serious bad debt problems for hospitals and other providers. In addition to providing a basic benefit package, third-party payors should provide coverage of catastrophic costs resulting from illness and injuries of extreme length and/or severity.

As the basic benefit package is developed, the ad hoc committee should keep in mind that the original intent of health insurance is to share the cost of unpredictable health care costs among policyholders. Thus, the development of a package for catastrophic health care costs is just as important as the development of a basic benefit package for common and predictable charges. The ad hoc committee may recommend a floor at which catastrophic coverage will begin; this floor might be related to the individual's income, to the amount of coverage provided by the basic benefit package, to the point at which basic coverage is terminated, or to the premium amount.

Options for Long-term Care in the Basic Benefit Package
In general, the high expenditures by the elderly for long-term care often result from the need for custodial care rather than the need for health care services per se. Custodial care services are not usually covered by either public or private health care financing programs. Because of the lack of coverage for personal and custodial care, many patients spend down to impoverishment and eventually enter nursing homes for extended stays. The average cost of nursing home care exceeds $20,000 per year, and few of the aged have long-term care insurance or the financial resources to cover these costs.

Coverage for long-term health care services should include various options such as hospital care, nursing home care, hospice care, home care, respite care, and day care. Coverage for these long-term health care services should be financed through payment systems. The primarily social service aspects of long-term care—long-term custodial or institutional care and outpatient personal care—should be financed separately from health care services. The development of alternative payment methods to finance long-term health care and related social services will be difficult, and the ad hoc committee should give full consideration to the many legal and actuarial issues involved.

Four alternative mechanisms that might be used to provide payment for long-term care are private long-term care insurance, tax incentives, long-term care accounts, and social health maintenance organizations. Because of the potentially high risks involved in providing long-term care coverage, private insurers are proceeding with caution. Recent plans provide varying degrees of coverage for intermediate and custodial nursing home care as well as for nonskilled home care services. Annual premiums vary considerably by age of the insured, coverage, and payment liability. To avoid undue costs, many of these policies have numerous restrictions, such as limited length of coverage, exclusion of preexisting conditions, and prescreening for medical problems. Federal or state initiatives might be necessary to accelerate product development. Laws might be modified to allow for tax credits and/or deductions for personal care. The establishment of long-term care accounts, with tax incentives similar to those of individual retirement accounts, would shift responsibility for long-term care to the individual. This option would not be feasible for workers at or near retirement. Another alternative is social health maintenance organizations (SHMOs), which are prepaid plans that cover all services paid by Medicare as well as different levels of ambulatory and home care. There are currently four SHMO demonstration projects around the country, and each site sets its own copayment levels and benefit ceilings. SHMOs offer combined coverage for both personal and health care services and emphasize preventive services and noninstitutional care.

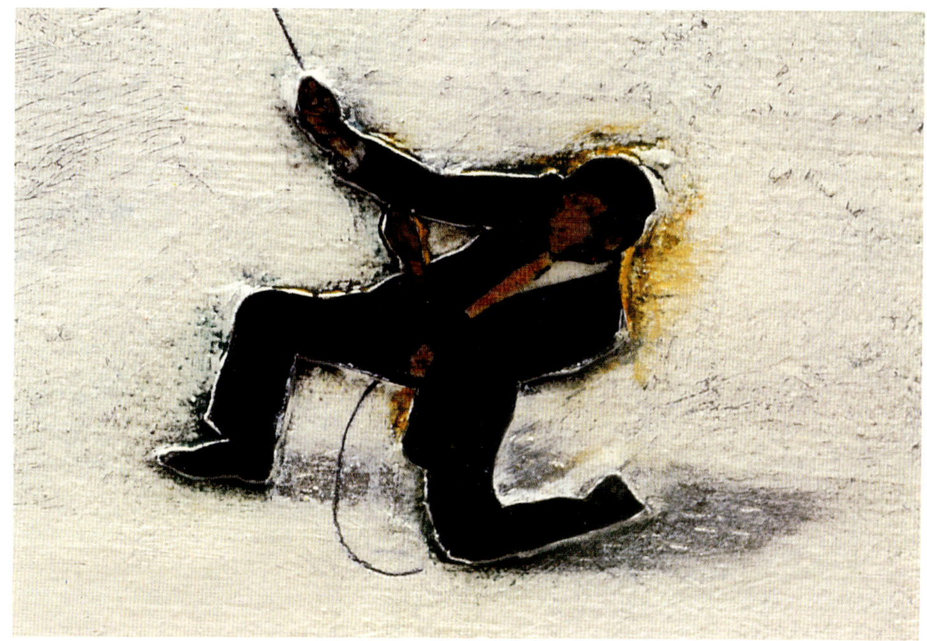

The competing objectives of providing quality health care, ensuring access, and containing costs must be balanced.

Recipient Cost-Sharing in the Basic Benefit Package

A cost-effective payment system that meets the dual purposes of providing broad access to quality health care services while encouraging health care recipients to use health care resources in a wise fashion requires appropriate financial incentives. These incentives should affect individual decision-making when insurance is purchased. Alternative insurance plans, with different schedules of deductibles, coinsurance, and premiums, should be available to beneficiaries so that they are aware of the financial tradeoffs associated with different plans. A number of studies indicate that deductibles and coinsurance affect the use of health care delivery mechanisms. Thus, third-party payment systems should use deductibles and coinsurance as financial incentives for health care recipients to use health care resources in an appropriate manner.

Although deductibles and coinsurance requirements can decrease wasteful expenditures and use of health care services, cost-sharing should not result in an undue financial burden for the health care recipient. Development of deductible, coinsurance, and catastrophic payment schedules should be coordinated with the development of the basic benefit package. Representatives from the health care professions, public and private third-party payors, employers, unions, and the public should develop schedules of premiums, deductibles, and coinsurance for alternative benefit packages; develop a schedule of catastrophic cutoffs for different income groups; evaluate the impact of alternative configurations of cost-sharing and catastrophic cutoff levels on utilization patterns and expenditures on health care; and evaluate the potential problems of adverse risk selection. The findings of this group should be presented to the ad hoc committee developing the basic benefit package.

The Role of Healthy Lifestyles in a Cost-Effective Payment Program

As indicated in Chapter IV, the individual has the ultimate responsibility to avoid health-endangering behaviors. In the United States, noncommunicable diseases such as cancer and heart disease are the main cause of death. Personal habits, including smoking, overeating, or improper diet, contribute to the onset or severity of such conditions. Recipients of health care should recognize their own responsibilities for avoiding unhealthy lifestyles and should be prepared to bear the financial consequences of their decisions. Health care providers can be influential in urging individuals to pursue healthy lifestyles, and they should encourage health care recipients to engage in healthy lifestyles and should practice and promote preventive health care.

Until recently, third-party payors provided little if any financial incentive for health care recipients who pursued healthy lifestyles. Automobile and life insurance policies offer financial rewards to encourage responsible behavior as a means of containing costs and lowering risks. Likewise, third-party payors should structure health insurance premiums to reward insureds who pursue healthy lifestyles.

The promotion of healthy lifestyles can lead to improvements in health and longevity and can also be cost-effective by reducing health care expenses in later years.

Employers, employee groups, and third-party payors should sponsor the development and presentation of employee educational programs to promote healthy lifestyles among employees and beneficiaries.

Role of Employers, Employee Groups, and Third-Party Payors in a Cost-Effective Payment System

Employers have begun to change the design and administration of health care plans. There has been significant growth in cost sharing by employees, many companies have expanded out-patient benefits, and a variety of incentives are provided to promote more efficient use of health care services. Employers, employee groups, and third-party payors should structure health care plans to provide necessary services to employees and beneficiaries without leading to unnecessary utilization of services. Savings may be realized if employees are given incentives to use health care services appropriately.

Consumers should have options to choose health plans that best meet their health care needs and financial situation. To foster freedom of choice and competition, employers, employee groups, and third-party payors should structure benefit programs which maintain access to licensed providers and various delivery systems. Guidelines for implementation of these two recommendations should be included in the charge of the ad hoc committee established to implement the basic benefit package.

Role of Providers in a Cost-Effective Payment System

Providers play an important role in determining how, when, and to what extent health care services are used. Current financial incentives tend to reward providers for utilization rather than nonutilization of health resources. Moreover, providers face little financial risk when making decisions regarding treatment options. Third-party payment mechanisms should be structured to place providers at some degree of financial risk with respect to their decisions regarding the use of health care resources. There are some mechanisms— case management approaches, primary physician IPA-HMOs, and capitation—which can be used to place providers at risk. Alternative mechanisms that could affect provider behavior to a greater extent should be reviewed. Providers may direct patients to inappropriate health care settings; e.g., minor surgery may be performed on an inpatient basis rather than in a less expensive outpatient setting. Payment differentials to providers should be used as incentives to encourage providers to direct health care recipients to the most cost-effective treatment settings. Representatives from business, third-party payors, and providers should develop guidelines for payment mechanisms and differentials.

Several studies suggest that educational programs may enhance the cost-effective delivery of health care. As part of their education and training, health professionals should participate in programs that sensitize them to the impact of cost in their treatment decisions. These educational programs should be incorporated into the curriculum at the undergraduate and graduate levels, and accreditation agencies should include such coursework in their accreditation criteria.

Defining the Role of Government

The government's role in health care—as third-party payor, as direct provider of health care services, and as regulatory agent—has steadily increased in importance since World War II. Presently, the government funds and administers the country's largest third-party payment program—Medicare—and the country's largest direct provider program—the Veterans Administration (VA) medical program. Substantial segments of the population would have inadequate or no access to health care services if the system operated in a purely competitive environment, and the government has intervened to varying degrees to ensure equitable access to services. The government's health care programs and policies ultimately affect all aspects of the health care delivery system. The most recent example of the impact of governmental policies can be seen in the extension of Medicare's prospective payment system into the Medicaid program and into private third-party payment mechanisms. The government also acts to protect the public through quarantine laws and regulations governing the safety and efficacy of drugs and medical devices.

Only after 1935, with the passage of the Social Security Act, did the government begin to play a major role as both payor and provider of health care services. At that time, the federal government began a major program of grants-in-aid to the states to promote the health of mothers and children. However, from 1935 to 1965, the federal government's role as provider and third-party payor was secondary to that of states and localities, except for care of the military, merchant marines, and veterans. Not until 1966, with the passage of Medicare and Medicaid, did the federal government begin to play a major role as payor for health care services for nonmilitary civilians. These programs were created to increase access to health care services for the elderly and the poor.

Subsequent to the passage of these two programs, the federal government's expenditures on personal health care rapidly escalated, going from $5.5 billion in 1965 to $112 billion in 1984. In recent years, both programs have become targets of cost-containment efforts. The Omnibus Budget Reconciliation Act of 1981 included numerous Medicare and Medicaid spending cuts, and provided for a waiver of Medicaid freedom-of-choice requirements. Likewise, the Tax Equity and Fiscal Responsibility Act of 1982 included spending cuts in both programs, and required contracts for utilization and quality control peer review. The Social Security Amendments of 1983 instituted a new Medicare payment system for hospital inpatient services based on prospectively determined rates for each of 467 diagnosis-related groups (DRGs). The Deficit Reduction Act of 1984 included further reductions in Medicare spending, instituted a 15-month physician fee freeze, and implemented a new Medicare participating physician program. The federal government's role has shifted over the years from that of regulator of public health and safety, to direct provider and payor of health care services for large segments of the population, and cost regulator for those health care services now provided.

State and local governments also make substantial contributions to personal health care costs. States are increasingly involved in cost-containment efforts. A number of states have established prospective hospital rates (i.e., rate-setting programs) to control hospital expenditures. These programs range from mandatory rate-setting by a legislatively established public agency to advisory budget review by nongovernmental associations. They also differ in the types of payors that are subject to rate-setting. In some states, for example, only Medicaid programs are subject to these programs, while in other states all payors are subject to them.

In general, the role of government in health care has been constrained to some degree through cost-containment strategies and through efforts to shift responsibility from the public to the private sector. The participants of the Health Policy Agenda believe that an appropriate balance needs to be maintained between the public and private sectors with regard to payment for health care; that guidelines concerning the level of federal, state, and local government involvement must be developed to encourage the most efficient use of health care services; and that regulatory policies should only exist to the extent that they ensure public safety, access to health care, cost containment, and fair competition. To this end, recommendations are made regarding the role of government as a third-party payor, as a direct provider of health care services, and as a regulatory agent.

Restructuring the Medicare Program. As currently structured, the Medicare program provides for the financing of health care services for the aged, the disabled, and those with end-stage renal disease (ESRD). Benefits under Medicare's two parts—hospital insurance (HI) or Part A and supplementary medical insurance (SMI) or Part B—began in 1966. Hospital insurance covers inpatient care in a hospital or skilled nursing facility and home health visits, while supplementary medical insurance covers a variety of medical services and supplies furnished by physicians or others in connection with physicians' services, outpatient hospital services, and home health services.

The HI trust fund is financed primarily through a tax on a portion of current earnings in employment covered under Social Security; approximately 90% of HI income is from payroll taxes. Additional but small amounts come from general tax revenues, voluntary premiums, and interest income. The SMI trust fund is financed from two primary sources—monthly premiums paid by or on behalf of enrollees and federal general tax revenues. Originally, the SMI premium was to cover one-half of program costs—enrollees and the government were to share the bill equally. However, by law the premium could be raised by no more than the percentage increase in Social Security benefits; because SMI costs increased over the years at a much faster rate than Social Security benefits, taxpayers have been contributing to an increasing share of SMI funds.

By 1983, federal revenue contributions for the aged amounted to three times as much the amount paid in monthly premiums, and beginning in 1984 the SMI premium was set to equal one-fourth of actuarily determined program costs.

Total Medicare benefit payments have grown from $4.6 billion in 1967, the first full year of its operation, to $62.9 billion in 1984. In terms of real growth (correcting for the general rise in the Consumer Price Index), the annual compound rate of growth over this same period was 9.1% for the total program, 8.6% for HI, and 10.3% for SMI. HI expenditures have always been substantially greater than SMI; HI now accounts for about 70% of total Medicare benefit payments.

The long-term solvency of both trust funds has been examined on a regular basis in the past few years. Predictions that the HI trust fund would be depleted prompted Congress to institute the prospective payment system in late 1983. Although the average length-of-stay was expected to fall under this new payment system, the actual decrease experienced is more pronounced than anticipated. Admissions to hospitals have decreased, the number of short-stay hospital beds has fallen, and occupancy rates are the lowest since data have been available on this measure. To constrain the rate of growth of SMI outlays for a period of time, the Deficit Reduction Act placed a freeze on Medicare maximum payment levels.

The SMI trust fund is designed to avoid the possibility of bankruptcy, but the Medicare Board of Trustees is concerned about the accelerating expenditures in this program. However, it is more than concerned about the future of the HI trust fund—it is alarmed. The most recent projections of the Medicare Board of Trustees indicate that this fund could be depleted sometime between 1993 and 2011. Immediate action is required to address this crisis; if this problem is ignored, the nation may have to resort to using the short-term decision-making and crisis management processes that weakened the Social Security System between 1971 and 1983.

The following five recommendations are based on these principles: there should be no further erosion of existing Medicare benefits; changes in the Medicare programs should not adversely affect the quality of health care services; current reserves

The Medicare Board of Trustees is more than concerned about the future of the hospital insurance trust fund—it is alarmed.

should be augmented to protect future beneficiaries and the solvency of the two trust funds; and any increased costs should be borne by all (i.e., the general public, employers, participants, and providers). A coordinated approach, which improves the efficiency of Medicare and contains costs while ensuring access to quality health care services, is needed.

Preservation of Medicare as an Entitlement Program

The Medicare program was enacted as a social insurance program to provide health insurance coverage for the most vulnerable population subgroup in the country—the elderly—so that they might enjoy dignity in their later years. Medicare was subsequently expanded in 1972 to include the disabled and those with ESRD. The concept of Medicare as an entitlement program for the elderly, the disabled, and individuals with end-stage renal disease should be preserved, with a primary goal being the provision of cost-effective, quality health care. This will ensure that these individuals, who otherwise might be unable to obtain health care services because of the financial burden or because of an inability to obtain insurance through the private sector, will have needed health care services.

Quality Assessment and Utilization Review in Medicare

The government's authority to tax carries with it the obligation to expend public revenues as prudently as possible. Public concern about rising health care costs has fueled demands for effective cost-control measures, but implementation of cost controls without due consideration of the impact on the quality of health care will no doubt prove to be both shortsighted and detrimental. As an initial step to improve Medicare program efficiency, a small percentage of the Medicare budget should be devoted to utilization review and research in quality assessment. Although the quality of health care services is difficult to define and measure, there are a number of areas that should be investigated. Studies should be conducted on the variations in hospital utilization and practice patterns; the structure, process, and outcome measures that are used to evaluate quality of health care, including medical and surgical procedures related to the covered populations; the effects of various cost and reimbursement mechanisms on beneficiary and service utilization patterns; and utilization rates and cost considerations associated with the population that is dually eligible for both Medicare and Medicaid services.

Restructuring of Medicare Funding

The crisis in Medicare is not only financial in nature—it also has a human element in that the government has committed itself to ensuring health care services for older Americans, for the disabled, and for those with ESRD. However, under current funding arrangements, Medicare will not be able to fulfill this promise indefinitely.

The notion of the Medicare "trust funds" is often misunderstood. In particular, the HI trust fund depends on intergenerational transfers; money paid into the HI trust fund through payroll taxes on current workers and employers is not invested and kept in a trust fund for these workers until they reach age 65. Rather, money paid into the HI trust fund by today's workers is spent on benefits provided to today's beneficiaries. Benefits that today's workers may get from Medicare when they retire will have to be paid by the next generation of workers. To maintain an adequate amount of funds, the Trustees of the HI trust fund have adopted a general operating principle that annual income to this fund should be at least equal to annual outlays. The trust fund reserves must be equal to a minimum of one-half year's expenditures. The reserve is to be used as a contingency to protect against future income and outlays that may differ from forecasted levels. As previously indicated, 90% of the funding for the HI trust fund comes through payroll taxes, and thus the amount of money coming into this fund depends on the number of workers in covered employment, the payroll tax rate, and the wage base.

To prepare for anticipated demographic shifts in the population, measures should be implemented to increase the level of the reserves in the HI trust fund. One anticipated shift has already begun: the ratio of workers to cash beneficiaries under the Social Security retirement and disability programs declined from 4.0 to 1 in 1965 to 3.3 in 1985, and the ratio is projected to decline to 3.1 during the next 25 years. To help ensure health care benefits for future beneficiaries, Medicare trust fund reserves should be augmented through a combination of revenue increases, expenditure reductions, and program efficiencies. A number of options to maintain the solvency of the Medicare trust funds and to build the necessary reserve levels are presented below. Although these options are not acceptable to all constituents, they are among those most commonly suggested. A combination of revenue increases, expenditure reductions, and program efficiencies should guarantee the future solvency of Medicare and provide greater flexibility in adapting to changes in the costs of health care.

□ *Options for Increasing Revenues.* Sources of revenue which could be used to provide additional income for the HI trust fund of Medicare include increased payroll taxes on employers and employees, general tax revenues, excise taxes on tobacco and alcohol, taxes on employer contributions to health insurance or to self-insured health benefit programs, and taxes on the actuarial value of Medicare benefits. Any or all of these options could be used to broaden the tax base, or the revenue itself could be earmarked for the Medicare HI trust fund. Increasing the HI payroll tax on employers and employees—which is currently 2.9%—may stabilize the fund over the next 25 years, although it may have detrimental economic effects. The Medicare law could be modified to permit supplementation of HI payroll tax contributions with general tax revenues. Excise taxes on health-endangering products—cigarette and alcohol beverage taxes are the most commonly mentioned—could be dedicated to the HI trust fund; a further advantage of taxing these products is that higher taxes may discourage use and therefore reduce disease in later years. Finally, a personal income tax could be levied on employer contributions to health insurance, or beneficiaries could be taxed on the actuarial value of Medicare benefits.

□ *Options for Reducing Expenditures.* Reducing the rate of increase in costs for health care services is another alternative that should be considered as a means of maintaining the solvency of the Medicare trust funds. Even with Medicare, the elderly must pay substantial out-of-pocket costs, including expenditures for Medicare deductibles, premiums, and coinsurance, as well as expenditures for unassigned claims and uncovered services. Medicare beneficiaries over 65 years of age now spend about 15% of their income on medical care—the same proportion they spent prior to the establishment of the Medicare program 20 years ago. Furthermore, it is projected that average out-of-pocket expenditures by the elderly for health and medical care will increase to 19% of income by the year 2000.

Options to control expenditures under the Medicare program include limiting or restricting prospective payment reimbursement, reducing the average length-of-stay and admission rates in hospitals and other health care facilities, using capitation or vouchers, raising the Medicare eligibility age, and eliminating earnings limits for retirees. Prospective payment to hospitals could be limited either by including capital payments under DRGs or by restricting the DRG update factor. However, it is unclear to what degree the federal government can further restrict hospital reimbursement without adversely affecting access to and the quality of health care. Further reductions in the average length-of-stay and in admissions might be achieved through more aggressive utilization review and through the adoption of payment policies which favor outpatient services that prove to be less expensive than inpatient care; however, the optimum level of reductions may already have been achieved through the prospective payment system. The use of capitation or vouchers are other options for reducing expenditures. Many HMOs and competitive medical plans (CMPs) are now accepting risk contracts to provide care to Medicare beneficiaries. Indemnity insurers, employers, or unions could develop programs that would allow Medicare beneficiaries who do not want to join an HMO or CMP to select plans that combine Medicare coverage with so-called medigap insurance. A voucher system would allow enrollees to purchase coverage from one of a number of competing health plans. The option of raising the age of Medicare eligibility from 65 to 67 in tandem with the planned rise in the minimum age for retirement on full Social Security (to be phased in between 2000 and 2022) should be considered. Because changes in retirement age are not planned to begin until 2000, however, a more immediate option is to eliminate earnings limits for retirees; this would encourage employment of Social Security beneficiaries. And, because under current law employers would have to continue any health benefits to employees who continue working for them, income would continue to flow into both the Social Security and HI funds while reducing Medicare expenditures.

□ *Options for Increased Program Efficiency.* In addition to the options for increasing revenues and decreasing expenditures, there are a number of options to be considered to increase the efficiency of the Medicare program itself. These options include requirements for second opinions prior to elective surgery and authorizations for hospitalization, the adoption of a prospective payment system for outpatient hospital services, reductions in the geographic variations in the average length-of-stay in hospitals, reductions in excess hospital beds, reforms in payment for physicians' services, and increased use of allied health professionals in the health care delivery system.

In some instances, mandatory second opinions have been found to reduce the risks and costs of surgery. The potential benefits to Medicare of a mandatory second opinion program could be considerable; the Congressional Budget Office estimated that a program such as this could save Medicare more than $200 million over three years. Similarly, requirements for authorizations prior to hospitalization might serve to increase program efficiency and to direct patients to more appropriate sites of care. However, any guidelines developed in this area must consider the social and physical well-being of older persons, and should balance these individual considerations against the potential cost-savings. The adoption of a prospective payment system for outpatient hospital services might reduce costs; for example, at present hospitals receive higher payments for outpatient cataract surgery than they receive for more expensive inpatient care. Reducing geographic variations in the average length-of-stay in hospitals could also produce savings. Although the average length-of-stay has declined since the introduction of the prospective payment system, considerable variation in average length-of-stay among states persists. Hospital occupancy rates have declined dramatically over the past few years and now average less than 70%; in some areas of the country, occupancy rates are below 50%. Because the cost of hospital care is inflated by the fixed costs associated with unused beds, closure or consolidation of hospitals or conversion of excess beds to long-term care or rehabilitation beds could reduce overhead costs. However, any changes must be implemented in a manner to ensure continued access to care and should not cause serious disruption in the provision of services. Reforms in payment for physicians' services under Medicare could increase program efficiency by encouraging the delivery of medical care in the most cost-effective setting. Finally, the health care delivery system could be more effective with the appropriate use of allied health professionals.

Because it is difficult to predict accurately the actual savings that might be obtained through implementation of any one or a combination of these options, these proposals should be evaluated on the basis of their intrinsic worth. Sensible options should be considered even if the expected savings are relatively small. It would be wise to adopt several effective but modest options rather than an option that would produce large savings at the expense of the quality of health care. Many, if not all, of these options represent a departure from current operations. If they are adopted, a national campaign would have to accompany these innovations to foster their acceptance.

Equitable Redistribution of Costs

When Medicare legislation was enacted in 1966, the aged as a group were in much poorer economic circumstances than the nation as a whole. Measured by the official poverty index, based on the cost of a minimum but nutritionally adequate diet, 29% of the aged in 1966 were living in poverty. The relatively high level of poverty, coupled with a higher-than-average incidence of illness and disability and inadequate private health insurance coverage, were compelling reasons for amending the Social Security Act to include health insurance coverage.

The economic position of most elderly persons has risen considerably in recent decades. In fact, if all of the resources of elderly persons could be converted to a cash value, as a group their economic status on a per capita basis would closely approximate that of the nonelderly. However, as in other age groups, a wide range exists in the economic status of the elderly. While some older persons have substantial resources, a large number have practically none. Although the proportion of the elderly who were under the poverty level has improved, the absolute number of aged persons living in poverty (3.3 million people) is still substantial because of the growth in the aged population.

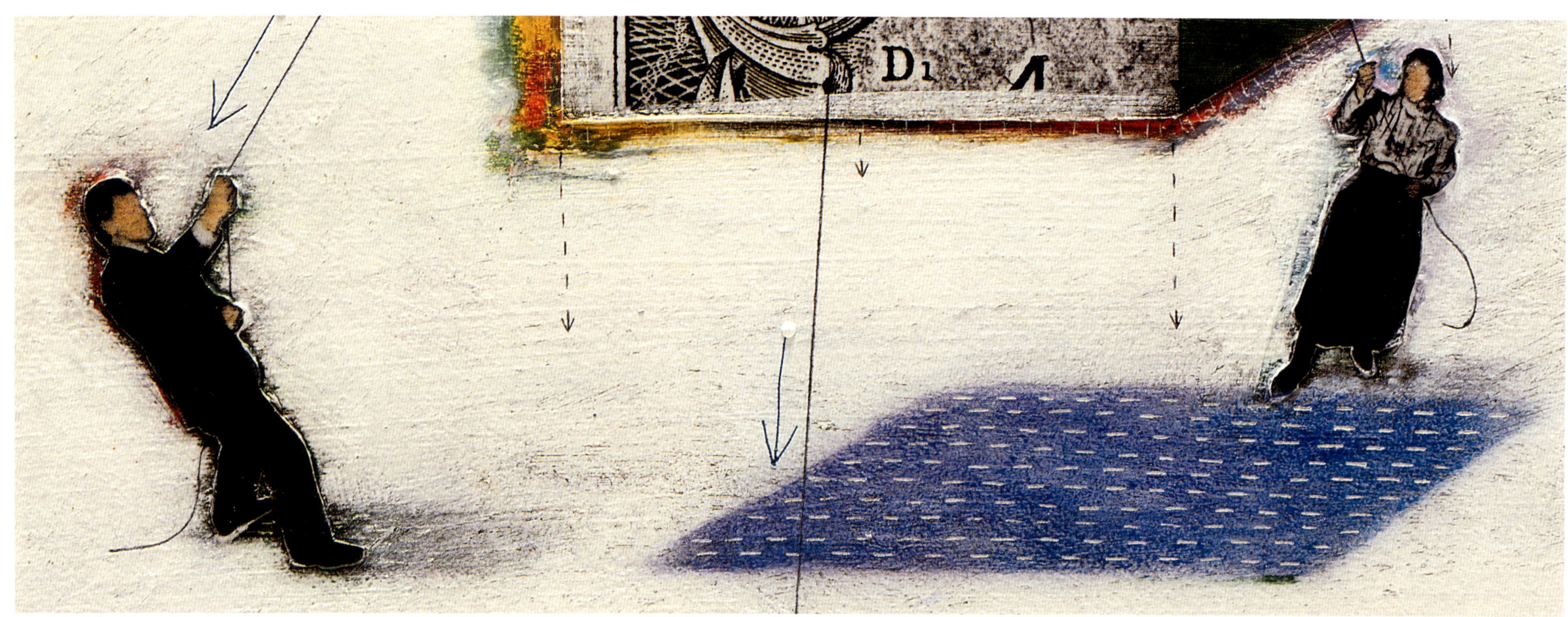

Providers should set initial prices for services, and reimbursement can then be subject to negotiation between the involved parties.

The variable economic status of the elderly needs to be examined in light of Medicare's cost-sharing requirements. To hold down program costs and to deter overutilization, the Medicare program from its inception required beneficiary cost sharing. Under HI, the patient is required to pay an inpatient hospital deductible in each benefit period. This deductible—$520 in 1987—approximates the cost of one day of hospital care. Copayments by beneficiaries are required after 60 days of hospitalization. Under SMI, in addition to paying a monthly premium—currently $17.90—the beneficiary must meet a deductible in the amount of $75 each year, a copayment for the charges above that, and the full liability for charges in excess of those recognized by Medicare as "usual, customary, and reasonable." The heaviest users of the Medicare program tend to be older and poorer; as expected, these individuals are unlikely to have private supplemental health insurance, and hence are generally unprotected against Medicare's cost-sharing requirements. It is estimated that elderly households with incomes of less than $10,000 will pay, on the average, nearly one-half of their income on out-of-pocket medical or health care charges and insurance premiums.

A study of copayments, deductibles, premiums, and tax mechanisms should be undertaken by government and private organizations to determine methods of equitably spreading the burden of Medicare beneficiaries' costs. When addressing the disparities in the residual financial burden of Medicare beneficiaries of varying economic means, policy-makers, the aged, and those who represent the aged should not prematurely dismiss a redistribution of costs among health care payors, including the aged themselves. Organizations representing the elderly, providers, and government should study how this might be equitably achieved. This topic is also addressed in "Designing a Cost-Effective Payment System" in this chapter.

Optional Supplemental Insurance

Americans are living longer, and they need to be financially prepared to meet their changing health care needs. To enable them to meet this obligation, the basic Medicare package should be supplemented by other resources, including private insurance, employer-sponsored health benefits, individual savings, and tax-deferred retirement income plans such as pensions, individual retirement accounts, and salary reduction plans. The viability of an additional tax-deferred individual medical account should also be explored. Those who are financially able to assume personal financial responsibilities for future health care needs should do so. Incentives should be developed to encourage individuals to purchase or obtain health insurance or to establish health care trusts to pay for health care costs, long-term care, and other potentially catastrophic health care costs. These trusts could be used, for example, to pay for extended care services or out-of-pocket medical or health expenses that Medicare does not cover. These options are discussed in further detail in "Designing a Cost-Effective Payment System" in this chapter.

Restructuring the Medicaid Program. Medicaid was enacted at the same time as Medicare; the goal of this program is to provide access to health care services for certain low-income persons. The program covers those groups of people who are eligible to receive cash payments under one of the existing welfare programs established under the Social Security Act, i.e., families with dependent children, the aged, the blind, and the disabled. In most cases, receipt of a welfare payment under either the Aid to Families with Dependent Children (AFDC) program or the Supplemental Security Income (SSI) program means automatic eligibility for Medicaid. Additionally, states may provide Medicaid to the "medically needy"—people who meet the criteria for categorical eligibility but who may earn up to 133% of the AFDC payment standard for the same size family in that state or who spend down to that level. Under general federal guidelines, states set income and asset standards for cash assistance and Medicaid eligibility, and the degree to which individual programs cover the poverty population varies considerably from one state to another.

Every state participating in the Medicaid program—states participate at their option, and Arizona is the only state that does not participate in this federal program—must offer certain basic services, such as hospital inpatient and outpatient care, skilled nursing home facility services, physician services, family planning, rural health clinic services, and periodic screening, diagnosis, and treatment for individuals under 21 years of age. States may provide a number of other services if they elect to do so, such as drugs, eyeglasses, intermediate care facility services, inpatient psychiatric services, physical therapy, and dental care. States also determine the scope of services; that is, they may limit the number of physician visits covered or the days of hospital care.

Since the Medicaid program began, the AFDC population has been the largest component of the program. To be eligible for cash assistance under AFDC, a family with children must have an income below a state-specified amount, and the children must be deprived of parental support or care because of the death, incapacity, or continued absence of a parent. Other needy children—those who are in foster homes, or have their adoptions by a public agency—may also be covered under state Medicaid programs. To be eligible for SSI payments, income and resource tests as well as program criteria must be satisfied. The federal government sets a uniform national payment level that may be supplemented by the states. However, states do not have to cover automatically all SSI cash recipients in their Medicaid programs.

Medicaid is jointly financed with federal and state funds; federal financial participation varies with states' per capita income, and now ranges from 50% to 78% of program payments. The program itself is administered by the states. Payment for health care services is made directly to the providers of care with reimbursement methods varying from state to state. States may require cost-sharing by Medicaid recipients, but they may not require recipients who are categorically eligible to share costs for mandatory services. Most state Medicaid programs have "buy in" agreements with Medicare; under this arrangement, Medicaid assumes the responsibility for the Medicare cost-sharing obligation of persons covered under both programs (the "dually eligible"). For services that Medicare does not cover, such as drugs and long-term nursing home services, Medicaid has the primary responsibility.

The number of Medicaid recipients has remained essentially the same over the past ten years. But the growth in Medicaid expenditures in many states has escalated, in many cases at a rate exceeding the growth in state revenues. Much of the increase in expenditures can be attributed to the growth in spending for long-term care services.

To control the growth in spending, states were allowed—under the Omnibus Budget Reconciliation Act of 1981—to institute a variety of programs to decrease costs by limiting the Medicaid provision that guarantees freedom of choice of provider and by reducing the number of persons eligible for Medicaid. Additionally, the Tax Equity and Fiscal Responsibility Act of 1982 permitted states to impose a nominal copayment, with certain limitations, to reduce program outlays and to instill cost-consciousness on the part of the recipient.

Total Medicaid benefit payments have grown far less rapidly than Medicare payments. From 1975 to 1984, Medicaid expenditures increased from $12.2 billion to $34.3 billion (during this same period, Medicare expenditures rose from $15.6 billion to $62.9 billion). Although the children and adults in the AFDC category represent about 70% of all Medicaid recipients, they account for only 25% of Medicaid expenditures; the SSI categorically eligible individuals account for a little less than 30% of Medicaid recipients, but these individuals account for more than 70% of Medicaid outlays. Medicaid plays a major role in the financing of nursing home care, and in 1984 it covered almost 44% of these expenditures. Because Medicare is the first payor for hospital care, expenditures on inpatient hospital care account for a much smaller proportion of the Medicaid dollar (about 25%) when compared to the proportion of Medicare dollar (about 65%). As previously indicated, there is considerable variation in state Medicaid expenditures, and it is difficult to find a single best measure to index this variation. Analyses of expenditures per person in poverty, with poverty levels adjusted for differences in cost-of-living across states, reveal that seven states had Medicaid expenditures per person in poverty of less than $500 and eight states had per person in poverty expenditures of $1,500 or more.

Uniform Medicaid Standards for Eligibility, Benefits, and Payment Mechanisms
Because it is governed by both the rules and regulations of separate state public assistance programs and federal Medicaid laws and regulations, Medicaid eligibility for all categories of assistance is exceedingly complex. Similar kinds of needy persons do not have equal access to Medicaid coverage throughout the country. For example, in 1983, 11

states set limits on preoperative days or weekend admissions, 16 set limits on the number of inpatient hospital days covered, and five imposed no limitations on inpatient hospital services other than those in federal regulations. Varying levels of benefits reflect the degree to which different state governments can afford to provide health care services to the needy; generally, poorer states provide lower levels of benefits than wealthier states. The current system for federal Medicaid funding, under which there is a direct matching of state funding, amounts to a federal subsidization of wealthier states because of their greater capacity to provide care for the poor.

Medicaid should be revised to establish national standards that result in uniform eligibility, benefits, and adequate payment mechanisms for services across jurisdictions. This would not require that Medicaid eligibility standards, benefits, and payment mechanisms be identical among states; rather, there should be uniformity. For example, Medicaid eligibility requirements could vary from state to state as long as income levels are adjusted to account for the fact that the purchasing power of a dollar in a"high cost" state is less than in a"low cost" state. In other words, those individuals who are eligible for assistance should be those in need of assistance, even if their actual income varies by location.

Expansion of Medicaid to Include the Medically Indigent
As previously indicated, states may provide Medicaid to the "medically needy"—people who meet the criteria for categorical eligibility but who may earn up to 133% of the AFDC payment standard; also included are individuals who may, because of their medical bills, spend down to the medically needy standards. By including a spend down provision, a state opens up Medicaid eligibility to categorically related people of any income level if their medical bills are large enough.

A rough gauge of the extent to which Medicaid covers the poverty population of all ages is the comparison between the number of Medicaid recipients and the number of persons below the poverty level. The gap between these two measures has been widening since 1978; the ratio of these two numbers reached a peak in 1977—0.92—and then began to decline; it now stands at 0.64. It is estimated that there are about 14 million individuals below the poverty line that are not covered by Medicaid. Medicaid eligibility standards should be expanded to include the medically indigent; i.e., those needy individuals who are not eligible for Medicaid because they do not belong to a categorically needy group. Payment for Medicaid benefits for the medically indigent should be based on ability to pay. Eligibility could be determined using a sliding scale based on income. Some of the administrative problems attendant on coverage of the short-term indigent and medically indigent could be reduced by establishing six-month eligibility reviews for these groups, with a presumption of eligibility maintained for this period. Standardization of eligibility and benefits, with extension of eligibility so that coverage is based on need rather than population group, should provide access to needed care for the majority of those individuals unable to pay for services.

"Test of Performance" Criteria for Delivery and Payment Mechanisms under Medicaid
Delivery and payment mechanisms in the Medicaid program should be subject to "test of performance" criteria to ensure that they are sufficient to guarantee appropriate access to quality and cost-effective care. Payment levels for Medicaid are generally lower than payments from other third-party payors. As a result, many providers are reluctant to participate and thereby restrict access for beneficiaries. The establishment of criteria to ensure that payment levels are adequate to encourage participation by providers would be helpful.

Funding and Administration of Medicaid
As indicated above, there should be uniform standards for Medicaid eligibility, benefits, and payment mechanisms, Medicaid eligibility should be expanded to include the medically indigent, and "tests of performance" criteria should be used to ensure adequate participation among providers in the Medicaid program. These recommendations will require some modifications in the Medicaid program, but Medicaid should continue to be funded jointly by federal and state governments. Administration should be the primary

responsibility of the state with federal oversight as needed. Some shifting in the balance between federal and state financing might be appropriate; for example, states might elect to be the primary payor for long-term care services, with the federal level responsible for short-term care services.

The Government as a Provider of Health Care Services. The federal government has long assumed the responsibility for providing health care services for the armed forces, veterans, and other special populations, such as American Indians and Alaskan natives. Military facilities serve more than nine million servicemen on active duty, their dependents, and retired military personnel at hospitals and medical and dental clinics at U.S. military installations around the world. For those who cannot be accommodated at military hospitals or clinics, health care services are paid for at civilian facilities through the Civilian Health and Medical Program of the Uniformed Services (CHAMPUS). Veterans with either service-connected or nonservice-connected disabilities who are over 65 years of age or who are unable to pay for health care services are eligible for free or subsidized hospital, ambulatory, and nursing home care. The majority of veterans do not meet the eligibility criteria, and many of those who are eligible elect to use community facilities instead, presumably because they prefer the non-VA facilities and have private or public health insurance to finance the costs. Thus, despite its extensive network of medical services, the VA assists only about three million veteran patients per year, or about 10% of the veteran population. Eligible dependents and survivors of some veterans may receive medical care under CHAMPUS, and the VA shares the cost of the medical benefits with these dependents. Finally, the Indian Health Service (IHS) provides preventive, curative, rehabilitative, and environmental health care services to about one million reservation Indians and Alaskan natives through its hospitals, health centers, and health stations. The IHS also contracts with private providers to deliver additional health care services.

Cost-Effective Provision of Health Care Services

Individuals who are eligible for health care services provided by the federal government through the DOD, the VA, or the IHS almost always receive that treatment in government facilities. These recipients, unlike private sector recipients, have little choice of provider. To increase individual choice in obtaining health care from the most appropriate and cost-effective providers, individuals eligible for health care services through government providers should have the option to use private providers at government expense when these private providers are cost-effective. While government-provided health care for active duty military personnel and veterans is necessary to maintain national security and to meet national obligations, there should be a concomitant concern for making the most effective use of the nation's health care system. Cost-effective private alternatives to government providers should be made available. The DOD, the VA, and the IHS should extend their efforts to seek contractual arrangements with private providers who can deliver cost-effective health care services. Because the comparative cost of public and private care is difficult to ascertain without uniform cost-accounting and billing systems, the DOD, the VA, and the IHS should develop these types of systems.

Health Insurance for Medically-Uninsurable Individuals

About one million people are either unable to obtain health insurance coverage or are able to obtain health insurance only at extremely high rates because of poor health status, previous medical history, or employment in a medically hazardous occupation. Although this number is relatively small in proportion to the total population, it is of sufficient magnitude to warrant attention.

To address this problem, several states have enacted legislation authorizing the creation of risk-sharing or reinsurance associations that offer health insurance at a reasonable cost to those individuals who are considered to be high risks or uninsurable by conventional underwriting standards. Other approaches include the offering of liberal open-enrollment periods by individual carriers, with premiums limited to a specified excess over standard rates; use of risk pools by individual carriers for reinsurance; or the formation of more than one risk pool by subgroups of carriers within a state.

Each state should establish a program to ensure that health insurance cover-

While the United States has made significant strides in ensuring access to services for children and youth, inadequate coverage and gaps in coverage still exist.

age is available to medically uninsurable individuals at a reasonable cost. The National Conference of Commissioners of Uniform State Laws should be asked to develop uniform state legislation to establish programs to ensure adequate health insurance coverage at a reasonable cost for those who would otherwise be unable to obtain coverage because of medical considerations. This legislation should define how the risk will be apportioned among all participating groups. Should the premiums collected from beneficiaries be insufficient to cover the costs of participating insurance carriers, state governments should fund the difference through direct cash grants to the risk pool, tax credits, or deductions.

The Government's Role as a Facilitator of Health Care Services. As the costs of health care have risen, many employers have sought to reduce their expenditures for employee health benefits. One method that is increasingly prevalent is the self-funding of health benefit plans by employers; this mechanism provides group coverage for employees with benefits financed entirely through the internal resources of the employer rather than through purchasing insurance from commercial carriers or Blue Cross/Blue Shield. Recent surveys indicate that about 50% of all health benefit plans are self-funded by employers. By the 1990s, the value of these plans will exceed the combined value of all commercial plans and will approximate that of the combined Blue Cross plans.

Regulation of Self-Funded Health Benefit Plans

While self-funded health benefit plans provide a means for employers to control health care costs, there are two problems with them. Under the Employee Retirement Income Security Act of 1974, all state laws relating to self-funded benefit plans except for insurance, banking, and securities regulation laws, were superseded or preempted. At this time, there are no specific federal controls governing self-funded health benefit plans. As a consequence, self-funded health benefit plans need not be part of state risk pools for the medically uninsurable, nor are they subject to state insurance solvency requirements. Businesses that self-fund their health benefit plans should be subject to certain basic regulations; to protect the public welfare, the federal government should exercise its

authority to regulate self-funded health benefit plans so that they are subject to participation in state risk-pooling mechanisms and are subject to solvency standards. Federal legislation should be enacted to permit the federal government to exercise appropriate regulation of self-funded group health benefit plans. Plans maintained by employers in bankruptcy should be placed under the administration of the Bankruptcy Court and should have the rights of a secured creditor. Federal legislation may also be needed to permit workers to continue in the plan at their own expense.

Public and Private Coverage for Preventive Child Health Services

While the United States has made significant strides in ensuring access to health services for all children and youth, inadequate coverage for services and gaps in coverage still exist. Neither private insurers nor employers provide adequate coverage for child preventive health services, and this has led to increased medical costs and to unnecessary health problems for children. For example, as a cost-saving mechanism, many insurers increase the front-end deductibles that are generally applied to the health care services used before hospitalization; while this may reduce the incentive for overuse of hospital services, it also creates economic disincentives for child health care. Furthermore, because "well visits" are considered to be routine, most insurance plans do not allow the costs for such services to be applied toward the deductible. The net result is that only 16% of payments for primary pediatric care come from third-party payors, including Medicaid. This places an undue burden on young families who must pay for the remaining expenses.

The results of preventive care may not be as easily appreciated as the results of treatment for illness, but preventive health care can improve health behavior and reduce risk factors in patients. The key to preventing disease and promoting good health in children is child health supervision, which is a mixture of preventive care, assessment of growth and development, anticipatory guidance, evaluation of general health, and diagnosis and treatment of hidden and overt conditions. This type of supervision discourages contagious disease and reduces the incidence of child abuse, illegitimate pregnancies, venereal disease, and hypertension.

Representatives from these groups should seek to modify federal laws to encourage the
use of preventive child health services. For example, taxpayers might be able to deduct
all out-of-pocket pediatric preventive care expenses, or employers might be granted a tax
credit for offering certain "well child" benefits. Health benefit plans could finance child
health care to encourage child health supervision and office care for illness, thereby
reducing unnecessary and expensive use of emergency-room and hospital services. Such
a program would lead to lower health insurance costs for employers and young families
and, more importantly, to better health care for children.

Adequate access to health care services for children and youth remains an
important social policy in this country. The government's role in child health has been
critical; noteworthy accomplishments include the implementation and expansion of Medicaid, the formation of community health centers, the growth of targeted maternal and
child health services under Title V of the Social Security Act, and the development of
Project Head Start. However, gaps in coverage persist. Over 25% of American children
are uninsured all or part of the year, and the effects of gaps in coverage are particularly
profound for children up to the age of two years and for adolescents and young adults
between 18 and 24 years of age. Since the late 1970s, the percentage of children in
poverty has increased. Eligibility standards for major welfare programs, especially AFDC,
have not kept pace with inflation, and Medicaid reimbursement rates in some states are so
low that they act as disincentives to pediatricians to provide services to children.
Coupled with these problems, there is duplication in programs, fragmentation of services
offered by different agencies and providers, bureaucratic entanglements at the federal
and state levels, and a lack of adequate data. As a result, the nation has failed to achieve
the level of health among children that other nations have achieved and that twentieth-
century scientific and medical knowledge make possible.

 The federal government should
devise an improved system of data collection to be used as the basis for uniform reporting
by all states and other jurisdictions. There should also be increased supervision of state
programs by the federal government, including more detailed and more frequent reviews
of child health service data.

Evaluation of Government Regulations

Examples of legislation that result in regulations that markedly affect health care services
include the Tax Equity and Fiscal Responsibility Act of 1982, which included major
revisions to the Medicare law to encourage the growth in the number of HMOs and
other comprehensive medical plans enrolling Medicare beneficiaries; the 1983 amendments to the Social Security Act, which established the prospective payment system
under Medicare; the Deficit Reduction Act of 1984, which instituted a physician fee
freeze and a new Medicare participating physician program; and the Emergency Extension Act of 1985, which extended the freeze on Medicare hospital reimbursement and
payment rates for physicians.

Other significant changes are taking place in the organization and delivery of
care. As the health system becomes more competitive, cross-subsidies and cost-shifting
are disappearing. This creates a problem for community hospitals, many of which provide
considerable amounts of uncompensated care to the uninsured. When the costs of
uncompensated care cannot be easily allocated across payors, institutions must either
reduce the amount of uncompensated care they provide or find other sources of
revenues. This may have a detrimental impact on access to needed health care services,
and some governmental intervention may be needed.

The general role of the government in regard to health care services should be
to foster a climate that allows effective and efficient delivery of services. At the same
time, government should be responsible for enforcing antitrust laws and for protecting the

public against fraud and abuse while avoiding undue regulation which might inhibit the delivery of health care services. Government regulations having an impact on the health care system should be evaluated on a regular basis to ensure that they are still needed and that they are consistent with the goals of ensuring access to health care services, ensuring fair competition in the delivery of health care services, and encouraging the efficient provision and use of health care services. The Office of Management and Budget should be encouraged to establish a program whereby federal regulations pertaining to the health care system are evaluated on the basis of their necessity in protecting the public interest and their potential for producing anticompetitive practices.

Summary

To provide for a cost-effective payment system, the roles of health care recipients, public and private third-party payors, health care providers, business, and labor were delineated in this chapter. The role of government as a provider, payor, and regulator in the health care delivery system was also discussed.

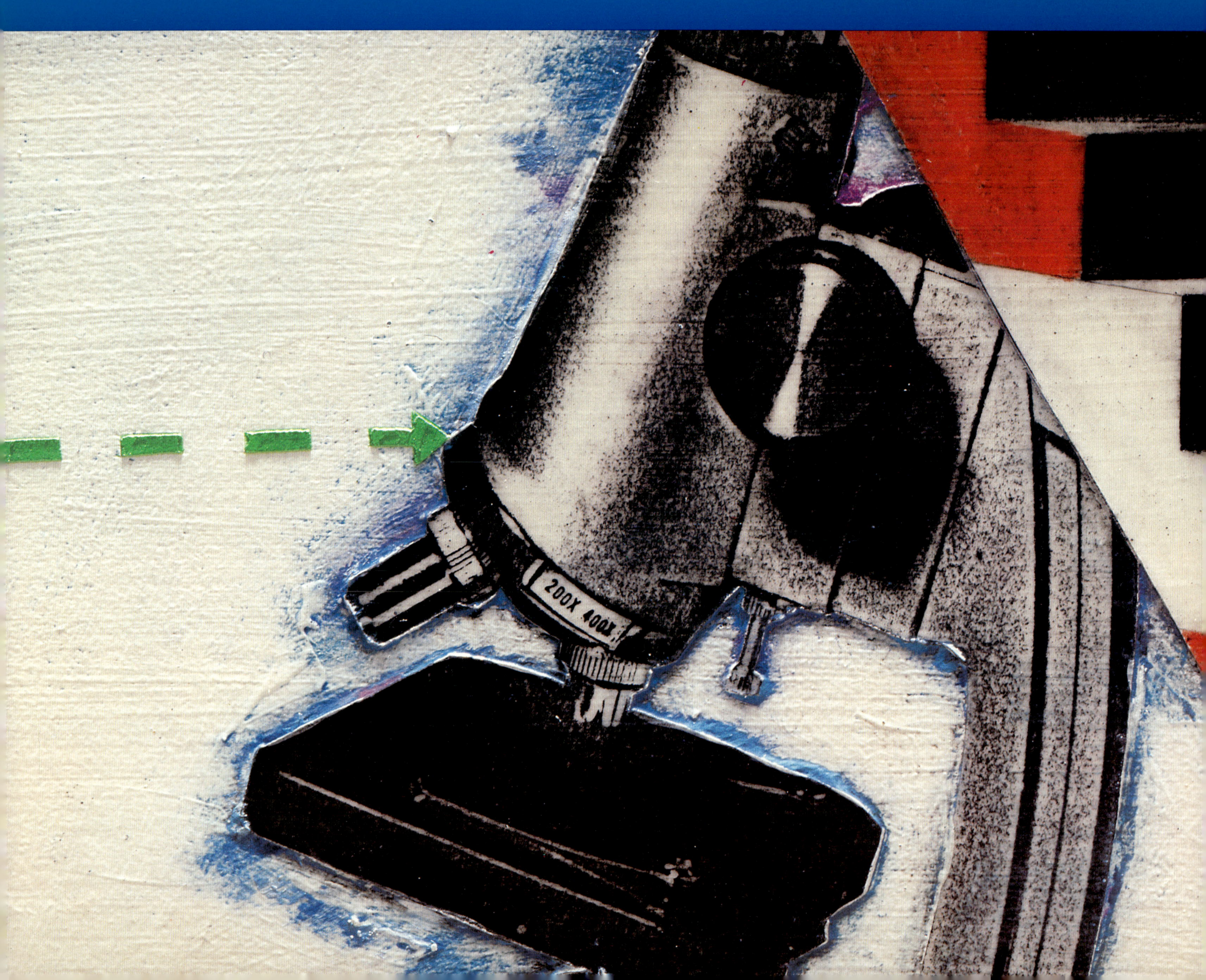

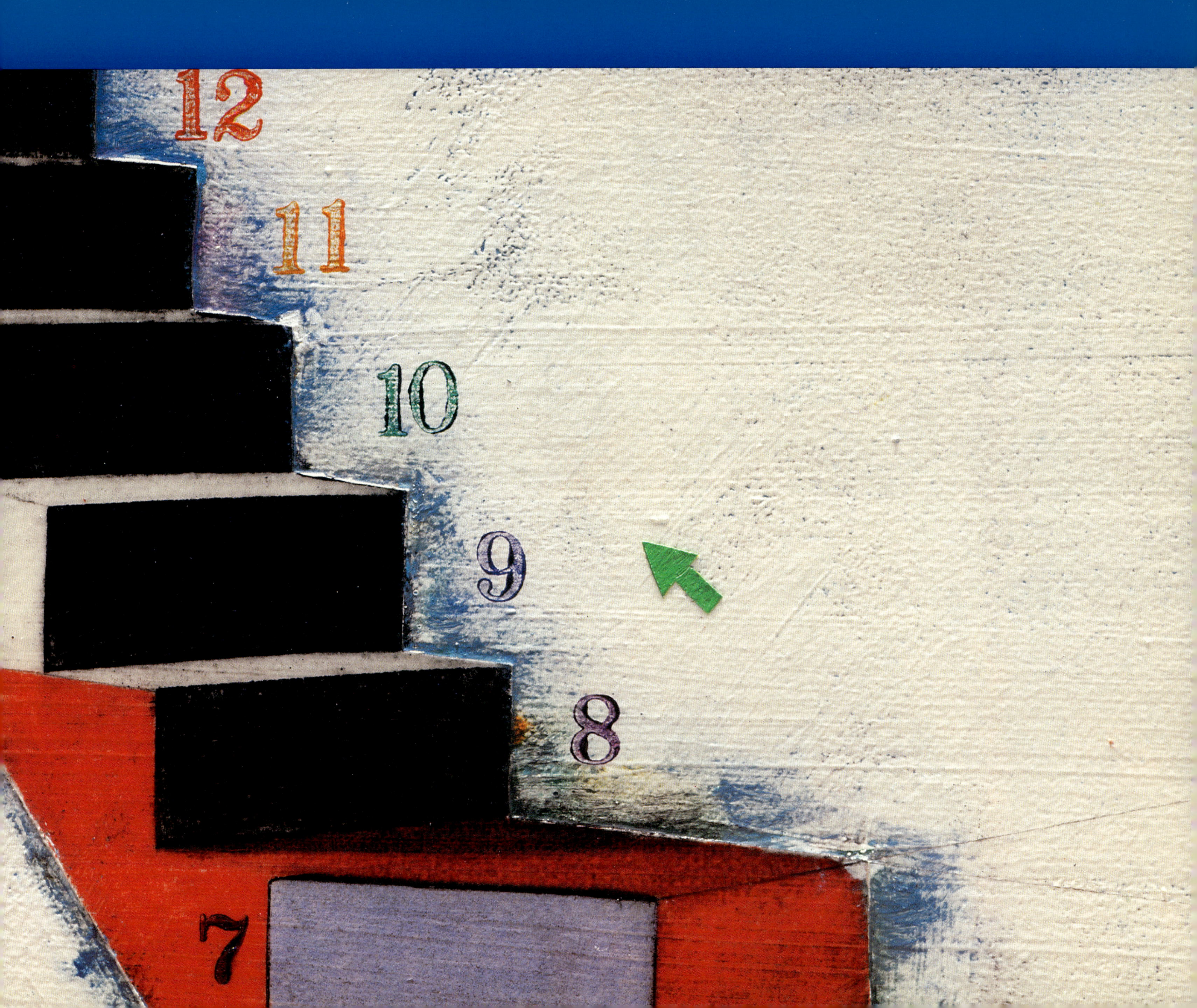

Biomedical research plays a crucial role in unraveling the underlying causes of complex disease states, in developing preventive, curative and rehabilitative measures, and in delineating lifestyles that promote good health. In this century, there have been striking reductions in mortality and morbidity because of past national investments in research. For example, from 1951 to 1976 there was a 99% drop in reported cases of polio—in 1951 there were over 28,000 cases of polio and by 1976 this number had dropped to 14. The development of the vaccination against measles has also had a major impact on morbidity; from 1963 to 1981 it is estimated that about 50,000,000 cases of measles were averted and about 16,000 cases of mental retardation were prevented. Advances in drug therapy also enhanced medicine's ability to treat such disorders as duodenal ulcers and manic-depressive illness. Cost reductions in medical care associated with the introduction and use of the drug cimetidine in the treatment of ulcers may exceed $20 billion. The discovery that lithium possessed an antimanic effect and the subsequent use of the drug in psychiatry has saved an estimated $4 billion in the last ten years by restoring productivity to people with manic-depressive illnesses.

The value of past national commitments to biomedical research is clearly apparent today as resources which have been dedicated over the past 40 years are mobilized to deal with the AIDS crisis. Faced with a new disease which cripples the body's ability to defend itself against viruses, bacteria, and cancer, those elements of the research community trained in the fields of immunology and virology first directed their efforts at uncovering the cause of this disorder. Because of past efforts, in a relatively short period of time a new virus, human immunodeficiency virus, was discovered as the causative agent. Further research led to the development of a sensitive and specific assay for the virus, which has allowed the screening of donated blood and plasma. With the number of diagnosed cases of AIDS estimated at a quarter of a million by 1991 and with an accompanying annual health care cost of between $8 and $16 billion, biomedical research is a vital resource in the development and testing of a vaccine to prevent the further spread of the virus and in the development of effective treatment for those with the disorder.

Biomedical research has immeasurably improved our nation's health. We must make a strong, continuous commitment to research—our promise for the future.

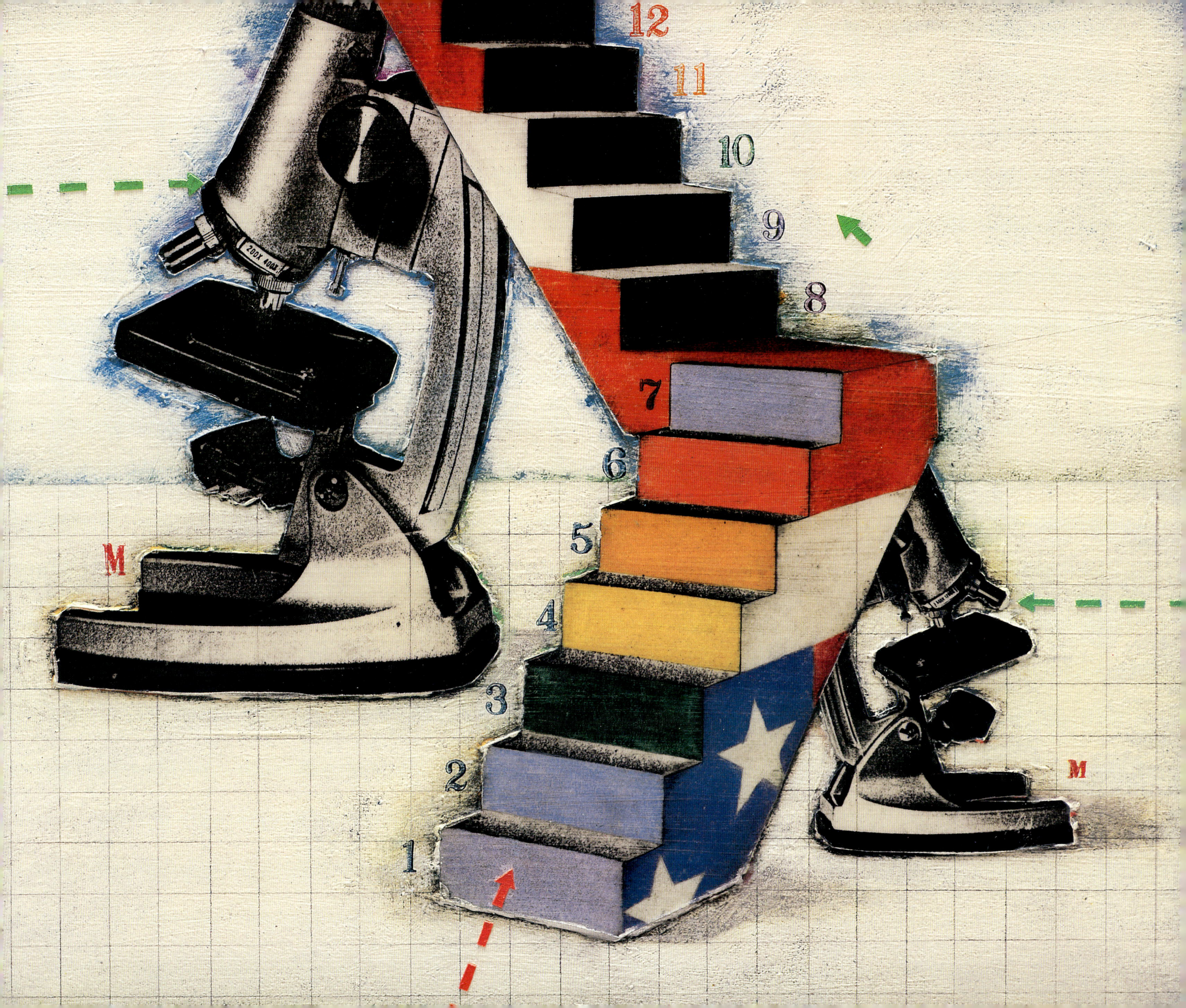

12
11
10
9
8
7
6
5
4
3
2
1
M
M

While accurate figures are difficult to obtain, there is sufficient information to indicate that research is both cost-effective—over the past 75 years, it is estimated to have saved the nation from $200 to $400 billion as a result of reductions in sickness and postponement of premature death—and important to the national economy. It has been estimated that the commercialization of biomedical research discoveries contributes considerably to the gross national product. If the potential applications of recombinant DNA technology are achieved, about $40 billion worth of products may be produced by the year 2000. Further, the preeminence of the country's biomedical research effort has important implications for national defense as it represents a vast intellectual resource.

Looking to the future, biomedical research is essential to the continued improvement in the health of the American people, and the nation must have a strong and long-term commitment to it. Biomedical research takes years of patient and often frustrating experimentation by many different research laboratories in both the private and public sectors of the scientific community. Whether an idea originates in a university laboratory or starts with basic product research conducted in the private sector, findings are disseminated to the entire scientific community, where each new finding serves as a basis for deeper understanding of human disease and functioning.

A variety of problems facing the research community need to be addressed. Competing national priorities—such as the defense budget and the need to resolve budget deficits—have an impact on the amount of money that is devoted to research projects and personnel. In fact, funding for biomedical research grants has fluctuated from year to year, and over the past five years, there has been a lack of growth in federal funding. This lack of stability in funding may influence a research scientist—often someone who has spent over ten years in training—to pursue a career elsewhere. The lack of growth has exacerbated already existing problems in the career opportunities for young investigators, in the maintenance of a stable research environment for established investigators, and in the renewal of facilities. Substantial increases in federal funding are necessary to attract and maintain the talented scientists to meet the nation's present and future health care needs.

Society seems to recognize, implicitly and explicitly, the value of medical science. Biomedical research contributes to good health, economic well-being and the scientific preeminence of the nation. Even in light of tight federal budgets, 70% of the American people believe that the government should increase its funding for basic research by a sizeable amount. A major concern for the remainder of this decade and the next is the commitment of the federal government to the availability, training, and support of biomedical researchers. At the same time, private industry, philanthropic organizations, voluntary health agencies and private foundations should supplement federal government funding for biomedical research. Special emphasis should be placed on the continued development of university-industry cooperative research ventures. These ventures serve to improve the communication between basic and applied research scientists and facilitate the transfer of findings of basic research to practical applications in the clinical setting.

Ethical and societal considerations in biomedical research also need to be addressed. While the application of scientific knowledge frequently results in immediate health benefits in preventing, diagnosing, and/or curing disease, the proliferation of knowledge and the application of this knowledge through technology have stimulated public concern in certain areas, such as fetal research and gene therapy. Public agencies and private groups have gathered to address the biological, medical, ethical, and legal aspects of research advances, and such discussion should be continued. Some of these discussions have addressed the use of animals in research. To maintain the faith of the public that the highest standards of care for research animals are being exercised, the research community must reaffirm its commitment to the humane treatment of animals in research.

Biomedical research is supported by both the private and public sectors. The American people need to be well-versed in the progress being made so that they can participate in public policy debates and decisions. Research findings may also affect the decisions of individuals regarding their own health care. Communication between the research community and the public is critical, for only an informed citizenry will continue to support the goals of biomedical research and apply its findings wisely to its own health care.

Availability of Funding for Research

Financial support for biomedical research comes from a variety of sources. In 1985, the government, industry, and private organizations together committed almost $13 billion to this effort. The government—federal, state, and local—provided about 58% of this money, industry provided about 39%, and private nonprofit foundations, voluntary health organizations and others provided the remaining 3%. This seems to be—and is—a great deal of money. To put this figure in perspective, however, it should be noted that research and development costs for health alone represent only 12% of the nation's total support for all types of research and development costs in all fields of science and technology.

In general, the absolute amount of money provided by the federal government for health-related research and development has increased over the years, but the proportion of funds as compared to total health expenditures per year has decreased. The proportionate decrease in federal funding for research and development has been balanced to some extent by increased funding from industry, particularly pharmaceutical companies. At first glance this increased industrial investment seems to bode well for biomedical research; but private industry funds only 10% of *basic* biomedical research, while the federal government funds about 90%. Thus, basic research (as opposed to applied research) is more vulnerable to decreased federal expenditures.

The level of funding for biomedical research is affected by many factors, including competing national priorities, available scientific opportunities, and the identification of acute or chronic public health concerns that may necessitate concentrated research efforts. Certainly some minor fluctuations in the level of funding are to be expected, but stable funding sources are essential to maintain and advance scientific knowledge and health care services.

Federal Funding for Basic and Applied Biomedical Research

Growth in research funding is needed to ensure that a substantially greater percentage of scientifically promising ideas can be explored, the need for intellectual resources and personnel can be met and replenished, research facilities and scientific instrumentation can be modernized, and the research environment of academic institutions can be stabilized.

Growth in basic and applied research funding is needed to meet the challenges of the remainder of this decade, the next decade, and the next century. Federal funding of basic and applied medical research should be increased at an annual rate of 10% (after inflation) for the remainder of the decade, and funding in the 1990s should be at a level sufficient to ensure appropriate growth in the nation's biomedical research enterprise. The major recipients of these increases should be the National Institutes of Health, the Veterans Administration, and the Alcohol, Drug Abuse and Mental Health Administration. Real growth of 10% per year after inflation (as computed by the Consumer Price Index) is achievable even in the context of present budget-cutting measures. For the 1990s, "appropriate" growth is defined as real growth above the rate of inflation; but this growth should be realistic, and the competing needs to exploit research opportunities and to address other national priorities should be balanced.

General tax revenues should continue to be the source of federal funding for biomedical research. The use of the recommended increases in federal funding to fortify

Less than 20% of the existing equipment in the biological and medical sciences used for academic research is "state of the art."

the nation's biomedical research enterprise should be implemented in two parallel phases. The first phase should concentrate on the restoration of the physical resources (facilities and instrumentation) needed to conduct biomedical research. According to a National Science Foundation study, less than 20% of the existing equipment in the biological and medical sciences used for academic research is "state of the art." Furthermore, many research facilities that were built in the 1960s under a National Institutes of Health matching fund program are now in dire need of modernization. Deficiencies in biomedical research instrumentation identified by the ongoing National Science Foundation study should be addressed by allocation of sufficient funding, and intramural programs at the National Institutes of Health should be strengthened.

The second phase should focus on the rejuvenation of intellectual resources, with an emphasis on increased funding of meritorious grant applications, modification of the renewal grant application system, and support of clinical research faculty under institutional grants. The specifics are discussed below.

Federal Funding of Approved Grant Applications for Biomedical Research

There has been a consistent decline in the funding of grants judged by the peer review process at the National Institutes of Health (NIH) to be of sufficient scientific merit to be approved and eligible for funding. During the first five years of this decade, the percentage of approved grants that are funded by the NIH has slipped from about 50% in 1979 to about 37% in 1984. Repeated and unpredictable reductions in the fraction of total NIH and the Alcohol, Drug Abuse and Mental Health Administration (ADAMHA) dollars available for funding grants have led to expenditures at levels below those recommended by peer reviewers. Annual fluctuations in the funding of a number of new and competing renewal awards have the potential to destabilize research careers because of the unpredictability of funding original high quality projects. The National Institutes of Health, the Alcohol, Drug Abuse and Mental Health Administration, and other granting agencies should fund 40% of the approved grant applications each year for the remainder of the decade. The level of 40% funding should be reexamined with respect to the conditions, such as scientific opportunities and the state of the economy, that exist in FY 1990.

Private Industry Support of Basic and Applied Biomedical Research

Although private industry cannot be directed to invest in research, an environment can be provided to stimulate its interest in investment, both to enhance its own financial interests and to ensure the continued well-being of the American people. Such an environment can be created by the provision of patent, tax, and licensing incentives for research and development, and by efficiency in regulatory processes. Appropriate measures to reform patent, tax and licensing laws, as well as measures to enhance the efficiency of regulatory processes, should be adopted by the federal government to encourage private industry involvement in basic and applied biomedical research.

The marketing exclusivity afforded by patent protection is a major incentive for private industry to invest funds in research and development. This incentive is particularly important to the pharmaceutical industry, for whom the overall average cost of bringing a new chemical entity to the market has reached $97 million in 1986. In an effort to improve the pharmaceutical companies' investment and also to provide new incentives for the development of generic drugs, the Competition and Patent Term Restoration Act of 1984 was enacted by Congress. Under this law, a pharmaceutical patent may be extended up to five years beyond the prescribed 17 years by matching year-for-year the amount of time spent waiting for FDA approval. The effective patent life after approval, however, must not exceed 14 years.

Implementation of tax credits should be limited to circumstances where other incentives and methods for stimulating industrial investment in biomedical research and development have failed. Any tax credit legislation that is developed should take these three factors into consideration:

□ Only increased investments in research and development by a particular company that exceed the industry-wide investment should result in a tax credit for that company.

□ The indexing of the base amount should be formulated so that credits are not awarded for merely keeping pace with inflation.

□ Research and development expenditures that qualify for the tax credit should be defined precisely to reduce instances in which firms merely redefine activities as research and development to take advantage of the credit.

Lobbying efforts and explicit expressions of support in oral or written testimony should be provided during any legislative initiative involving tax credits for research and development. Support by nonprofit organizations is particularly desirable because such organizations will be viewed as not having a vested interest in the extension of tax credits.

Mechanisms to extend patents and federal licensing agreements that stimulate investment should be used. In some cases, extension of exclusive licenses can be granted if companies agree to conduct additional research and development on the use of a particular drug to treat other medical problems. Further improvements in the FDA's drug approval process should be supported. Reform measures that enhance incentives for significant investment in research and development, sustain competition in the marketplace, facilitate further research on new uses of marketed products, and maintain high standards for the protection of the public should be supported.

Availability of Professionals for Research

The training and continued support of basic researchers and clinical investigators is essential to the advancement of the nation's health care system. Health science education and training programs are critically dependent upon programs and faculties at 270 nonfederal teaching hospitals. The teaching faculty of the academic medical center is the focus of a system that provides the base for highly specialized tertiary care and clinical research into the discovery of disease mechanisms and the delivery of new services.

The federal government makes annual commitments to support research while the academic medical center makes long-range decisions on faculty size and research facilities. However, changing federal priorities, constraints on limited funds, and hospital cost-containment programs have led to a growing concern about the short- and long-term training and maintenance of biomedical researchers. First, there is concern that the present number of physicians entering research training programs is inadequate. Second, the pool of future PhD biomedical researchers may not be sufficient for the personnel needs of both academia and the rapidly expanding private biotechnology

effort. Third, annual fluctuations in federally funded research grants discourage long-term research commitment by new and established investigators. Finally, the maintenance of clinical research faculty at academic medical centers is threatened by economic conditions that necessitate the diversion of faculty time from the conduct of research to the delivery of health care.

It is imperative that basic and clinical biomedical research scientists be available in sufficient numbers to assure the maintenance of the standards and quality, as well as the unparalleled output, of the American biomedical research effort. Further, the high quality of basic and clinical biomedical research faculty at academic medical centers must be maintained both by protecting their research time and enhancing their multidisciplinary research environment.

Determination of Personnel and Training Needs for Biomedical Research

In 1974, Congress assigned the National Academy of Sciences (NAS) the task of determining the national need for biomedical and behavioral research personnel. In addition, it was to assess the research training programs offered through the NIH; the Alcohol, Drug Abuse, and Mental Health Administration (ADAMHA); and the Division of Nursing of the Health Resources and Services Administration (HRSA). The Institute of Medicine of the NAS formed the Committee on National Needs for Biochemical and Behavioral Research Personnel to determine personnel needs for research and training.

The Committee on National Needs determines training needs by the marketplace demand for trained professionals. Although the number of available academic positions has been the primary determinant in training considerations, the Committee continues to include in its recommendations consideration of nonacademic positions. Because of the approximately nine years of training required to produce PhD and MD investigators, the biennial market-based analysis does not adequately assess the future personnel needs in rapidly developing research areas. With its primary focus on academic positions, market analysis ignores the growing opportunities resulting from discoveries in basic biomedical science.

In its determination of personnel and training needs, the Institute of Medicine of the National Academy of Sciences should consider the future research opportunities in the biomedical sciences as well as the marketplace demand for new researchers. This approach would allow an integration of the market-based analysis with one based on research opportunity. The latter analysis would estimate the number of researchers needed to explore scientifically promising avenues of research. The market-based analysis should be used as a secondary measure to fine-tune the recommendations of the opportunity-based analysis. The NIH, ADAMHA, and the Committee on National Needs of the Institute of Medicine are urged to consider research opportunities when determining personnel needs. This proposal should be supported at all public hearings concerning research training.

Research Opportunities and Careers for Physicians in Biomedical Research

Physician researchers are important for the education of new physicians and for continued advances in health care. Surveys indicate that the decision to pursue a research career occurs most often during medical school, and research opportunities and role models are often influential in career choice.

However, there are indications that interest on the part of medical school students in research is decreasing. This can be attributed to personal economic factors and the instability of research funding and training awards. Additional factors include lessening of the high regard in which scientific research was once held and curriculum changes resulting in less time for student involvement in research projects.

Because of their importance to research, the number of physicians in research training programs should be increased by expanding research opportunities during medical school through the use of short-term training grants and through the establishment of a cooperative network of research clerkships for students attending less research-intensive schools. In addition to the funding measures previously described, research opportunities during medical school should be promoted independently by medical schools themselves, by the use of an expanded National Research Service Short-Term Training Program, and by programs like the Howard Hughes Medical Institute-NIH Research Scholars program. In addition, an interuniversity program of research clerkships should be established that is of sufficient length to expose interested students to various phases of research and to influence positively the student's career choice. Support should be given to those students with biomedical research interests who attend less research-intensive schools, and interuniversity clerkship programs should be assured adequate funding by participating universities and by government and private sources.

The number of physicians in research training programs should be increased by providing financial incentives for research careers. Federal loans should be forgiven for those medical school graduates who enter research careers. To qualify for loan forgiveness, a physician would be required to complete at least two years in an NIH or other research training fellowship program. A total of four years of research training and/or a faculty position would be sufficient for forgiveness of the entire federal loan. Arrangements between federal programs to allow medical student loan debts to be repaid with full-time research under National Research Service Awards (NRSA) should be supported.

The National Health Service Corps (NHSC) scholarship program should continue to allow research commitment as fulfillment of obligation. In order to fulfill their NHSC obligation, medical graduates must first receive research training under NRSA for a minimum of two years. Following completion of research training, each subsequent year spent on full-time research pays back each corresponding year under the NHSC program. The NHSC-NRSA pathway to research careers already exists and its continuation should be supported.

The compensation of research fellows should at least be comparable to the salary of clinical residents. The number of Physician Scientist Awards should be increased and medical students should be made aware of the existence of this avenue of research career development.

PhDs and Biomedical Research

The 1983 report of the Institute of Medicine indicated that, in the short-term, the production of PhDs in the biomedical sciences was in balance with the marketplace demand for their services. However, the long-term balance into the 1990s is in question due to a number of interrelated events. The report indicates that the number of PhDs finding jobs outside academia has been increasing in recent years and is expected to continue as a result of explosive growth in biotechnology. Furthermore, the projected rise in the number of established scientists reaching retirement age in the next two decades will create additional demand for PhDs to fill these vacant positions.

The current annual production of PhDs trained in the biomedical sciences should be maintained into the next decade. The federal government should be committed to stable, long-term funding increases to the NIH and ADAMHA so that the present number of PhD trainees does not decline.

Nurses, Dentists, and Other Health Professionals in Biomedical Research Training Programs
Nurses, dentists and other health professionals all have a role to play in biomedical research in their respective fields. At the present time, a solid core of well-trained nurse investigators has not yet been developed, and since 1970 there has been a precipitous drop in the number of dentists receiving postdoctoral research training. While there are currently no federal research training programs specifically for pharmacists, the NIH and other agencies fund numerous research projects in pharmaceutical sciences and medicinal chemistry, and postgraduate programs are becoming increasingly available. Optometry schools do have research training programs, and they are eligible for Biomedical Research Support Grants and predoctoral and postdoctoral research training grants from the federal government. Research training for allied health professionals varies among allied health specialties, and research experience is frequently obtained in conjunction with medical and other health professions faculty. There are increasing numbers of graduate programs in allied health, but more basic research training is needed.

The numbers of nurses, dentists, and other health professionals in research training programs should be increased. In the field of nursing, the emphasis of the NRSA fellowship program should be on predoctoral support to increase the pool of researchers and to provide research faculty. The number of predoctoral and postdoctoral NRSA training awards should be increased, with a maximum of 15% of these awards at the postdoctoral level.

To increase the pool of dental investigators, the Dentist Scientist Awards and other NIH training programs should be assured continued and adequate funding.

NIH training programs should continue to include support for a research-related clinical component.

Graduate programs in pharmacy should be supported and strengthened. Emphasis should be given to providing research experience to interested pharmacy students in the graduate as well as undergraduate years. Pharmacists should be encouraged to apply for NIH research and training awards. Pharmacist researchers should also take advantage of training grants offered through private agencies and industry.

While optometry schools do have research training programs, there is a substantial need for persons so trained. Since there are currently no federal sources of research training support for predoctoral allied health professionals, the government should make research training programs already in place available to these individuals. To enable allied health professionals to compete more successfully for federal research grants, allied health curricula should include elements of research training.

Private Industry Support for Biomedical Research
Research and training in medical science ultimately benefits all constituents of the industrial community. Increased support for research and training in medical science should be a goal for all constituents of the industrial community. The life and health insurance industries are examples of industries with a logical link to biomedical research. These industries have had a special affinity for medical research for reasons of self-interest and public service, and they have a laudable record of supporting the training of MD/PhD investigators.

Members of the industrial community should increase their philanthropic financial support to the nation's biomedical research enterprise. Concentration of support on the training of young investigators should be a major thrust of increased funding. Constituents include but are not limited to those in life and health insurance, computers, petrochemicals, and other representatives of industry that derive a benefit from biomedical research.

The pharmaceutical and medical device industries should increase substantially their intramural and extramural commitments to meeting postdoctoral training needs. A system of matching grants should be encouraged in which private industry would supplement NIH- and ADAMHA-sponsored Career Development Awards, NRSAs, and other sources of support.

Philanthropic, Voluntary Health Agency, and Private Foundation Support for Biomedical Research

The benefit of philanthropic and voluntary contributions can best be described by providing examples of a few of the largest charitable organizations. The American Heart Association provided $48 million for research in 1983, and local American Heart Association affiliates supported cardiovascular researchers with $20 million. In 1984 the American Cancer Society funded the training of over 500 clinical fellows in more than 100 hospitals nationwide. The American Diabetes Association provided $2.8 million in 1983-1984, and the American Lung Association provided over $925,000 in 1982-1983 to fund new investigators. Private foundations have also advanced research activity for selected disorders by providing stable and in some cases lifetime financial support to faculty. The American Heart Association funds a limited number of clinical investigators, and the American Cancer Society funds a similar number of professors of clinical oncology.

Philanthropic foundations and voluntary health agencies should continue their work in the area of training and funding new investigators. Private foundations and other private organizations should increase their funding for clinical research faculty positions.

Funding for and Modification of the Renewal Grant Application System for Biomedical Research

The process involved in applying for grant support can be time-consuming and frustrating. Substantial faculty time is expended preparing the grant proposal and unfunded applications are revised and resubmitted to NIH, ADAMHA, or another funding source. Generally this effort is unproductive with regard to research activity. Additional time is required of the review group to prioritize grant applications.

Longer grant periods provide greater stability for the research community and make possible the funding of projects that require extensive laboratory and clinical facilities. Long-range support is necessary for research that requires time to collect detailed data and to assemble and train a highly qualified cadre of clinicians, technicians, consultants, and graduate and postgraduate students.

Although the average length of research grants awarded by the NIH has increased, tight federal budgets have continued to restrict the length of research grants. While shortening the period of research support leads to greater fiscal accountability, it also has led to increasing competition between new and renewal applications. NIH and ADAMHA should modify the renewal grant application system by lengthening the funding period for grants that have received high priority scores through peer review. The NIH and ADAMHA should review their policy regarding the funding of renewal grants. The length of funding for renewal grants should be increased to a range of five to seven years for those grants that receive a high priority rating from peer review.

Funding for Institutional Grants for Biomedical Research

The support of individual scientists with research project grants has been the first priority of federal support to medical science. In 1960, Congress passed authorization of the general research support fund which permitted the National Institutes of Health to allocate as much as 15% of the research budget to institutional grants. This was the forerunner of the Biomedical Research Support Grants (BRSG) program. These grants are awarded to a variety of institutions, including medical schools, graduate schools, and hospitals.

The BRSG program offers alternative means of supporting institutional research and providing clinical faculty more time for research projects. By law, NIH is allowed to spend up to 15% of its budget for institutional research grants, 15-fold more than it currently spends. The support of clinical research faculty from the NIH Biomedical Research Support Grants (institutional grants) should be increased from its current 1%. The level of funding for institutional grants should be increased as part of the recommended overall 10% increase in the annual NIH budget for the remainder of the decade. Increases in institutional grants should not be made at the expense of the direct NIH research grants.

Federal and Nonfederal Funding for Biomedical Research at Academic Medical Centers
There has been a decline in funding for research training at academic medical centers in
the past decade. In the early 1970s, such funding constituted about 12% of the NIH
budget, and this figure has now declined to under 5%. In addition, since 1966, the real
level of federal support to the ADAMHA has dropped markedly, even as research
opportunities and available scientific personnel have expanded. During the period of liberal
financing for biomedical research, many academic medical centers increased their
medical school faculty both in the basic sciences and in the clinical departments. As the
research dollars began to level off, a considerable number of researchers were shifted
to the hospital budget or were subsidized from practice plan revenues. The outlook for
continuance of hospital support is jeopardized by competition in the health care system
and by the shift to the prospective payment system under Medicare. Centers that
rely heavily on practice plan income will soon find that many of their faculty are so busy
practicing that they have little time for research, and perhaps even less for students.

The academic medical center, which provides the multidisciplinary research
environment for the basic and clinical research faculty, should be regarded as a vital
medical resource and be assured adequate funding in recognition of the research costs
incurred. The federal government and the American public should be convinced of the
importance of these centers. Federal and nonfederal funding should be assured for the
maintenance of the research environment and for support of research faculty.

University-Industry Cooperative Research Ventures

The biomedical research community has become increasingly interested in developing
university-industry research partnerships. These cooperative ventures improve the communication between basic and applied research scientists and facilitate the transfer of the
findings of basic research to practical applications in the clinical setting. Additional
advantages include the increased funding that is available to the university and the
availability to industry of the vast intellectual resources of the university.

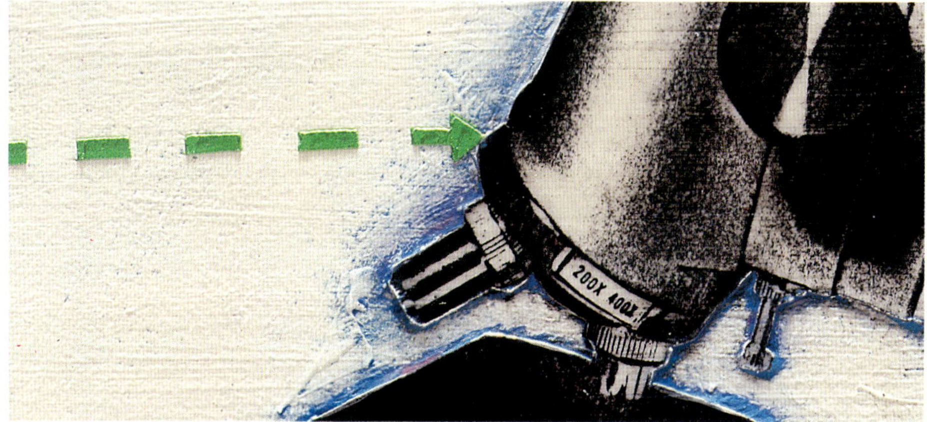

*Informed consumers will continue to
support the goals of biomedical research
and will apply findings to their own
health care.*

A variety of university-industry research relationships have been established over the years and many have proven to be successful. Relationships have ranged from undirected corporate contributions to universities to long-term research partnerships, which usually involve detailed contractual agreements to govern planning and management of research projects.

The success of such ventures depends heavily upon the delineation of guidelines that ensure the integrity and productivity of the university's research effort while providing benefit to the industrial sector. University involvement in these ventures has raised some questions, however. There are potential problems concerning dilution of the university's primary responsibility to educate; conflicts of interest on the part of the university or its departments, faculty, or students; communication of research results; and the public's perception of the independence of university research. These issues need to be resolved at the local level by responding to the individual circumstances and needs of the academic and industrial institutions involved in the projects.

The participants of the Health Policy Agenda believe that university-industry research partnerships should be recognized as key resources in maintaining our international advantage in the development of health care technology. University-industry cooperative research ventures should be encouraged, as this type of interaction has a synergistic effect on the creativity and productivity of the research efforts of both parties.

Guidelines Governing University-Industry Cooperative Research Ventures
It is important that all parties involved in a cooperative venture—universities, industry, and individual researchers alike—have a clear perception of the goals and objectives of each party in the venture. There should be a clear delineation and explicit expression of guidelines concerning the planning, implementation, and management of the cooperative research venture. For the maintenance of a cooperative research environment, all members of the community, the university, and industry should understand if and how such cooperative ventures will affect their individual goals. Academic institutions and industrial firms should establish explicit guidelines, policies, and goals for cooperative research ventures that will best accommodate the interests and integrity of both organizations. The public should have access to and be aware of these goals; public support of research deserves such accountability. Public involvement can help to substantiate the argument that in the long run cooperative ventures benefit society as a whole. In the university, members of the administration, faculty, and student body should have a clear understanding of the benefits to be derived from industry-sponsored research and should have the opportunity for input into the development of guidelines. Industrial management and researchers should also have a clear understanding of industry and university roles to maximize the benefit derived by the company and advance the mission of the university. The extent of industrial input will be determined by the company's formal policy-making process.

At no time should the higher goals of research—the expansion and free communication of knowledge and promotion of the greater societal good—be compromised to fulfill the narrower interests of a segment of the research community. The mission of academic institutions should not be compromised in any manner through participation in cooperative ventures.

Constituents of the industrial, academic, and governmental research communities participating in a research partnership should undertake a clearinghouse activity to provide information about the issues, resources, and mechanics that are involved in formulating an agreeable and effective working partnership. This clearinghouse should be available to all constituents of the research community, especially to less research-intensive universities and small businesses desiring to augment their research capabilities.

Faculty Conflict of Interest in University-Industry Cooperative Research Ventures
In cooperative ventures between university researchers and industry, the distinction between an investigator's academic work and commercial interests may become blurred. A number of universities participating in university-industry relationships have established conflict-of-interest policies which require faculty members to disclose equity interests and managerial involvement in businesses. Although none of the policies prohibit faculty from engaging in nonuniversity professional work, the policies do mandate disclosure to

and approval by a dean or department chairperson. Such policies are properly developed to inhibit at the outset the formation of inappropriate relationships between university scientists and industry sponsors.

Academic policies relating to faculty members involved in cooperative research ventures should address potential conflict-of-interest problems. Faculty members should disclose the nature of and time spent in university-industry research ventures. When their major orientation becomes commercial development rather than teaching and research, faculty members should take a leave of absence or leave the university to pursue their dominant interest. Faculty should reaffirm their primary mission of teaching and research since full disclosure prevents exploitation of graduate students for personal or industrial gain and ensures that the exchange of ideas and new research is in the traditional academic spirit.

In some cases, it may be appropriate to place a ceiling on the amount of money an investigator can personally receive, with the remainder to be distributed to the university, department, and/or school in which the research is conducted. Mechanisms such as these, in addition to annual disclosure of equity holdings, should help preserve the primary responsibility of faculty members to teaching and research.

Use of Patent Rights, Licensing Rights, and Proprietary Information in University-Industry Cooperative Research Ventures

The major purposes of the patent protection system are to serve as an inducement to commercialize an invention and to provide the impetus for further exploration of ideas and advancement in health care technology. The holding of a patent by the university affords the university the overall control of the commercialization process—including protection against any delay or withholding by an industrial concern—for a particular invention. It provides assurance that society will ultimately benefit from inventions derived from research for which it has directly or indirectly provided much support.

As is true of the patent protection system, the appropriate use of licensing arrangements can enhance technological innovation and thus improve health care. The licensing arrangement suitable for a particular university-industry cooperative venture in biomedical research will vary according to the circumstances of the individual research agreement. If the cooperative venture involves a university with a consortium of industrial firms, the university may favor the granting of a nonexclusive license to retain the right to permit broader use of the invention protected by the patent. In the case of a one-on-one research partnership, the industrial firm usually desires the option to obtain an exclusive license for any inventions that might emanate from interaction with a university. As long as the open communication of scientific information and the appropriate advance of technology continue, the exclusive license is an appropriate arrangement for a university.

Regardless of the nature of the partnership arrangement, patent and licensing rights emanating from university-industry cooperative ventures should accrue to university, investigator, and industry by a mechanism agreed upon in advance. The details concerning the use of patent and licensing rights resulting from cooperative research ventures should be resolved between the universities, industries, and individuals involved in the projects. In general, the patent for discoveries or innovations should be held by the university when the major portion of the work or resources allocated to do the work emanate from the university setting. Licensing arrangements should be based on the type of partnership involved in the venture.

It is also the responsibility of the university to resolve problems that might arise from the use of proprietary information. It is not necessary to preclude the use of proprietary information for the initiation of university-industry cooperative ventures, as in all likelihood this might eliminate many cooperative efforts that would otherwise produce valuable scientific information. However, the degree to which a research project depends on proprietary information should be a prime consideration during the planning stages of a university-industry cooperative venture. Proprietary information can rightfully be viewed as being excluded from full disclosure of research results and, thus, its confidentiality should be maintained by both parties. The ultimate purpose of the use of the proprietary information in a university research effort should be to generate new knowledge that can be freely disseminated and published. The use of proprietary information should be minimized in order to lessen any coincident or future constraints on faculty in developing their own careers and pursuing their own interests.

Dealing with students who are asked to sign confidentiality agreements is a potential problem. Although private firms may require university investigators to sign confidentiality agreements prohibiting disclosure of trade secrets, if students sign such agreements they may be faced with undue restrictions on the types of future employment they may seek. Students should be exempted from signing confidentiality agreements prohibiting disclosure of proprietary information. Universities should try to insulate students from the proprietary information of industrial sponsors; access to this data should be limited to faculty and staff. Considerations regarding patents or disclosure of proprietary information should not be impediments to the granting of a degree.

Income in University-Industry Cooperative Research Ventures

In general, the acquisition of substantial equity, direct control, or direct ownership in a private for-profit research firm by a university involved in a cooperative venture with that firm should be viewed as presenting conflict-of-interest problems. Especially in the initial stages or during difficult periods, the private firm might drain resources from what should be dedicated to the primary mission of the university. Universities should not engage in research at the expense of the educational mission of the institutions. However, university administrators should keep in perspective the contribution that participation in cooperative ventures can make to the achievement of the mission of the university.

A striking example of the possible intrusion of the profit motive is provided by the proposal at Harvard in 1980 that the university have a substantial equity share in a Harvard-formed biotechnology company. This proposal was rejected after much debate by the faculty on the grounds that the level of involvement and resources necessary to run a successful company would compromise the overall educational and research missions of the university.

A related topic is the distribution of any monetary profits that may occur as a result of a cooperative research venture. The distribution of monetary gain within the academic setting has raised questions regarding distributive fairness for both researchers involved in the project and other members of the university community. The university community functions best as a whole, and thus some recognition of the contributions, albeit indirect, of some departments far removed from the research arena is in order. Monetary profits emanating from cooperative ventures should accrue to the university, investigators and industry by an agreeable mechanism. Distribution of profits within the university setting should recognize those programs or individuals who have invested their time, energies and resources. Conditions of distribution of profits should be negotiated at the local level by the parties involved.

Communication and Publication of Research Findings in University-Industry Cooperative Research Ventures

The free and open communication of research results is a basic tenet of any scientific undertaking in a university setting. The publication of important research findings often represents the culmination of many years of intense devotion to a research problem. Thus, the freedom to express such findings is essential to career fulfillment. On a practical level, publication of research results is the most frequently utilized measure of research competence and, thus, forms the basis for career advancement.

It is critical that the university retain the right to publish or communicate any new information resulting from scientific endeavors. An integral component of publishing or communicating research results is to acknowledge the source of research support. Attribution of institutional support in all professional communications is necessary to ensure that peer reviewers, the scientific community, and the public can fully evaluate the validity, applicability, and utility of research findings.

The free and expeditious communication of research findings to the scientific community should be a major objective of academia and industry. Reasonable delays for review of patentable subject matter and for filing of a patent application should be permitted. The university and the industrial sponsor, in developing the contractual agreement for a cooperative venture should give careful consideration to the specification of the terms under which publication of research results will occur. Members of the university faculty should be provided ample opportunity to participate in the delineation of such terms in order to protect their own interests as well as those of students and the university as a whole.

Federal Support for University-Industry Cooperative Research Ventures

Analyses of university-industry cooperative ventures indicate that such programs have had a significant positive impact on individual scientists and their respective organizations. The need for the federal government to assist in the establishment of models for these types of efforts has diminished because of the success under the National Science Foundation's initial grants to initiate the Industry/University Cooperative Research Projects (IUCR) program. However, there is a need for the federal government to encourage the participation of small business in these kinds of ventures. Small businesses have traditionally been a major source of technological innovation across a broad variety of industrial fields, including health care. In fact, small businesses produce more innovations per dollar invested and more innovations per employee than large companies.

The federal government should encourage the participation of small businesses in cooperative research ventures, and should continue to support starter programs for such projects. Federal government support for such ventures should proceed from a close scrutiny of the merits of the scientific undertaking, and not from a mandatory expenditure of an allocated sum.

Although the United States currently holds a world leadership position in the development and commercialization of biotechnology, Japan, West Germany, the United Kingdom, Switzerland, and France have been identified as major competitors. Neither Japan nor the European countries have nearly as many or as well-financed university-industry relationships, but governments in these countries are placing increased emphasis on such partnerships.

The key participants in our nation's biomedical research efforts must evaluate the quality of university-industrial ventures to ensure the most efficient use of the resources of the federal government, private industry, and academia. The federal government should be charged with conducting an ongoing analysis of the productivity and capacity of the nation's biomedical research enterprise, with the university-industry partnership as the focal point of the analyses. The mechanism of this partnership should be evaluated to assure that the state of the art between the academic and industrial research communities is being maintained. Such a study has been initiated recently by the National Science Foundation. It should be the responsibility of this agency and of the U.S. Department of Commerce to sustain this important evaluative activity.

State and Local Government Support for University-Industry Cooperative Research Ventures

In addition to the support for state university systems, state and local governments provide direct support for research in the university setting. In 1984, for example, state and local governments provided about 13% of the funds for research performed in the university setting.

In recent years, a number of state governments have been investing large sums of money to enhance the attractiveness of their universities for further investment by industry. An example of such efforts is New Jersey, which recently approved a "Jobs, Science and Technology Bond Issue." Money is being provided to advanced technology centers at New Jersey universities in biotechnology, hazardous and toxic substance management, food technology, industrial ceramics, and new high technology areas as they emerge.

State and local governments are a crucial link in the nation's biomedical research effort, and they should be encouraged to provide a legislative, economic, and research environment conducive to the establishment of university and industry cooperative ventures. State and local governments should be commended for their efforts to support research efforts at academic institutions. States should be further encouraged, using the National Science Foundation's Industry/University Cooperative Research Projects as a model, to establish additional cooperative ventures at their academic institutions.

Private Industry Support for University-Industry Cooperative Research Ventures

Because of past concerns that universities might lose control over the direction of research or that cooperative ventures might delay chances to improve health care, the research community in the academic setting avoided extensive involvement with private industry. But this dissociation from large scale cooperative ventures has all but disappeared in recent years. Increasing attention is being paid to the development of cooperative research ventures between private industry and universities in biomedical research, especially in the area of recombinant DNA technology. Private industry support of biomedical research performed in academia in 1984 accounted for about 4% of the funds invested by all parties. However, this figure does not include the money invested by pharmaceutical and medical device firms for screening, testing, and clinical studies in the university setting.

Private industry should increase its financial support of university-industry cooperative ventures in biomedical research. While it is unrealistic to expect that private industry will supply a major portion of the monetary support of university research efforts, the factors that motivate private industry to commit resources for collaboration with universities will endure, and their participation in cooperative research ventures should be encouraged. Private business organizations such as the U.S. Chamber of Commerce, the Business Roundtable, and the Pharmaceutical Manufacturers Association should be encouraged to mount campaigns to heighten the awareness of member organizations to the benefits derived from university research and to the service provided to society by such research.

Ethical and Societal Considerations in Research

The proliferation of scientific knowledge and the application of this knowledge through technology has stimulated public concern about the ethical and societal implications of biomedical research. The public is concerned because there is increasing reliance on public funds to conduct the research. In addition, there is growing interest on the part of the general public, the media, and elected officials in the discoveries emerging from the nation's laboratories. Finally, the intricacies of deciding whether individual technologies should be employed has resulted in reliance on public institutions, such as the courts, legislatures, and regulatory agencies, to resolve ethical issues involved in these decisions. Resolution of these issues should occur through broad societal participation.

The conduct of biomedical research involving human subjects is governed by codes, laws, rules and guidelines that have been developed over the last 40 years. A number of these guidelines were prompted by and developed after violations of the most basic human rights. For example, the Nuremberg Code was the result of the inhumane and unethical experimentation conducted by Nazi physicians on concentration camp prisoners. Several incidents involving human subjects—the injection of live cancer cells into chronically ill patients to determine the human body's ability to reject foreign cells (the Jewish Chronic Disease Hospital case); the administration of hepatitis virus to mentally retarded children (the Willowbrook State School case); and the withholding of penicillin from black men known to have syphilis (the Tuskegee Syphilis Study)—were influential in the formulation of the National Research Act of 1974. As a result of this act, the National Commission for the Protection of Human Subjects in Biomedical and Behavioral Research was established, and its deliberations and recommendations ultimately provided a basis for regulations governing research involving fetuses, pregnant women, the products of *in vitro* fertilization, children, and prisoners.

To carry on the work of this National Commission, Congress created the President's Commission for the Study of Ethical Problems in Medicine and Biomedical and Behavioral Research in 1978. The President's Commission produced a series of reports and recommendations for ethical reforms in health care and research involving human subjects which have recently led to implementation of uniform federal regulations. In general they have served to enhance public debate on compensation for research injuries, and have contributed to increased compliance with regulations concerning the need to report misconduct in research.

The most recent federal initiative in biomedical issues is the 1985 Health Research Extension Act. This act established a Biomedical Ethics Board that is responsible for appointing a Biomedical Ethics Advisory Committee. This Advisory Committee has been mandated to produce a report on research and developments in genetic research, including research involving recombinant DNA technology.

Other federal programs involved in ethical issues are the National Science Foundation's Ethics and Values in Science and Technology (EVIST) and the National Center for Health Services Research and Health Care Technology Assessment. The National Institutes of Health has considered the possibility of developing a program to fund research studies in biomedical ethics, but the National Science Foundation is the only federal agency that currently funds this type of research.

A number of private organizations, such as The Hastings Center, Public Responsibility in Medicine and Research, and the American Association for the Advancement of Science's Committee on Scientific Freedom and Responsibility, also study ethical issues relating to biomedical research. Other centers include Georgetown University's Kennedy Institute of Ethics and Harvard University's Center for Health Policy and Management. Nearly every major university has some resource center for studying ethics.

Through public commissions, studies, court decisions, and other means, guidelines and regulations have been developed to protect the rights of human subjects in research. However, the current revolution in molecular biology is likely to lead to the development of a genetic map of the human species by the early 1990s. With such a blueprint, researchers will begin to systematically locate and identify genetic alterations that are responsible for or predispose one to such disorders as hypertension, cancer, diabetes, and schizophrenia. The ethical implications of this capability are now being discussed by researchers and other members of society.

Health care will be greatly improved if individuals who are genetically predisposed to cancer are identified, so that their lifestyles may be tailored to minimize their exposure to cancer-causing agents. On the other hand these individuals may suffer if this information is made available to health and life insurers and potential employers; restrictions on the rights and choices of these individuals is likely to occur. When the identification of defective genes is combined with the capability of synthesizing correct copies of those genes and delivering these genes to defective cells, a new therapeutic modality is introduced. This capability is called gene therapy and for certain disorders such as severe combined immunodeficiency or sickle-cell anemia, somatic cell gene therapy may be a reasonable therapeutic intervention. Certain disorders such as cystic fibrosis, Duchene muscular dystrophy, and Tay-Sachs involve genetic disorders affecting multiple genes or organs not easily accessible to this therapy. In these cases, gene therapy may be attempted on the ovum, sperm, fertilized egg, or early embryo to increase the chances of reaching the correct tissue. This approach has the potential of introducing the new gene into that portion of the chromosome destined for the germ line cells. The new gene will then become a heritable trait. Such an occurrence may raise important ethical concerns if gene therapy in germ line cells is used to correct these kinds of disorders.

As the mission of improving society's health is pursued, research activities should remain consistent with the moral and ethical values of society. Discussions of the ethical and societal implications of biomedical research should occur at a national level where all parties can be heard, and where those facing difficult and complex problems may turn for counsel and assistance.

Study and Discussion of Ethical Issues in Biomedical Research

Previous studies of ethical issues in biomedical research have developed general principles to guide the conduct of the investigator, granting agency, and research subject. But there are no handy formulas or cookbooks to consult when ethical or legal issues arise which have broad implications for society. The application of theoretical ethical principles to real situations is complex due to the number of uncertainties inherent in the decision-making process. The scientific community can and does address the technical and medical issues, but its expertise is insufficient to address all the ramifications of its work. Biomedical research has entered an age in which advances require the analysis and consideration of divergent viewpoints. Participation from all segments of society—ethicists, sociologists, theologians, lawyers, educators, government leaders—is required.

Private organizations and academic institutions should jointly develop a means to continue and enhance broadly based study and discussion of ethical and societal issues in biomedical research. It is important to build on the available expertise in bioethical studies currently located at academic and private research centers or within private organizations concerned with discussions of ethics in research. The advantage of joint activities by these groups is primarily one of freedom to address long-term ethical issues and to provide a national forum to discuss and debate bioethical issues without federal mandates, deadlines, or undue political pressures.

Organizations which have expertise in sponsoring conferences on ethical issues in biomedical research—such as the American Association for the Advancement of Science, Public Responsibility in Medicine and Research, and the Kennedy Institute of Ethics, among many others—could jointly develop a series of public workshops and conferences to be held in various regions around the country. Examples of research topics that have social, legal, and ethical implications and that could be addressed in such forums include intervention in human reproduction, artificial organs, organ transplantation, aging, and recombinant DNA technology. Meetings should be open to the public, with time set aside for public comment.

Funding of Bioethical Research Studies

The National Institutes of Health has been largely responsible for the progress that has been made in biomedical research, and as a natural extension of its activities, the federal government should provide the resources to support new initiatives within the NIH for the funding of research studies in bioethics. Various directors of the NIH have supported such activities but no action has been taken because of the lack of funds and an inability to find a base for the project. One possible base is the National Library of Medicine, but Congress will need to provide monetary assistance if it is located here.

Existing federal programs that fund bioethical research studies should be preserved. The National Science Foundation's Ethics and Values in Science and Technology program is an example of a federal program which funds studies on ethics in biomedical research. EVIST should be protected by highlighting this program's accomplishments, which include funding for projects on gene therapy, research fraud, and the use of animals in research.

Currently not one private foundation or organization has a defined program for funding research studies in biomedical ethics. As a result, many centers must constantly work to convince each foundation or organization that bioethics studies are an integral part of health care research. Private foundations should be encouraged to provide resources to support research studies in bioethics.

Uniform Federal Rules Governing Research with Human Subjects

As a result of the principles of the Nuremberg Code, the World Medical Association's Declaration of Helsinki, and the National Commission for the Protection of Human Subjects of Biomedical and Behavioral Research, all federal agencies engaged in human experimentation have formal rules and policies that serve to protect research subjects. While most of the regulations of various federal agencies conform to the core elements of Department of Health and Human Services regulations pertaining to review and informed consent, the adoption of a uniform set of federal regulations would decrease the burden of Institutional Review Boards, which are often faced with a variety of requirements "buried" in regulations of various federal bodies. Moreover, uniform regulations could eliminate the need for over 200 pages of redundant requirements contained in the Code of Federal Regulations and departmental policies.

A uniform set of federal regulations governing research with human subjects, based on the core regulations of the Department of Health and Human Services (as revised in 1985), should be adopted by all federal agencies. Because of the agreement for the adoption of uniform regulation among 22 federal agencies and bodies worked out by the Ad Hoc Committee on the Protection of Research Subjects, this recommendation might best be implemented with a directive from the Administration to all federal agencies. Uniformity should not preclude additions to Department regulations that do not conflict with the core regulations or that enhance the protection of research subjects.

Formation of Associations of Regional Institutional Review Boards

Institutions conducting federally-funded research on human subjects must first have that research reviewed and approved by an Institutional Review Board (IRB). Following IRB approval, the institution must forward assurances to the National Institutes of Health for final approval. Assurances must include statements to the effect that the rights and welfare of human subjects will be protected, and that the research study is subject to both initial and continuing review by the IRB.

This formal process assists in the protection of the rights of human research subjects, but certainly strict adherence to a set of regulatory rules is not all that is required—there must also be compliance with the "spirit" of these regulations. And, although the NIH can review the intention of the institution to comply with the standards, this activity is not the same as an evaluation of the performance. In fact, a study of IRB performance revealed wide variations in the comprehensiveness of IRB discussions, frequency of IRB-requested protocol modifications, completeness and clarity of informed consent, IRB self-evaluations, and researcher evaluation of the IRB.

Because the inspection of IRBs to assure compliance with federal regulations is too costly and time-consuming, the National Institutes of Health and the Food and Drug Administration, in conjunction with private organizations, conduct regional workshops and seminars on IRB performance. To capitalize on these efforts, associations of regional institutional review boards should be formed to enhance IRB performance through the development of educational site visits and local workshops. Site visits or seminars conducted by colleagues provide a rich characterization of the major strengths and weaknesses of IRBs, especially if the purpose of these visits is educational rather than investigational. The associations of regional IRBs can be used to promote educational activities and to provide access to expert consultation through seminars, workshops, and site visits. Protection of human subjects in ambulatory settings should also be discussed in these forums.

Role of Institutions in Monitoring Research Conduct and Investigating Research Misconduct

The responsibility for developing and implementing a system of research-monitoring lies with the institution conducting the research. The system must be accountable to both public and private supporters of research. At many institutions, procedures to monitor the conduct of clinical research involve institutional review boards and quality assurance units. Monitoring basic research, such as oversight of grant applications, is usually handled at the departmental level. Departmental review can prevent unintended errors in the proposed research or serious overlaps with existing projects.

In addition to monitoring research conduct, institutions must be committed to the identification of misconduct (poor or unethical research) and to the expeditious investigation of allegations of misconduct. They need to establish channels for reporting research misconduct as part of the monitoring process.

Although the diversity of institutions conducting research precludes a uniform approach, each institution should have a system both for monitoring the conduct of biomedical research and for investigating and reporting allegations of research misconduct. In general, monitoring can be carried out by departmental chairmen, quality control offices, research grants offices, IRBs, or through joint action of all of these.

Institutional actions regarding misconduct should be prompt, based upon facts, and handled within the recognized administrative channels. The protection of both the reporter of the alleged misconduct and the reputation of the researcher under investigation should be assured. The investigation must adhere to the principles of due process. For allegations suggesting increased risk to the patient, the investigational process must be expeditious and must ensure that immediate corrective measures can be taken if necessary.

Institutions should report to the NIH or other funding agencies only when an institution has begun a formal investigation into charges of research misconduct. Institutions may conduct a preliminary inquiry without notifying granting agencies to determine the plausibility of the allegations and whether further investigation is necessary. Notification of the NIH of a formal investigation provides the agency with the option of participating; however, treatment of matters under investigation should be confidential.

Role of Investigators in Proper Research Conduct

Research investigators also have a critical role to play in ensuring proper research conduct. They need to maintain standards of excellence in designing research projects;

conducting the research, including the protection of human research subjects; and reporting the results of their research. The fulfillment of such standards ultimately depends on the personal integrity and honesty of the individual investigator and his/her adherence to established ethical guidelines. All investigators involved in research projects should be responsible for the clear articulation and enforcement of standards that ensure the integrity of scientific data and conclusions. Regardless of whether the research project is a result of individual or collaborative efforts, investigators should thoroughly understand the data and conclusions in research publications and studies. Investigators must be assured that research has been conducted under the most rigorous experimental conditions and that it has been reported in an objective, accurate, and comprehensive manner. Anything less weakens the usefulness of research to society.

Role of Students in Research Conduct

Following competition for admission to professional schools, students begin training under a faculty advisor whose professional advancement often depends on successful competition for grant support and on the number of scientific publications. In this high-pressure environment, students may be especially vulnerable to compromises in proper research conduct due to their relationship to their mentors. Exposure of the students to improper research conduct has the potential to erode their commitment to research.

Furthermore, some faculty advisors may coauthor publications with their students without thoroughly reviewing the data. As part of their formal training in research investigation, graduate, medical, and postdoctoral students should be instructed on the importance of adhering to the ethical and scientific requirements in research conduct and in the reporting of research results. Students should become familiar with publications which provide examples of problems that may arise to compromise the proper conduct of research. Institutions could establish a mechanism for confidential consultation on student concerns relating to research standards. Finally, and perhaps most importantly, the principle investigator-advisor should take the lead role in setting high standards for research.

The Use of Animals in Research

The ultimate outcomes of the debates on the use of mammalian animals in the research process will have a considerable impact on the progress that can be made in health care. Current estimates of the number of animals used for biomedical research vary, but a recent national survey sets the figures at 17 to 22 million, the vast majority of which are rats and mice. About 180,000 dogs, 50,000 cats, and 56,000 monkeys are used. These animals are involved in experiments largely and ultimately aimed at improving the health care available to human beings. Data are currently being collected in an effort to determine whether the use of particular animals can be reduced or altogether eliminated. Unfortunately, though, it appears that while alternatives (e.g., mathematical models, computer simulation and *in vitro* biological systems) may be appropriate in some types of research, animals remain indispensable for other types of research. For many aspects of human biology, mammalian models provide the best avenue for studying specific diseases; even proposals that cell and tissue culture systems or mathematical models could replace animals fail to consider the need to ultimately validate data in the intact animal. Certainly there is no question that researchers—and we as a society—have an obligation to minimize pain and suffering in other species. But if researchers are prevented from validating scientific data on animals, an important part of the research process will be adversely affected. Additionally, the research community would be hard-pressed to fulfill its ethical responsibility to minimize risks for human research subjects.

Because of these concerns, the public and the research community have become involved in discussions about the care and use of animals in research projects. Many of the regulatory requirements governing human experimentation, such as institutional committees which review the research protocols, have been applied to animal research. In fact, the past 20 years represent a period of significant change in the regulation of animal research in this country. In 1966, the first major act governing the humane use of animals in research, the Laboratory Animal Welfare Act, was passed by Congress; this act was amended several times and is now simply known as the Animal

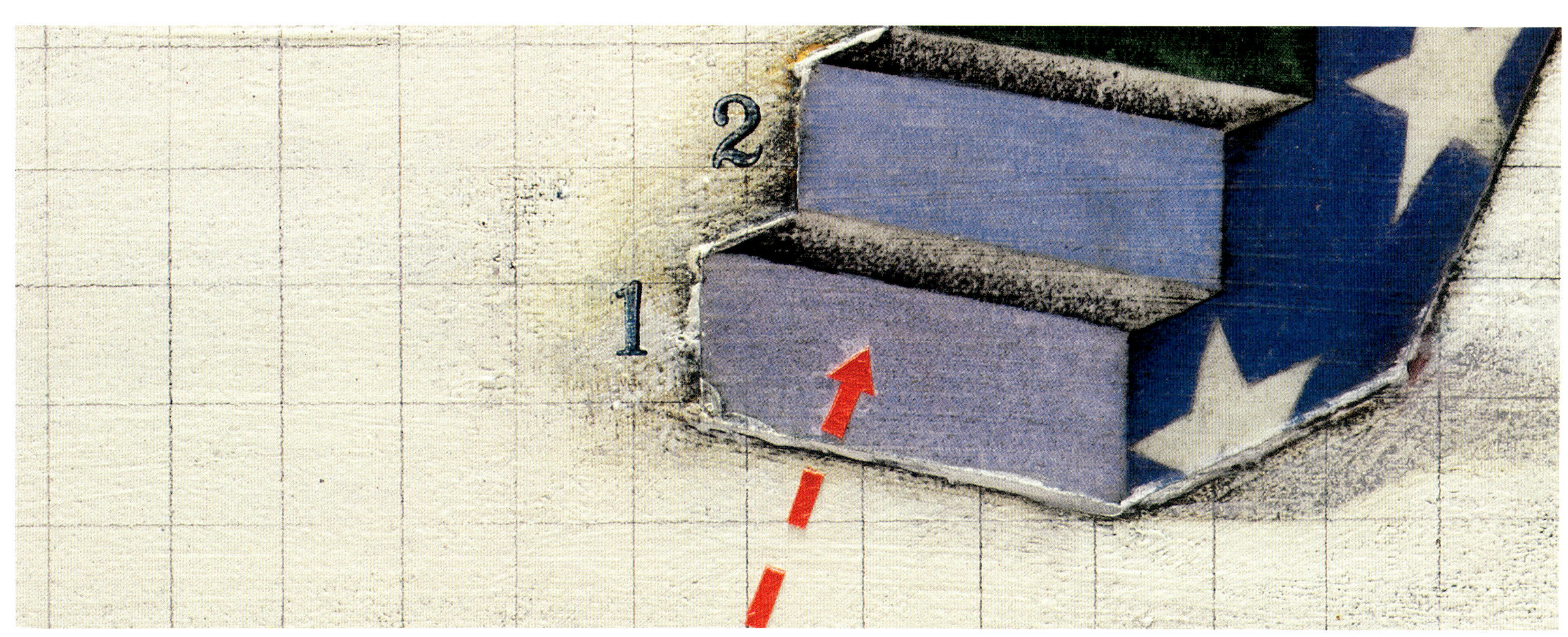

Increases in funding are necessary to attract and maintain talented scientists to meet the nation's future health care needs.

Welfare Act. Briefly, this act requires that research facilities establish an animal review committee with outside member participation. Research facilities must also provide training for researchers, technicians, and others involved in animal care to promote humane practices in animal maintenance and experimentation, to minimize pain or distress, and to reduce or eliminate the use of animals in research.

The first federal guidelines on the care of animals in research were those contained in the National Institutes of Health's "Guide for Laboratory Animal Facilities and Care," published in 1963; this document was amended five times and is now known as the "Guide for the Care and Use of Laboratory Animals." Eventually, this guide was used to develop the Public Health Service "Policy on Humane Care of Laboratory Animals by Awarded Institutions." Under this policy, institutional assurances and the establishment of institutional animal care and utilization committees are required for each institution applying for Public Health Service funds for research involving animals. Finally, the Health Research Act of 1985 included a directive to the National Institutes of Health to develop alternatives to the use of animals in research.

The ethical debate over the use of animals in research is unlike the debate over the use of humans in research—the latter debate is generally predicated on the assumption that all human beings have equivalent moral value, whereas the debate on the former is complicated by the broad range of positions on what the moral status of animals should be. Animal-welfare groups are particularly active in promoting the passage of legislation that would repeal state and local laws permitting the release of animals from pounds to be used in research. Repeal of such laws is a top priority of the Humane Society of the United States, which suggests that the research community use purpose-bred dogs and cats as they do rats and mice. Currently, nine states have outlawed the use of animals from pounds within their states. The biomedical and behavioral research community has initiated a coordinated approach to its opposition in the form of such organizations as the National Association of Biomedical Research and the Foundation for Biomedical Research. A top priority of the latter organization is the education of the public about the use of animals in research and the enlistment of practicing physicians,

voluntary health organizations, and professional societies in this effort.

The great majority of researchers and the public believe that animals are necessary for certain types of research and that they should receive some type of moral consideration. To maintain the faith of the public that the highest standards of care for research animals are exercised, the research community must reaffirm its concern for humane treatment of animals by strengthening the oversight of animal use, and by being responsive to public participation in the review of animal research as required by the Animal Welfare Act and Public Health Service policy.

Investigator and Institutional Responsibility for Humane Care and Treatment of Research Animals

In the great majority of animal experiments, researchers, veterinarians, and institutional committees have assured the humane treatment of animal subjects. But it also needs to be acknowledged that guidelines have not always been followed. To ensure that research animals receive humane care and treatment, researchers and institutions must recommit themselves to the strengthening of animal review committees. Failure to provide credible review of animal research protocols may result in additional cases of animal pain and suffering, and almost assuredly in further regulatory action with correspondingly disruptive consequences for research.

Researchers should include in their protocols a commitment to ethical principles that promote high standards of care and humane treatment of all animals used in research. Further, they should provide animal review committees with sufficient information so that effective review can occur. For their part, institutions should strengthen their animal review committees to provide effective review of all research protocols involving animals.

While the law is clear regarding the composition and purpose of the committee, the investigator and the research institution have the final responsibility for developing an effective committee. To establish an effective review of animal research protocols, the researcher should provide the committee with information on the types and numbers of animals that are planned for the research project, and the rationale for their use based upon scientific necessity and ethical guidelines. The committee must develop processes for reviewing initial research protocols involving animals, as well as monitoring of ongoing research. Finally, the animal care and utilization committee should have the full support of the administration and the authority to suspend research when the investigator fails to respond to committee inquiries or objections.

Humane Care and Treatment of Research Animals

Society in general recognizes the importance of animal research and supports biomedical research; however, it is concerned over the potential for pain and suffering in research animals. Strengthening the role of research institutions in monitoring the use of animals and enforcement of the Animal Welfare Act amendments and Public Health Service policy are measures that have been taken to address concerns, and they seem generally acceptable to both the general and research community. However, legislation that forbids the use of pound animals or restricts the use of certain types of animal research is not in the public interest because it leads to reductions in the level and types of scientifically valid research. The appropriate and humane use of animals in biomedical research should not be unduly restricted. Local and national efforts to inform the public about the importance of the use of animals in research should be supported. The general public needs to understand that research is a slow process requiring the use of a variety of models, including animals. It is appropriate that animals be treated in a humane fashion, but their critical link to medical progress must also be recognized.

The most effective way to prevent restrictions on the use of animals is to prevent abuse of animals by strengthening institutional oversight through public, veterinary, and researcher involvement. Additionally, the research community should continue its public educational efforts through such organizations as the Foundation for Biomedical Research. Health care professional organizations should develop effective public awareness programs to educate the public at the community level of the benefits derived from animal research. When restrictive legislation is introduced, the research community and health care professionals should be prepared to counter misinformation on the use of research animals based on sound scientific and ethical considerations.

Alternatives to Animal Research

In the early stages of research, both nonmammalian and mammalian cell or tissue culture systems have provided the first scientific basis for understanding a process or function of a structure. Advances in immunobiology have occurred through research utilizing cell culture. This approach has been responsible for furthering knowledge regarding the regulation of cell function and proliferation, the nature of cell-to-cell interactions, and the mechanism of carcinogenesis. Mathematical modeling is potentially useful in most disciplines of biomedical research but may have its greatest utility in conjunction with experimentation. The development of research models cannot be approached on the assumption that suitable alternatives to animal research can be found in all cases.

Nonetheless, the development of suitable alternatives to the use of animals in research should be encouraged among investigators and supported by government and private organizations. The selection of alternatives ultimately must reside with the research investigator. To assist the researcher in the development or adoption of a nonanimal model, NIH should develop a program to increase the awareness of researchers of potentially useful alternatives and should fund research and training in the use of invertebrate animal alternatives. The NIH, professional scientific organizations, and animal welfare groups could sponsor symposia at which investigators discuss the scientific merit of various alternatives to animal models. The scientific approach would be directed by the research investigator and not dictated by rigid protocols from without. In addition, the NIH should develop a data base of information on alternatives and provide a clearinghouse for such information.

Communication among the Research Community, the Media, and the Public

Given the investment that the nation has made in health research and development, the American public is entitled to know what kinds of research it supports through tax revenues and to receive progress reports on this research. The media regularly covers progress that is being made in AIDS research, for example, and it also covers other health stories on a regular basis. Media coverage of these issues has no doubt enhanced the public's awareness of health practices, medical science, and biomedical research.

In general, more cooperation is needed between the scientific community and the media to improve the reporting of biomedical research findings and to enhance the quality of health care information disseminated to the public. To facilitate the public's ability to make informed personal and societal health care decisions, the level of understanding of the scientific process should be improved. This, in turn, will also lead to a fostering of realistic expectations of science and health care. The scientific community should realize that the media can be a valuable ally in relaying information to the public, for only an informed public will continue to support the goals of biomedical research.

Public Understanding of Science

The formulation of the nation's biomedical research policy and the information required to make informed health care decisions are both highly dependent upon the public's understanding of basic scientific information. However, it seems that society's understanding of basic scientific principles falls considerably short of its interest in major scientific breakthroughs. In a national survey conducted in the late 1970s, for example, only 7% of the respondents had a clear understanding of science and scientific constructs.

The scientific understanding of the American public should be improved to foster realistic expectations and knowledgeable support of scientific undertakings and to assist in the formulation of informed health care decisions. Improvements in the public's understanding of science should begin with the reform of science education in the schools. This effort should be aimed at reversing the following trends: the declining enrollments in science courses, the declining mathematical ability among students, the general lack of preparation in science and math, and the shrinking number of trained science and math teachers. The National Science Foundation (NSF) has already made some progress in reforming science curricula, and it should be assured adequate funding to continue its work. The private sector should be encouraged to form partnerships with the NSF to share the costs of reform. State and local governments and local school systems should also participate in the evaluation and improvement of science education.

Reform of the health education curricula in the schools should be the responsibility of federal and state governments, local and state school systems, and boards of education; this topic is addressed in greater detail in the section on "Health Information and Education" in Chapter IV.

Communication of Research Findings to the Public

In general, the findings of research are reported to the public on a widespread basis through the "popular" media, such as newspapers, magazines, and television. Each party in this communications link — researchers, the media, and the public — has a role to play to ensure that findings are presented and interpreted accurately. To present accurate and understandable information, those parties engaged in biomedical research should determine how to handle inquiries from, and how to communicate effectively with, the media. Health care professionals, scientists, and institutions do not and cannot always anticipate the demands of the media as they cover news events of great interest to the public, such as artificial heart implants and AIDS research findings. In cases such as these, a proactive rather than reactive approach on the part of researchers could be helpful in facilitating the orderly flow of information to the media and to the public. Advance planning reduces confusion and allows the media and the public to receive full and reliable information. Seminars on developing effective communication skills and media relations should be offered to designated spokesmen by hospitals, institutions, and health care professions organizations.

Increased cooperation is needed between the scientific community and the media to improve the reporting of biomedical research findings and to enhance the quality of health care information that is disseminated to the public. Most members of the scientific community have developed good rapport with the media, and more relationships such as these are needed. To improve the quality of scientific reporting, the research community should develop a clearer understanding of how the media works. For example, inadvertent distortion or errors may be made by the media because of impending deadlines, editorial processes, or space limitations. Conversely, the media should develop a better understanding of the world of science. For example, the media are accustomed to factual reporting of information, but this is often not possible when writing about science. There are very few real scientific breakthroughs, and many researchers are reluctant to discuss preliminary research findings that have not yet been subjected to the peer review process.

Frequent roundtable discussions, seminars, and symposia should be organized to provide for an exchange of information between journalists and scientists, so that each group can have a better understanding of the other's profession. Such discussions might not eliminate all of the tension between the scientific community and the media, but they would provide each group with an opportunity to air their grievances, to understand their differences and, ultimately, to improve biomedical communication.

Although most biomedical research reporting is factually correct, at times research findings are not presented in an economic, social, or political context. For example, insufficient consideration may be given to synthesizing related elements into a broader context that includes potential costs or the social ramifications of an innovative technique, or there may be too much emphasis on "expert" opinions with little emphasis on reporting the views of those individuals in related fields who may have varying perspectives. Additionally, because decisions regarding health care may be based on information reported in the media, it is essential that the media verify health information through the appropriate channels before it is published. Media reports may, for example, lead patients to discontinue the use of a drug and thereby jeopardize their health.

Both scientists and journalists should communicate biomedical research findings accurately and in an appropriate context. Journalists should include information on the limitations of research and should be cognizant of the emotional content of the health news they report. Announcements of research findings should be handled with restraint by the news media. Physicians and other health care providers and their professional organizations should encourage health and science writers to check their information with them prior to publication. Journalists should also seek experts to interpret and verify the research being reported, but the opinions of individuals in related fields who may have different perspectives on the research should not be neglected.

News reports should include information concerning the design of the study, including but not limited to the number of patients involved, the length of the study, and the criteria for entry in the study. Information of this type is especially important in the reporting of preliminary research findings, since it enables individuals to critically evaluate findings before making any changes in their own health care and treatment.

Responsibility for the dissemination of correct and thorough information on the limitations of biomedical research findings rests primarily with the scientific community. Research results distributed to the media should always include information on the limitations and applicability of the study. At news conferences announcing research results, the complete scientific paper (or a version prepared by the authors for release to the media) should be made available to newswriters and reporters; the media kit should also contain background information on the disease or product. Providing complete information to the media would facilitate greater accuracy in reports of health care. Omission of information concerning the limitations of research, and in particular omission of information concerning preliminary or investigative treatments may only heighten the anxiety of desperately ill patients and their families. With the assistance of the scientific and health care communities, news organizations, reporters, and other journalists should develop internal review criteria for evaluating when scientific results have sufficient validity to warrant news coverage. For example, findings from a study involving a very small number of patients should be evaluated to determine if the research justifies coverage and to what extent.

Almost all health care stories have an emotional impact. The AIDS epidemic, artificial heart implants, organ transplants, and the Baby Fae xenograft are examples of emotionally charged stories recently covered by the news media. The media should balance their need to sell newspapers or commercial air time with the higher goal of informative and accurate reporting that does not prey on public emotion. The media should report on the aspects of health that are inherently interesting without resorting to sensationalism. The health care and scientific communities also have a responsibility not to overemphasize preliminary research results when such emphasis is unwarranted.

Role of the Peer Review Process in Communicating Research Findings

Scientific findings are frequently announced in the popular media prior to being subjected to review by colleagues, or peer review. The release of preliminary research results to the media occurs for a variety of reasons, including the researcher's enthusiasm over the research findings, the desire to establish scientific priority by attaching one's name to a research finding before competitors do so, competition resulting from the involvement of academic scientists in industrial biotechnology, or an obligation to sponsoring agencies or organizations. Sometimes the media report these findings as medical breakthroughs when the research has not yet undergone rigorous peer review or has not yet been published in scientific literature. In some cases, these breakthroughs may actually be insignificant, and therapeutic implications for the general population may not be well-defined.

Journalists generally receive a great deal of information concerning preliminary research results at medical and scientific meetings, which serve as forums for investigators to receive criticism and suggestions from peers on their ongoing research. Most organizers of such meetings arrange news conferences for the media, and advance copies of manuscripts may be given to the media. However, the media should recognize the preliminary nature of the work and should not present these preliminary findings as definitive.

Additionally, academic institutions, private industry, individual scientists, and funding agencies should not publicly announce results of biomedical research until they have received critical review by others in the scientific community. Peer review and publication of research findings do not guarantee scientific truth, but this research is no doubt of better quality than research that has bypassed the traditional channels of scientific communication. Those engaged in biomedical research should recognize that bypassing the established systems of peer review and publication does not contribute to good medical science or good science reporting.

Continuing Education for Medical and Science Writers

Many journalists who regularly cover medical and scientific issues do not possess specialized training in these areas. This is not to say that science writers are not well-educated— almost 90% of science journalists working in television or for major newspapers are college graduates and about 40% have completed some graduate work. Nonetheless, most health reporting skills are often developed on the job.

Journalists, like the public, should understand the nature of science and the workings of the scientific community. Medical and science writers should be encouraged to participate in continuing education seminars sponsored by public and private organizations to assess and broaden their skills and to increase their scientific knowledge. Journalists can develop skills by covering science and medical issues, attending media conferences and scientific meetings, and interviewing investigators and other authorities in biomedical science. Participation in seminars sponsored by private sector organizations and government agencies also helps journalists.

A number of private sector organizations foster the continuing education of science and medical writers by sponsoring conferences that highlight recent research findings or by providing background information on scientific issues. Voluntary health organizations also contribute to the continuing education of medical and science writers by presenting and discussing research results and sponsoring informative seminars on specific health problems. These organizations should continue to sponsor conferences and journalists should be encouraged to attend in an effort to improve the quality of science reporting.

The NIH, ADAMHA, and FDA currently sponsor seminars for medical and science writers to elicit more accurate reporting of health issues. The health care and scientific communities and the media should be made more aware of the existence of science writers seminars sponsored by government health agencies. Government health agencies should receive adequate funding to present science writers seminars. Government agencies that do not currently sponsor seminars (such as the Centers for Disease Control, the National Center for Health Services Research and Health Care Technology, and the medical research branches of the Veterans Administration and Department of Defense) should consider doing so. Interagency conferences should be created to avoid duplication of efforts as well as to provide a broad perspective on health issues.

Pharmaceutical and medical device manufacturers often sponsor informational seminars for health care providers on diseases for which they market products. Such seminars provide information on the etiology, diagnosis, and treatment of a disease and offer a forum for practitioners to exchange ideas on treatment. They also provide an opportunity for manufacturers to promote new products and to impart knowledge on health care problems to the health care community. The pharmaceutical and medical device industries should consider broadening these symposia to include media journalists, or creating separate seminars to educate the media about new products. Although media conferences and media kits already provide journalists with product information, that information may not always help the reporter to understand the disease and its prevalence, prevention, and treatment. The pharmaceutical and device industries should finance seminars and conduct them regionally. Eminent physicians, researchers, and other health care professionals should be invited as discussants. By sponsoring symposia for journalists, industry would more fully contribute to the knowledgeable, accurate, and balanced reporting of the results of biomedical research by the media.

Summary

The training and ongoing financial support of basic researchers and clinical investigators are essential to the advancement of the nation's health care system. While the pluralistic support system for biomedical research must be maintained, advantage should also be taken of new opportunities as they arise, such as cooperative research ventures between universities and industries. The proliferation of scientific knowledge and the application of this knowledge will continue to stimulate concern about the ethical and societal implications of biomedical research. These concerns must be addressed, both by the research community and by society as a whole. Only a fully informed public can be expected to support the goals of biomedical research.

Summary of Recommendations

Financing Undergraduate Education

1. The pluralistic system of financial support for undergraduate education for the health professions should be maintained. (p. 11)

2. The federal government should continue its support of undergraduate education for the health professions, especially to enhance access to the professions for minority and disadvantaged students and to supply professionals to underserved areas. The role of the Armed Forces, the Public Health Service, and the Veterans Administration in health professions education is important and should be continued. State and local governments should continue to support undergraduate programs of education for the health professions. (p. 11)

3. Public and private programs of undergraduate education for the health professions should actively solicit contributions from alumni and from private foundations. (p. 12)

4. While income from patient care should be used to support undergraduate education programs for the health professions, disproportionate reliance on this source of funding should be avoided. (p. 12)

5. Undue reliance on tuition and fees to support undergraduate education for the health professions should be avoided. (p. 12)

6. Student financial aid at the undergraduate level for health professionals should be based on demonstrated need. (p. 13)

7. Undergraduate programs for health professions education should consider financial aid trust funds as a means of increasing funding for student financial aid, including scholarships. (p. 13)

8. When possible, the costs of undergraduate education should be reduced; cost-containment measures include eliminating duplication of classes and facilities, controlling the length of education programs, reviewing the use of preceptorships as a teaching strategy, and contract education. (p. 13)

9. A consistent, comparable data collection strategy on the costs of undergraduate education should be used by all health professions. (p. 14)

Financing Clinical Graduate Education

10. A system of financing clinical graduate education that includes support from patient care revenues, including payments from Medicare and major insurance carriers, as well as specific subsidies, should be maintained. Federal, state, and local governments, as well as private foundations and private industry, should provide some share of support for clinical graduate education as part of their support for health professions education. The role of the Armed Forces, the Public Health Service, and the Veterans Administration in clinical graduate education should be continued. (p. 15)

11. Additional patient care costs associated with educational programs should continue to be included in payments made by Medicare and by insurance carriers. Direct patient payments should also pay for these costs. (p. 16)

12. Teaching hospitals that engage in patient care activities including research, tertiary care for severely ill patients, and uncompensated care, should be reimbursed by all payors in both the public and private sectors. (p. 16)

13. Stipends should be paid to trainees in professions requiring lengthy education when the trainee provides patient care services. When calculating the value of services, the teaching responsibilities of clinical graduate trainees should be considered. (p. 16)

14. A study of potential cost-saving innovations in programs of clinical graduate education, including, when feasible, the shortening of the duration of education, should be undertaken by professional organizations responsible for such training. (p. 16)

15. Medicare and other third-party payments should be made for the number of years of residency training required for admission to basic specialty board examinations or for five years. Rules concerning payments for residency training should be changed to permit payments for such training provided in ambulatory settings. The welfare of the public requires continued training of medical and surgical subspecialists. (p. 17)

Minorities in the Health Professions

16. Each educational institution should accept responsibility for increasing its enrollment of members of underrepresented groups. (p. 19)

17. Programs of education for health professions should devise means of improving retention rates for students from underrepresented groups. (p. 19)

18. Financial assistance, including scholarships, and financial counseling should be provided to minority students who are in need; financial aid should be based on a demonstration of need. (p. 20)

19. Health professions organizations should support the entry of disabled persons to programs of education for the health professions, and programs of health professions education should have established standards concerning the entry of disabled persons. (p. 20)

20. Financial support and advisory services and other support services should be provided to disabled persons in health professions education programs. Assistance to the disabled during the educational process should be provided through special programs funded from public and private sources. (p. 20)

21. Data must be collected about underrepresented groups in health professions education as a means of improving recruitment and educational activities. (p. 21)

22. Programs of health professions education should join in outreach programs directed at providing information to prospective students and at enriching educational programs in secondary and undergraduate schools. In addition, health professions organizations, especially the organizations of professional schools, should establish regular communication with counselors at both the high school and college level as a means of providing accurate and timely information to students about health professions education. (p. 21)

23. Health professions organizations must support programs directed at strengthening preschool, elementary, and secondary education legislative activities at state and federal levels. (p. 22)

Graduates of Foreign Health Professional Schools

24. Any United States or alien graduate of a foreign health professional educational program must, as a requirement for entry into graduate education and/or practice in the United States, demonstrate entry-level competence equivalent to that required of graduates of United States' programs. Agencies recognized to license or certify health professionals in the U.S. should have mechanisms to evaluate the entry-level competence of graduates of foreign health professional programs. The level of competence and the means used to assess it should be the same or equivalent to those required of graduates of U.S. accredited programs. (p. 23)

25. All health care facilities, including governmental facilities, should adhere to the same or equivalent licensing and credentialing requirements in their employment practices. (p. 24)

Educating Competent and Caring Health Professionals

26. Programs of health professions education should foster educational strategies that encourage students to be independent learners and problem-solvers. Faculty of programs of education for the health professions should ensure that the mission statements of the institutions in which they teach include as an objective the education of practitioners who are both competent and compassionate. (p. 25)

27. Admission to a program of health professions education should be based on more than grade point average and performance on admissions tests. Interviews, applicant essays, and references should continue to be part of the application process in spite of difficulties inherent in evaluating them. Admissions committees should review applicants' extracurricular activities and employment records for indications of suitability for health professions education. Admissions committees should be carefully prepared for their responsibilities, and efforts should be made to standardize interview procedures and to evaluate the information gathered during interviews. Research should continue to focus on improving admission procedures. Particular attention should be paid to improving evaluations of personal qualities. (p. 26)

28. Faculty of programs of education for the health professions must place greater emphasis than they have in the past on educating practitioners who are skilled in communications, interviewing and listening techniques, and who are compassionate and technically competent. Faculty of health professions education should be attentive to the environment in which education is provided; students should learn in a setting where respect and concern are demonstrated. The faculty and administration of programs of health professions education must ensure that students are provided with appropriate role models; whether a faculty member serves as an appropriate role model should be considered when review for promotion or tenure occurs. Efforts should be made by the faculty to evaluate the attitudes of students toward patients. Where these attitudes are found lacking, students should be counseled. Provisions for dismissing students who clearly indicate personality characteristics inappropriate to practice should to be enforced. (pp. 26-27)

29. In spite of the high degree of specialization in health care, faculty of programs of education for the health professions must prepare students to provide integrated patient care; programs of education should promote an interdisciplinary experience for their students. (p. 28)

30. Patient relations and ethics are appropriate subjects for continuing education; educational providers should increase the offering in these fields. (p. 28)

Boundaries of Practice for Health Professionals

31. Each state should establish a well-staffed and adequately financed bureau of health professional licensure for the purpose of administering and coordinating the work of the individual licensure and certification agencies or boards. That bureau should be overseen by a blue ribbon commission including representatives of the professions and the general public. The commission should be charged with mediating disputes regarding the boundaries of practice permitted under certification and/or licensure, the standards of certification and/or licensure, and the appropriateness of disciplinary actions taken by the individual licensing and certification agencies or boards. (p. 30)

32. Public and private third-party payment programs for the services of health professionals are required to define which services are treated as covered benefits. It should be an objective for public and nongovernmental programs alike to define those benefits so that essentially identical services are covered when appropriately and legally rendered by any category of health professional. (pp. 30-31)

33. The health professional who coordinates an individual's health care has an ethical responsibility to ensure that the services required by an individual patient are provided by a professional whose basic competence and current performance are suited to render those services safely and effectively. In addition, patients also have a responsibility for maintaining coordination and continuity of their own health care. (p. 31)

As a supplement to strengthen state licensure of health professionals, standard-setting and self-regulatory competency assurance programs should be conducted by and coordinated among health professions associations, certifying and accrediting agencies, and health care facilities. (p. 32)

Supply and Distribution of Health Professionals

35. A national consortium of concerned organizations and groups should collect, analyze, and synthesize data concerning the need and demand for, as well as the supply and distribution of, health professionals, by profession and by specialties within professions. Projections concerning the future supply of, and the need and demand for, health professionals should be developed by the consortium based on such data, and these projections should be made available to any interested parties. The consortium should be advisory rather than regulatory in nature. Issues related to supply should not be limited to aggregate numbers alone, but should assure adequate representation of groups that are currently underrepresented, such as minorities. (p. 33)

36. Licensure, certification, and accreditation should not be used for the purpose of regulating the supply of health professionals. (p. 34)

37. Appropriate agencies of government, as well as business, labor, and health care professional and institutional associations should collect appropriate data on the distribution of health care professionals relative to the unmet needs of communities throughout the country. Methods that are used to calculate the requirements for services of health professionals should incorporate the health care needs of the underserved. In the short-term, priority should be placed on funding mechanisms and organized systems of delivery to make professional practice in underserved communities more attractive than it currently is. In the long-term, the nation's education and training programs should place a high priority on attracting students who want to serve minority and underserved populations, whether such students are from minority groups or from the general population. Local and national leadership groups concerned about the needs of underserved populations should advocate major changes in financing and delivery mechanisms and in education to achieve an equitable distribution of health care professionals. Health care professional associations, third-party payors, and state and federal governments should stimulate grassroots pressure for modifications in financing and delivery mechanisms and in education. (p. 34)

38. Health professions' curricula should emphasize the needs of underserved populations, including the poor, minorities, the chronically ill and disabled, and the geographically isolated. Decisions regarding the financing of health professions education should be based in part on the data and analyses of the national consortium on the supply and distribution of health professionals. (pp. 34-35)

Maintaining Competence of Health Professionals

39. Health professionals are individually responsible for maintaining their competence and for participating in continuing education; all health professionals should be engaged in self-selected programs of continuing education. In the absence of other financial support, individual health professionals should be responsible for the cost of their own continuing education. (pp. 35-36)

40. Professional schools and health professions organizations should develop additional continuing education self-assessment programs, should prepare guides to continuing education programs to be taken by practitioners throughout their careers, and should make efforts to ensure that acceptable programs of continuing education are available to practitioners. (p. 36)

41. Only those health professionals who fail to meet the requirements of a recognized health professional organization should be required to report participation in continuing education directly to a state licensing board. (p. 36)

42. Health professions organizations and faculty of programs of health professions education should develop standards for competence. Such standards should be reviewed and revised periodically. (p. 36)

43. When reliable and cost-effective means of assessing continuing competence are developed, they should be required for continued practice. (p. 37)

Moral and Ethical Issues in the Use of Health Care Technologies

44.   The criteria on which to base professional recommendations for the application or withdrawal of health care technology should be developed by the individual health care facility in which the technology is to be used, and should be consistent with professional and ethical considerations. Each health care facility should establish a permanent ethics committee, composed of health professionals and lay representatives from the general community, to develop the criteria. Each facility should, on an ad hoc basis, convene ethics committees to advise health professionals and patients regarding the application of criteria to individual cases. In those cases in which a technology is used outside of a health care facility, local consortia of health professionals and lay people should be created to develop criteria governing the application or withdrawal of health care technology. (p. 44)

45.   Recommendations by a health professional to apply or withdraw a health care technology in the diagnosis or treatment of an individual patient must be based on clinically valid criteria consistent with professional and ethical standards. In particular, such decisions should not be based on the patient's chronological (as opposed to biological) age, sex, race, ethnic origin, current wealth or probable future income, but should take into consideration the quality of life resulting from application or withdrawal of the technology. (p. 45)

46.   The health care professional responsible for managing and coordinating an individual's health care should have the responsibility for determining whether application of a technology is clinically appropriate and consistent with the criteria established by the health care facility. That health care professional is also responsible for communicating recommendations, including the rationale for such recommendations, to the patient. The decision to use or not to use the technology should be made jointly by the health professional and the patient or his or her representative. When the decision to withdraw or deny a technology cannot be made by the patient or his or her representative and the health professional, either party should have the right to seek the counsel of an ethics committee. (p. 45)

47.   Competent terminally ill individuals should have the freedom to make their own decisions regarding the withholding or withdrawal of treatment. Appropriate individuals should be encouraged to develop guidelines for the withholding or withdrawal of treatment and state legislatures should be encouraged to pass "right to die" legislation. (p. 45)

48.   In making decisions as to whether to commit resources to the development of capital-intensive technology in a given area, the appropriate balance between individual and societal rights should be considered. Such decisions should take into consideration the recommendations and findings of local and regional planning entities as to the need for such technology in relation to the need for alternate services that might be offered and the appropriate distribution of the technology itself. (p. 46)

The Allocation of Privileges to Use Health Care Technologies

49.   Each health profession has the responsibility to identify the technologies for which its practitioners have the training, competence, and need to use in delivering health care services. Professional associations should arrive at these determinations openly, based on scientifically valid standards and criteria, and should inform the public accordingly. (p. 48)

50.   Each health care facility should decide which professionals (both as a class and individually) are allowed to use each technology in the facility, subject to the facility's licensure requirements and the standards developed by health professional associations. Such decisions should be consistent with the professional practice acts in the state. (p. 49)

51.   Health professional associations should establish mechanisms to ensure that health professionals providing technology in offices or other out-of-facility health care settings are qualified to use such technology safely and effectively. (p. 50)

52.   Privileges to use technologies classified as "investigative" should be restricted to those health professionals and facilities that can demonstrate sufficient experience in using related technologies; guarantee a critical mass of candidates for whom use

of the technology is clinically appropriate; devise a research protocol that can
meet recognized scientific standards; and demonstrate willingness to share data
for collaborative studies, while insuring confidentiality of individual patient
information. (p. 50)

Definition of Health Care Facilities

53. A health care facility should be defined as "a formally organized and legally
     constituted entity that arranges or contracts for the provision of health care and
     shares public accountability for the quality, accessibility, and costs of such care
     with the health professionals who provide or direct the care." (p. 52)

Licensure of Health Care Facilities

54. Omnibus and uniform principles that incorporate minimum standards should
     be developed to be used by states as a basis for their individual facility
     licensing acts. (p. 55)

55. All nonfederal health care facilities should be subject to licensure by the state in
     which they operate. State governments should provide adequate staffing and fund-
     ing to support the implementation and enforcement of licensure laws. The federal
     government should ensure that its health care facilities meet the licensure require-
     ments of the states in which they operate, or comparable federal standards. (p. 55)

Supply and Distribution of Health Care Facilities

56. Local communities or regions should exercise the responsibility for assessing their
     needs with respect to the type, size, scope, and location of health care facilities.
     State governments should have mechanisms to ensure that needs of the underserved
     are being met satisfactorily and that wasteful duplication and costly excess
     capacity are minimized. (p. 56)

57. The role of the federal government in planning the supply and distribution of health
     care facilities should be limited to providing planning incentives and resources to
     states and communities for their activities. (p. 57)

58. It is the responsibility of the governing body of health care facilities to ensure that
     the primary goal of facilities is to serve community need. (p. 57)

Planning and Delivery of Health Care Services

59. Planning agencies should utilize policies, educational programs, and incentives to develop and maintain individual lifestyles that promote good health. The planning process should identify incentives for the providers and participants in the health care system to encourage the development and introduction of innovative and cost-effective health care services. Government at all levels, as a provider, purchaser, and consumer of health services, should play an integral role in the planning process, including the provision of adequate funding and ensuring that government policies and/or regulations facilitate and do not unduly restrict the planning process. The authority to impose sanctions on those who take actions that are inconsistent with developed plans should be separated from the planning process. Funding for the planning process should be developed by the participants. (p. 63)

60. The planning process should seek to ensure the availability and the coordination of a continuum of supportive health care services for special populations in senior citizen centers, day care and home care programs, supervised life-care centers, nursing homes, hospitals, hospices, and rehabilitation facilities. (p. 64)

Access to Health Care Services

61. Decisions concerning the use of health care services, including the selection of a health care provider or delivery mechanism, should be made by the individual. (p. 65)

62. Both the public and private sectors should be encouraged to donate resources to improve access to health care services. Where appropriate, incentives should be provided for those in the private sector who give care to those who otherwise would not have access to such care. In addition, existing shortcomings in the current public system for providing access need to be addressed. (p. 65)

63. Health care facilities should have or should establish review bodies (such as hospital ethics committees) to resolve conflicts over access to scarce health care technologies. In the event that a conflict over delivery of scarce health care technologies cannot be mediated satisfactorily, individuals should be able to seek redress through appropriate appeal mechanisms. (p. 67)

The Transfer of Technology

64. All providers, payors, manufacturers, health care facilities, governmental units, and consumers of health care have an obligation to contribute to an orderly process of technology diffusion. The nature of each group's involvement should be based on the characteristics of the technology, which include safety and effectiveness, potential for societal benefit, and cost. (p. 69)

65. The availability and application of technology should never be limited in the health care sector because of cost alone, but continuing analysis of cost-effectiveness and cost-benefit should always be a major factor in the continued availability and utilization of a given technology. Public and private payors should make coverage available for any costly technology that can be demonstrated to improve health or quality of life and that is cost-effective. Coverage decisions by payors should be based on clear criteria for clinical indications and contraindications. (p. 70)

66. Third-party payors should support and promote limited diffusion of new technologies and regionalization of all technologies that are costly or resource-intensive. Third-party payors should accomplish this by limiting payment to those providers that demonstrate, according to professionally-developed standards, that they possess (1) a critical mass of potential patients for whom the technology is appropriate; (2) the resources to use the technology at a volume sufficient to achieve clinical proficiencies; and (3) an institutional commitment to maintain adequate standards of proficiency. (p. 71)

67. Third-party payors and professional associations should jointly determine, based on a technology's resource costs relative to other technologies, the payment level for a new technology. (p. 71)

68. Health care facilities should use processes that incorporate data regarding safety, effectiveness, cost, and conditions of use; and these factors should be balanced with the institution's mission, community need, delivery capacity, and financial feasibility in decisions regarding the acquisition of costly or resource-intensive technology. (p. 71)

69. Third-party payors should contribute to the acquisition of technologies that may
be expensive but that improve the quality of care; they should also contribute
to clinical research for the development, refinement, and evaluation of new
and established therapies. (p. 73)

70. Health care professionals and their organizations should ensure that the results
of biomedical research and of technology assessment are communicated in an
accurate and timely manner to both the research and the practicing communities.
Specialty societies, health care professional organizations, and local and state
medical societies should intensify their efforts to disseminate information to their
members on the effective use of technology. (p. 73)

71. The peer review system used by professional journals should be strengthened by
health professionals and their organizations. (p. 74)

72. Health care professionals should employ a variety of methods, including formal
continuing medical education and self-directed studies, to acquire the necessary
knowledge to use technology appropriately. (p. 74)

73. To enable them to use a health care technology, individual consumers have a
right to receive sufficient information from suppliers of health care technology,
providers of health care, and relevant governmental agencies. Consumers have an
obligation to comply with the instructions for the use of health care technologies.
Providers should make available sufficient information to allow self-administration
of low-risk technologies, and consumers should exercise their preferences for
these technologies either independently or in conjunction with the appropriate
health care professional. (p. 74)

74. In addition to assuring safety and efficacy, federal regulatory agencies should be
given the additional charge of assessing the long-term effects of their activities on
the development of new technologies. These agencies should be given the necessary
resources to perform this activity. (p. 75)

75. Manufacturers of health care technologies and the Department of Health and Human
Services and its branches should continue to cooperate in the research of rare
disorders and in the development of technologies for rare disorders. Additionally,
manufacturers should maintain the availability of currently utilized investigational
and marketed products. The federal government should improve the interagency
coordination of research efforts and product regulation. (p. 75)

76. The Food and Drug Administration (FDA) and other appropriate government
agencies should be allocated greater resources with which to strengthen postmarketing surveillance programs. With regard to the FDA, pharmaceutical and
device manufacturers should modify their postmarketing surveillance activities
to augment FDA activity. (p. 76)

77. Manufacturers and suppliers of health care technologies should ensure that
promotional material and marketing strategies provide accurate and balanced
information regarding the risks, benefits, and uses of products to be used in
health care. (p. 76)

Health Information and Education

78. Individuals should seek out and act upon information that promotes appropriate use of the health care system and that promotes a healthy lifestyle for themselves, their families, and others for whom they are responsible. Individuals should seek informed opinions from health care professionals regarding health information delivered by the mass media. Self-help and mutual aid groups are important components of health promotion/disease and injury prevention, and their development and maintenance should be promoted. (pp. 82-83)

79. Employers should provide and employees should participate in programs on health awareness, safety, and the use of health care benefit packages. (p. 83)

80. Employers should provide a safe workplace and should contribute to a safe community environment. Further, they should promptly inform employees and the community when they know that hazardous substances are being used or produced at the worksite. (p. 84)

81. Government, business, and industry should cooperatively develop effective worksite programs for health promotion and disease and injury prevention, with special emphasis on substance abuse. (p. 84)

82. Federal and state governments should provide funds and allocate resources for health promotion and disease and injury prevention activities. (p. 85)

83. Public and private agencies should increase their efforts to identify and curtail false and misleading information on health and health care. (p. 85)

84. Health care professionals and providers should provide information on disease processes, healthy lifestyles, and the use of the health care delivery system to their patients and to the local community. (p. 86)

85. Information on health and health care should be presented in an accurate and objective manner. (p. 87)

86. Educational programs for health professionals at all levels should incorporate an appropriate emphasis on health promotion/disease and injury prevention and patient education in their curricula. (p. 87)

87. Third-party payors should provide options in benefit plans that enable employers and individuals to select plans that encourage healthy lifestyles and are most appropriate for their particular needs. They should also continue to develop and disseminate information on the appropriate utilization of health care services for the plans they market. (p. 87)

88. State and local educational agencies should incorporate comprehensive health education programs into their curricula, with minimum standards for sex education, sexual responsibility, and substance abuse education. Teachers should be qualified and competent to instruct in health education programs. (p. 88)

89. Private organizations should continue to support health promotion/disease and injury prevention activities by coordinating these activities, adequately funding them, and increasing public awareness of such services. (p. 88)

90. Basic information is needed about those channels of communication used by the public to gather health information. Studies should be conducted on how well research news is disseminated by the media to the public. Evaluation should be undertaken to determine the effectiveness of health information and education efforts. When available, the results of evaluation studies should guide the selection of health education programs. (pp. 88-89)

Informed Consent and Decision-Making in Health Care

91. Health care professionals should inform patients or their surrogates of their clinical impression or diagnosis; alternative treatments and consequences of treatments, including the consequence of no treatment; and recommendations for treatment. Full disclosure is appropriate in all cases, except in rare situations in which such information would, in the opinion of the health care professional, cause serious harm to the patient. (pp. 89-90)

92. Individuals should designate surrogate decision-makers to act for them in the event of incapacity, and should provide instructions regarding their care. When a patient is incapable of making health care decisions, such decisions should be made by a

surrogate acting pursuant to the previously expressed wishes of the patient, and when such wishes are not known or feasible, the surrogate should act in the best interests of the patient. (p. 90)

Confidentiality of Health Care Records and Information

93. A patient's health record should include sufficient information for another health care professional to assess previous treatment, to ensure continuity of care, and to avoid unnecessary or inappropriate tests or therapy. (p. 92)

94. Conflicts between a patient's right to privacy and a third-party's need to know should be resolved in favor of patient privacy, except where that would result in serious health hazard or harm to the patient or others. (p. 93)

95. Holders of health record information should be held responsible for reasonable security measures through their respective licensing laws; it should be grounds for disciplinary action not to utilize proper security measures. Third parties that are granted access to patient health care information should be held responsible for reasonable security measures and should be subject to sanctions when confidentiality is breached. (p. 93)

96. A patient should have access to the information in his or her health record, except for that information which, in the opinion of the health care professional, would cause harm to the patient or to other people. (p. 94)

97. Disclosures of health information about a patient to a third party may only be made upon consent by the patient or the patient's lawfully authorized nominee, except in those cases in which the third party has a legal or predetermined right to gain access to such information. (p. 94)

Meeting Public Health Care Needs through Health Professions Education

98. Faculties of programs of health professions education should be responsive to the expectations of the public in regard to the practice of health professions. Faculties should consider the variety of practice circumstances in which new professionals will practice. Faculties should add curriculum segments to ensure that graduates are cognizant of the services that various health care professionals and alternative delivery systems provide. Because of the dominant role of public bodies in setting the standards for practice, courses on health policy are appropriate for health professions education. Additionally, governing boards of programs of education for the health professions, as well as the boards of the institutions in which these programs are frequently located, should ensure that programs respond to changing societal needs. Health professions educators should be involved in the education of the public regarding health matters. Programs of health professions education should continue to provide care to patients regardless of the patient's ability to pay and they should continue to cooperate in programs designed to provide health practitioners in medically underserved areas. (p. 96)

99. Faculty and administrators of health professions education programs should participate in efforts to establish public policy in regard to health professions education. Educators from the health professions should collaborate with health providers and practitioners in efforts to guide the development of public policy on health care and health professions education. (pp. 96-97)

Assessment of the Quality of Health Care Services

100.   Health care professionals and providers conducting quality of care evaluations should examine the process, structure, and outcome of health care services. Using the results of research on quality assessment, quality assurance, treatment outcomes, and technology evaluation, health care professionals should develop criteria to evaluate patient care. (p. 103)

101.   Multidisciplinary research to assess the quality of health care should be conducted. This research should concentrate on patient outcome relative to the structure and process of health care delivery, and should be broad enough in scope to be applicable to a multitude of health care settings. Research findings should be used to evaluate and improve quality assurance programs used by health care professionals and facilities. (p. 103)

102.   Educational programs that assist people in making informed choices about their personal health and about the appropriate uses of both self-care and professional care should be established. (p. 104)

Quality Assurance in Health Care

103.   Accountability through quality assurance mechanisms should be part of every system of health care delivery. Quality assurance activities must be expanded into nontraditional settings, new practice configurations, and specifically into the areas of chronic illness and long-term and ambulatory care. This effort must be a unified interdisciplinary approach with consumer participation where appropriate. The cost of quality assurance programs and activities should be considered a legitimate element in the cost of care. (p. 105)

104.   All health care facilities should be required to undertake or continue risk management programs. (p. 106)

105.   To fulfill its fundamental responsibility to maximize the quality of services, each health care facility should establish, through its governing body, a formal structure and process to evaluate and enhance the quality of its health care services. This should be accomplished by participation of the professional staff, management, patients, and the general public. Every health care facility licensed or certified to provide any kind of health care should be required by its licensing or accrediting body to establish a formal committee to coordinate all quality assurance activities that occur among the various health care professions within the facility. (p. 106)

106.   Voluntary accreditation programs with standards that exceed those of state licensure and that focus on quality of care issues should be offered to all health care facilities. Various agencies that accredit health care facilities should develop a formal interagency structure to coordinate their activities and to resolve any interorganizational problems that may arise. (p. 107)

107.   Public and private payment programs should limit their coverage for services provided in health care facilities to those that meet standards of acceptable quality, should structure their reimbursement to support the improvement of quality, and should provide information on quality for the benefit of their subscribers. (p. 107)

108.   Educational programs on quality assurance issues for health care professionals should be expanded through the inclusion of such material in health professions education programs, in preceptorships, in clinical graduate training, and in continuing education programs. (p. 107)

109.   Educational programs should be developed to inform the public about the various aspects of quality assurance. Health care facilities and national and local health care organizations should make information available to the public about the factors that determine the quality of care provided by health care facilities, and about the extent to which individual health care facilities meet acceptable standards of quality. (p. 108)

110.   The analysis of utilization patterns should take economics into consideration but not at the expense of delivering quality health care services. Government and private sector peer review groups should evaluate variations in the utilization of health services and should provide information about the characteristics of health care practices within the hospital staff, the local community, and the geographic region to health care professional groups and the public. (p. 108)

111. Research should be undertaken to assess the effects of peer review programs and payment mechanisms on the overall quality of health care. (p. 109)

112. There should be a coordinated and cost-effective system for data collection, analyses, and dissemination on a national level to improve quality assurance activities on the local level. (p. 109)

Qualifications of Health Professionals

113. State legislatures should develop a mechanism to consider the need for new health professional licensure laws; additionally, they should review existing health professional licensure laws to determine which should be strengthened to protect the public and which should be repealed because they are no longer necessary. (p. 111)

114. Private certifying organizations should be encouraged to continue certification programs for all health professionals and to communicate to the public the qualifications and standards they require for certification. Decisions concerning recertification should be made by the certifying organizations. (p. 111)

115. Working with state licensing and certifying boards, health care professions should use the results of quality assurance activities to ensure that substandard practitioner behavior is dealt with in a professional and timely manner. Licensure and disciplinary boards, in cooperation with their respective professional and occupational associations, should be encouraged to work to identify "deficient" health care professionals. (p. 112)

Professional and Societal Responsibilities Regarding Patient Injury

116. Tort system modifications should be evaluated to determine the extent to which they provide expeditious, fair, and reasonable compensation in a cost-effective manner for injuries that occur as a result of negligence. (p. 116)

117. A demonstration study of a patient compensation fund, which would replace the tort system as the initial entry point into the system, should be undertaken by a state or group of states. In this demonstration study, a broadly representative panel should make expeditious determinations about compensation for injuries arising from medically related events. Payments should be made according to a predetermined schedule based on the severity of the injury and/or should include limitations on the compensation for pain and suffering. The patient compensation fund should be jointly financed by the public and private sectors; the initial portion of awards should be paid by the public sector, subject to a cap per case and reduced by the value of collateral sources. In the event that the injured or the defending party is not satisfied with the determination made by the panel, then that party should have the option to reject the panel's decision and to sue under state law, subject to more stringent standards established to parallel the compensation system (i.e., when a plaintiff rejects the panel's award, tougher tort law standards would be triggered, and when a defendant rejects the panel's award, current tort law standards would govern the case). A substantial monetary penalty should be imposed when the result of a lawsuit is less favorable to the party that rejected the panel's decision. If both parties accept the determination of the panel, then access to the tort system would be waived. A report, which includes a study of the costs, the number and types of cases, any cost-shifting, and the degree of satisfaction of those involved in the system, should be prepared as the basis for future decisions. (p. 116)

118. State licensure/disciplinary boards should be given full and extensive disciplinary powers within constitutional limits. Members of state licensure/disciplinary boards should be granted immunity for actions performed in good faith, and they should be indemnified at state expense against any legal actions brought under either state or federal law when they are acting in good faith in performance of their duties. (p. 117)

119. Health care professional associations and health care facilities should be required to notify state licensing/disciplinary boards when disciplinary action is taken against a health care professional. (p. 117)

120. Health care professionals should report personal knowledge of any conduct that they reasonably believe constitutes grounds for disciplinary action to the state licensing/disciplinary board. (p. 117)

121. State licensing/disciplinary boards should be required to review judgments and settlements against health care professionals who have been judged negligent by the courts or who have settled claims which exceed a predetermined amount. (p. 118)

122. Information systems should be expanded to allow prompt transfer among jurisdictions of pertinent licensure and disciplinary information about health care professionals. (p. 118)

123. In the case of allied health professions, malpractice decisions and disciplinary actions of licensing boards and certification agencies should be communicated to a central clearinghouse. Health care facilities should have access to the resources of the clearinghouse to screen prospective employees, and the public should be able to use the clearinghouse to gather data to make informed health care decisions. (p. 118)

124. State licensure/disciplinary boards should be adequately funded to allow for appropriate investigation and disposition of complaints regarding quality of care and/or the competence of health professionals. (p. 119)

Ethical Considerations in Health Care

125. When making treatment decisions that involve ethical choices, health care professionals and patients (or their authorized representatives) should strive for a high level of mutual understanding and shared decision-making. (p. 120)

126. The establishment of ethics committees at health care facilities to provide ethical guidance to protect patients' rights and responsibilities should be encouraged. (p. 121)

127. The inclusion of ethics in the curricula of health professions education programs and emphasis on ethical concerns in the traditional peer review process should be encouraged. (p. 122)

Assessment of Health Care Technology

128. The primary goal of the assessment process should be the evaluation of the safety, efficacy, and conditions of use of existing and new health care technologies. Evaluations of the cost-effectiveness of such technologies should also be conducted, but as a separate process so as not to affect the evaluation of safety and efficacy. Health care technology should be evaluated on a continuing basis after its introduction, particularly if it is expensive or has potential for inappropriate applications in health care. The applications of the technology and the relationship between benefits and costs, both in general and with respect to specific patients, should be assessed through professionally-developed standards of utilization and peer review. (pp. 123-124)

129. An expanded and more organized system should be established for the assessment of health care technology. Individual organizations should continue to pursue assessment activities that further their organizational and societal goals. Additionally, a public and private technology consortium should be established to evaluate, synthesize, and disseminate assessment data and to administer an independent Council for Research in Health Care Technology Assessment. (p. 124)

130. Adequate funding for the administrative and organizational expenses of the public and private consortium and the Council for Research in Health Care Technology Assessment should be borne equitably by all voting members. (p. 124)

Health Services Research and Evaluation

131. Health services research should be regularly evaluated for reliability, validity, and timeliness, and health services research findings should be used in the development of national health policy. (p. 125)

132. The National Center for Health Services Research and Health Care Technology Assessment (NCHSR-HCTA), in conjunction with an Advisory Board, should be responsible for identifying informational needs and for determining the types of information to be collected to meet those needs. When appropriate, uniform standards for data collection to guide health services research activities should be established. Additionally, the work of the NCHSR-HCTA should be coordinated with all public sector research activities, including liaison with the National Center

for Health Statistics, the National Committee on Vital and Health Statistics, and state health agencies. Finally, the Secretary of the Department of Health and Human Services should be responsible for assessing the validity and reliability of research activities and for correlating and disseminating health services research findings. (p. 126)

133. The National Center for Health Services Research and Health Care Technology Assessment (NCHSR-HCTA) should be adequately funded to support an appropriate number of research projects, educational programs in academic institutions, and graduate-level education. The National Center for Health Statistics (NCHS) should be funded to ensure the continuity and maintenance of its databases and survey activities. State health data systems should be funded at levels commensurate with their responsibilities to collect mortality and morbidity statistics that comply with national objectives and unite public health activities. All constituents of the health care industry should continue their investment in basic and applied health services research, and philanthropic foundations and organizations should continue their support of research and training in health services. (p. 126)

134. A central body should be designated to act as a clearinghouse for the linkage, indexing, storage, and dissemination of health services research data and information. Data and information should protect the confidentiality of consumers, health care professionals, and health care facilities. (p. 127)

Designing a Cost-Effective Payment System

135. Health care recipients should have free choice of health care providers from among available resources. The following information should be made available through appropriate channels to the public: each professional specialty group's standards of education and training, standards of practice, scope of practice, and initial and continuing standards of competence; licensure standards, scope of practice permitted by the license, and licensed practitioners; the treatment outcomes of health care providers, as well as the varied classifications of health care providers; and the prices of health care services offered by different health providers. (p. 134)

136. With the exception of those professionals subject to mandatory price freezes and those providers located in states with mandatory rate-setting programs, individual providers should be able to determine what their prices will be for services offered. (p. 134)

137. Health care recipients, individually and collectively, have the right and the responsibility to negotiate health care prices with providers when possible. (pp. 134-135)

138. Individual providers and third-party payors should have the right to enter into contracts with each other. They should be allowed to designate their own bargaining agents in the negotiation process, and bargaining should take place at the national, regional, state, and/or local level as appropriate to the third-party payors involved. Providers and third-party payors should have the right to negotiate both the level of reimbursement and the payment mechanism. (p. 135)

139. Health care providers should consider the financial circumstances of health care recipients and should accept reduced fees when warranted. (p. 135)

140. Health care professions should have a role in the review of exorbitant fees that may be charged by their respective practitioners. (p. 135)

141. A basic benefit package for all Americans should be defined to serve as the basis for private health insurance plans and for public programs that finance health care. (p. 135)

142. Third-party payors should provide coverage of catastrophic costs. (p. 136)

143. Coverage for long-term health care services should include various options such as hospital care, nursing home care, hospice care, home care, respite care, and day care. Coverage for these long-term health care services should be financed through payment systems. The primarily social service aspects of long-term care—long-term custodial or institutional care and outpatient personal care—should be financed separately from health care services. (p. 136)

144. Alternative insurance plans, with different schedules of deductibles, coinsurance, and premiums, should be available to beneficiaries so that they are aware of the financial tradeoffs associated with different plans. Third-party payment systems should use deductibles and coinsurance as financial incentives for health care recipients to use health care resources in an appropriate manner. Cost-sharing should not result in an undue financial burden for the health care recipient. (pp. 137-138)

145. Recipients of health care should recognize their own responsibilities for avoiding unhealthy lifestyles and should be prepared to bear the financial consequences of their decisions. Health care providers should encourage health care recipients to engage in healthy lifestyles and should practice and promote preventive health care. Third-party payors should structure health insurance premiums to reward insureds who pursue healthy lifestyles. Employers, employee groups, and third-party payors should sponsor the development and presentation of employee educational programs to promote healthy lifestyles among employees and beneficiaries. (p. 138)

146. Employers, employee groups, and third-party payors should structure health care plans to provide necessary services to employees and beneficiaries without leading to unnecessary utilization of services. To foster freedom of choice and competition, employers, employee groups, and third-party payors should structure benefit programs which maintain access to licensed providers and various delivery systems. (p. 138)

147. Third-party payment mechanisms should be structured to place providers at some degree of financial risk with respect to their decisions regarding the use of health

care resources. Payment differentials to providers should be used as incentives to encourage providers to direct health care recipients to the most cost-effective treatment settings. As part of their education and training, health professionals should participate in programs that sensitize them to the impact of cost in their treatment decisions. (pp. 138-139)

Defining the Role of Government

148. The concept of Medicare as an entitlement program for the elderly, the disabled, and individuals with end-stage renal disease should be preserved, with a primary goal being the provision of cost-effective, quality health care. (p. 141)

149. As an initial step to improve Medicare program efficiency, a small percentage of the Medicare budget should be devoted to utilization review and research in quality assessment. (p. 141)

150. To help ensure health care benefits for future beneficiaries, Medicare trust fund reserves should be augmented through a combination of revenue increases, expenditure reductions, and program efficiencies. (pp. 141-142)

151. A study of copayments, deductibles, premiums, and tax mechanisms should be undertaken by government and private organizations to determine methods of equitably spreading the burden of Medicare beneficiaries' costs. (p. 145)

152. The basic Medicare package should be supplemented by other resources, including private insurance, employer-sponsored health benefits, individual savings, and tax-deferred retirement income plans such as pensions, individual retirement accounts, and salary reduction plans. The viability of an additional tax-deferred individual medical account should also be explored. Incentives should be developed to encourage individuals to purchase or obtain health insurance or to establish health care trusts to pay for health care costs, long-term care, and other potentially catastrophic health care costs. (p. 145)

153. Medicaid should be revised to establish national standards that result in uniform eligibility, benefits, and adequate payment mechanisms for services across jurisdictions. (p. 147)

154. Medicaid eligibility standards should be expanded to include the medically indigent; i.e., those needy individuals who are not eligible for Medicaid because they do not belong to a categorically needy group. Payment for Medicaid benefits for the medically indigent should be based on ability to pay. (p. 147)

155. Delivery and payment mechanisms in the Medicaid program should be subject to "test of performance" criteria to ensure that they are sufficient to guarantee appropriate access to quality and cost-effective care. (p. 147)

156. Medicaid should continue to be funded jointly by federal and state governments. Administration should be the primary responsibility of the state with federal oversight as needed. (pp. 147-148)

157. Individuals eligible for health care services through government providers should have the option to use private providers at government expense when these private providers are cost-effective. Cost-effective private alternatives to government providers should be made available. (p. 148)

158. Each state should establish a program to ensure that health insurance coverage is available to medically uninsurable individuals at a reasonable cost. (pp. 148-149)

159. To protect the public welfare, the federal government should exercise its authority to regulate self-funded health benefit plans so that they are subject to participation in state risk-pooling mechanisms and are subject to solvency standards. (p. 149)

160. Government, employers, and private insurers should give serious consideration to providing health insurance coverage for preventive child health care services. Existing government programs for child health care should be coordinated to avoid duplication of services and gaps in coverage. (p. 150)

161. Government regulations having an impact on the health care system should be evaluated on a regular basis to ensure that they are still needed and that they are consistent with the goals of ensuring access to health care services, ensuring fair competition in the delivery of health care services, and encouraging the efficient provision and use of health care services. (p. 151)

Availability of Funding for Research

162. Federal funding of basic and applied medical research should be increased at an
annual rate of 10% (after inflation) for the remainder of the decade, and funding in
the 1990s should be at a level sufficient to ensure appropriate growth in the nation's
biomedical research enterprise. The major recipients of these increases should be
the National Institutes of Health, the Veterans Administration, and the Alcohol,
Drug Abuse and Mental Health Administration. (p. 157)

163. The National Institutes of Health, the Alcohol, Drug Abuse and Mental Health
Administration, and other granting agencies should fund 40% of the approved
grant applications each year for the remainder of the decade. (p. 158)

164. Appropriate measures to reform patent, tax and licensing laws, as well as measures
to enhance the efficiency of regulatory processes, should be adopted by the federal
government to encourage private industry involvement in basic and applied
biomedical research. (p. 158)

Availability of Professionals for Research

165. In its determination of personnel and training needs, the Institute of Medicine
of the National Academy of Sciences should consider the future research
opportunities in the biomedical sciences as well as the marketplace demand for
new researchers. (pp. 159-160)

166. The number of physicians in research training programs should be increased by
expanding research opportunities during medical school through the use of short-
term training grants and through the establishment of a cooperative network
of research clerkships for students attending less research-intensive schools.
The number of physicians in research training programs should be increased by
providing financial incentives for research careers. (p. 160)

167. The current annual production of PhDs trained in the biomedical sciences should
be maintained into the next decade. (p. 161)

168. The numbers of nurses, dentists, and other health professionals in research training
programs should be increased. (p. 161)

169. Members of the industrial community should increase their philanthropic financial
support to the nation's biomedical research enterprise. Concentration of support
on the training of young investigators should be a major thrust of increased funding.
The pharmaceutical and medical devise industries should increase substantially their
intramural and extramural commitments to meeting postdoctoral training needs.
A system of matching grants should be encouraged in which private industry would
supplement NIH- and ADAMHA-sponsored Career Development Awards, the
National Research Service Awards, and other sources of support. (pp. 161-162)

170. Philanthropic foundations and voluntary health agencies should continue their
work in the area of training and funding new investigators. Private foundations and
other private organizations should increase their funding for clinical research
faculty positions. (p. 162)

171. NIH and ADAMHA should modify the renewal grant application system by
lengthening the funding period for grants that have received high priority scores
through peer review. (p. 162)

172. The support of clinical research faculty from the NIH Biomedical Research Support
Grants (institutional grants) should be increased from its current 1%. (p. 162)

173. The academic medical center, which provides the multidisciplinary research
environment for the basic and clinical research faculty, should be regarded as a
vital medical resource and be assured adequate funding in recognition of the
research costs incurred. (p. 163)

University-Industry Cooperative Research Ventures

174. Academic institutions and industrial firms should establish explicit guidelines,
policies, and goals for cooperative research ventures that will best accommodate
the interests and integrity of both organizations. The mission of academic institutions should not be compromised in any manner through participation in
cooperative ventures. (p. 164)

175. Faculty members should disclose the nature of and time spent in university-industry research ventures. When their major orientation becomes commercial development rather than teaching and research, faculty members should take a leave of absence or leave the university to pursue their dominant interest. (p. 165)

176. Regardless of the nature of the partnership arrangement, patent and licensing rights emanating from university-industry cooperative ventures should accrue to university, investigator, and industry by a mechanism agreed upon in advance. The degree to which a research project depends on proprietary information should be a prime consideration during the planning stages of a university-industry cooperative venture. Proprietary information can rightfully be viewed as being excluded from full disclosure of research results and, thus, its confidentiality should be maintained by both parties. (p. 165)

177. Universities should not engage in research at the expense of the educational mission of the institutions. Monetary profits emanating from cooperative ventures should accrue to the university, investigators and industry by an agreeable mechanism. (p. 166)

178. The free and expeditious communication of research findings to the scientific community should be a major objective of academia and industry. Reasonable delays for review of patentable subject matter and for filing of a patent application should be permitted. (p. 166)

179. The federal government should encourage the participation of small businesses in cooperative research ventures, and should continue to support starter programs for such projects. The federal government should be charged with conducting an ongoing analysis of the productivity and capacity of the nation's biomedical research enterprise, with the university-industry partnership as the focal point of the analyses. (p. 167)

180. State and local governments should be encouraged to provide a legislative, economic, and research environment conducive to the establishment of university and industry cooperative ventures. (p. 167)

181. Private industry should increase its financial support of university-industry cooperative ventures in biomedical research. (p. 168)

Ethical and Societal Considerations in Research

182. Private organizations and academic institutions should jointly develop a means to continue and enhance broadly based study and discussion of ethical and societal issues in biomedical research. (pp. 169-170)

183. The federal government should provide the resources to support new initiatives within the NIH for the funding of research studies in bioethics. Existing federal programs that fund bioethical research studies should be preserved. Private foundations should be encouraged to provide resources to support research studies in bioethics. (p. 170)

184. A uniform set of federal regulations governing research with human subjects, based on the core regulations of the Department of Health and Human Services (as revised in 1985), should be adopted by all federal agencies. Uniformity should not preclude additions to Department regulations that do not conflict with the core regulations or that enhance the protection of research subjects. (p. 170)

185. Associations of regional institutional review boards (IRBs) should be formed to enhance IRB performance through the development of educational site visits and local workshops. (p. 171)

186. Each institution should have a system both for monitoring the conduct of biomedical research and for investigating and reporting allegations of research misconduct. (p. 171)

187. All investigators involved in research projects should be responsible for the clear articulation and enforcement of standards that ensure the integrity of scientific data and conclusions. Regardless of whether the research project is a result of individual or collaborative efforts, investigators should thoroughly understand the data and conclusions in research publications and studies. (p. 172)

188. As part of their formal training in research investigation, graduate, medical, and postdoctoral students should be instructed on the importance of adhering to the

ethical and scientific requirements in research conduct and in the reporting of
research results. (p. 172)

The Use of Animals in Research

189. Researchers should include in their protocols a commitment to ethical principles
that promote high standards of care and humane treatment of all animals used in
research. Further, they should provide animal review committees with sufficient
information so that effective review can occur. For their part, institutions should
strengthen their animal review committees to provide effective review of all research
protocols involving animals. (p. 174)

190. The appropriate and humane use of animals in biomedical research should not
be unduly restricted. Local and national efforts to inform the public about the
importance of the use of animals in research should be supported. (p. 175)

191. The development of suitable alternatives to the use of animals in research should
be encouraged among investigators and supported by government and private
organizations. The selection of alternatives ultimately must reside with the
research investigator. (p. 175)

Communication among the Research Community, the Media, and the Public

192. The scientific understanding of the American public should be improved to foster
realistic expectations and knowledgeable support of scientific undertakings and to
assist in the formulation of informed health care decisions. (p. 176)

193. Those parties engaged in biomedical research should determine how to handle
inquiries from, and how to communicate effectively with, the media. Increased
cooperation is needed between the scientific community and the media to improve
the reporting of biomedical research findings and to enhance the quality of
health care information that is disseminated to the public. Both scientists and
journalists should communicate biomedical research findings accurately and in
an appropriate context. Journalists should include information on the limitations
of research and should be cognizant of the emotional content of the health news
they report. (pp. 176-177)

194. Academic institutions, private industry, individual scientists, and funding agencies
should not publicly announce results of biomedical research until they have
received critical review by others in the scientific community. (p. 178)

195. Medical and science writers should be encouraged to participate in continuing
education seminars sponsored by public and private organizations to assess and
broaden their skills and to increase their scientific knowledge. (p. 178)

Appendices

Participating organizations that were represented on the Steering Committee were given an opportunity to submit formal comments on and dissenting opinions to the Health Policy Agenda.

It is clear from the wide diversity of comments and opinions that the participating organizations subscribe to a broad range of philosophies on how to best structure and manage a health care system. For example, some organizations prefer a system in which there is greater reliance on market forces, while others believe that more emphasis should be placed on centralized decision-making by the federal and state governments. There are varying views concerning the extent to which the health care system should focus on treatment of health problems as compared to health promotion and disease prevention. Opinions also differ on how to meet the health care needs of the American people with available resources.

Participating organizations sought solutions to these issues by balancing the views of their constituencies with the needs of the public at large, and the Steering Committee sought a consensus on the most appropriate balance. Although differences remain, they do not negate the value of the consensus, which can serve as the basis for ongoing pursuit of the Health Policy Agenda.

Comments and dissenting opinions are presented below. Please note that when reference is made to a specific recommendation, the number cited corresponds to the recommendation as it appears in the Summary of Recommendations.

The American Association of Retired Persons is deeply committed to the goal of improving the quality, affordability, and access to our health care system for all Americans. Our 24 million members have made health care reforms our top priority across the full range of our activities—in consumer education, promotion of healthier lifestyles, community based prevention programs, consumer representation on regulatory and review bodies, promotion of biomedical and health services research, as well as advocacy for public policy reforms in reimbursement, coverage, and quality assurance.

The Association is deeply alarmed at the direction of recent changes in our health care system, particularly as they affect older Americans. First, the overall cost of the health care sector has been increasing at twice the rate of overall inflation since 1982. Second, some so-called "savings" in Medicare and other insurance programs have actually been nothing more than additional cost-shifting to consumers and do not represent any savings overall. For those 65 and older, average out-of-pocket expenditures for health have increased 50% in just five years—from $1200 in 1981 to $1800 in 1986. Third, a growing number of Americans are losing health insurance coverage. Despite the recent economic recovery, Americans with inadequate or no health insurance protection have increased from 28.6 million in 1980 to over 35 million today. Fourth, disturbing signs of gaps in quality are developing, from inadequate services for post-acute patients to increasing reports of injury due to error, patient "dumping," and over-intensive treatment procedures related to financial incentives for both providers and beneficiaries.

The AARP has participated in the Health Policy Agenda for the American People (HPA) because of our commitment to join in a constructive dialogue with provider representatives exploring needed health care improvements. Unfortunately, only the American Public Health Association and the Consumer Federation of America have joined with AARP to bring the broader perspective of health care users and public health concerns to this dialogue. The Association joins with the statements by the APHA and the CFA in voicing a shared concern with the limited scope, lack of vision, and anti-public sector value orientation of the HPA report.

AARP must briefly identify five major concerns with the overall direction and tone of the HPA report.

1. The obligation of health care providers to reverse out-of-control price increases and to support strong steps toward a more efficient health care system is not sufficiently addressed. The primary factors behind rising hospital charges, for example, have been growing intensity of services per admission and inflation in hospital prices beyond overall inflation levels. These are matters within the control of health care providers, and they should be addressed first before asking other segments of the population to bear diminished services or greater financial sacrifice.

2. The need for comprehensive physician payment reform is not recognized. Physicians are the effective decision-makers regarding health care utilization for the most expensive forms of treatment, so marginal reforms that do not impact physician compensation are not likely to achieve significant savings. Medicare Part B must be comprehensively reviewed and reformed to integrate the objectives of optimum patient care, beneficiary financial protection, and program efficiency.

3. Competition is over-emphasized as a strategy to curb escalating health care costs. Market-based incentives may play an important role in an ideal market environment, but we are a long way from such an environment today. Even with meaningful provider-specific information and greatly strengthened quality assurance mechanisms, competitive strategies risk improvements for the healthy and well-off at the expense of those less attractive segments of the health care "market"—those most in need of greater protections. Our experience to date indicates that enlightened regulatory programs, such as state all-payor rate setting, have been more effective than so-called "competitive" situations in furthering cost-containment, quality assurance, and improved access goals.

4. The Association takes strong issue with the HPA report's inference that there should be a reduction in government's role in health care and that public programs should be "scaled down" to serve only the needy. As a result of this anti-public bias, the recommendation for improving coverage for chronic illness and disability lacks sub-

stance, and other essential improvements where public sector action would clearly be effective are downplayed. Despite projected financing problems, the role of government needs to be strengthened to develop a more effective public/private sector partnership in managing health benefit programs. Contrary to the HPA assumption, there is absolutely no significant public support today for any withdrawal or weakening of our social commitment to health care programs.

5. The emphasis on greater financial incentives or cost sharing for consumers threatens a further weakening of health insurance protections for those already burdened with excessive direct costs. For Medicare, which today covers only 45% of the average annual health care bill, the path to a stable and strengthened program lies in the direction of better managed and more informed care, not in the direction of further erosion in insurance protection or in retreat from the universal nature of social insurance implied in means-testing proposals.

While these concerns with the tone of the HPA report are serious ones, the Association is also strongly supportive of many of the specific HPA recommendations. In particular, AARP cites the following proposals as worthy of broad-based public support and prompt implementation.

1. The need for a greatly increased public commitment to research on quality assessment and utilization review. The Association is convinced that higher-quality health care is also more cost-effective, and that greater knowledge with regard to outcomes and variations in practice styles could have tremendously beneficial implications for patient outcomes and health costs alike.

2. The call for development of a basic benefit package, which would promote better consumer understanding of coverage and greater ability to shop for insurance, as well as improved coverage for the millions of employees with inadequate insurance arrangements today.

3. The recognition that the consumer must play a greater role, both individually and collectively, in resolving problems of cost, access and quality. This role includes both direct participation in health review and regulatory bodies and collective negotiation with providers, where appropriate. To be meaningful, consumer action must be founded upon provider-specific information as to pricing and performance.

4. The need to strengthen and standardize Medicaid coverage for low-income Americans of all ages, including the medically indigent. It is a national disgrace today that 14 million Americans in poverty are not protected by Medicaid. Barriers to care due to poverty only result in greater social obligation in the future. There is neither a financial nor an ethical basis for Medicaid's present limitations.

5. The recommendation that Medicare be strengthened financially through a balanced program to assure future generations of older Americans that the promise will be kept for them. Solutions to Medicare's financing problems will of necessity involve a comprehensive set of program reforms and increased revenues. We should not await a more imminent funding "crisis" to begin this work. Continued public confidence in one of our most essential social commitments is at stake.

In conclusion, the AARP reaffirms its commitment to the process of seeking solutions to financing problems facing health care today, but insists that corresponding improvements in affordability, quality and access must also be implemented. It is our firm belief that meeting this challenge will involve an unprecedented effort on the part of the public and private sectors, as well as individual consumers and providers. We hope that the Health Policy Agenda project represents just the beginning of this process.
Submitted by Robert B. Maxwell

The Health Policy Agenda deliberations and product represent a synthesis of different points of view, reasonable compromises, and, in some cases, re-examination of the validity of previously held views. The principles and recommendations deserve general support. Clearly no one organization will be able to support every recommendation.

We want to reinforce the theme that the rights of the payer must be respected in the development and implementation of health policy. Payer, in this sense, refers to the individual or organization which actually provides the money for services, most usually a business or labor group or a unit of government.

We believe that the rights of the payer include: the right not to be assessed through charges for the care of individual for costs which are properly the responsibility of society as a whole; the right to design the benefit package through a process of free negotiation, with the understanding that in this process there are trade-offs, some of which may involve modifying health benefits for the sake of other desired benefits, particularly at a time when many families have more than one wage-earner, and thus access to more than one health benefit program; and the right to determine the degree to which the payer will accept fiscal responsibility for specific technologies or innovative means of delivery.

We also believe that in the absence of market discipline, some well-intentioned proposals may have adverse effects. For example, the report contemplates that all payers meet the cost of research and uncompensated care in teaching hospitals. If, in an era of provider competition, teaching hospitals must look to patient services as the primary source of revenue for these functions and if, therefore, collateral sources of funding are not developed, it is entirely possible that this inflation of the true cost of patient care in these institutions will make them uncompetitive in selective contracting situations, and jeopardize their ability to attract paying patients as they pursue their missions.

The proposal to provide additional funding to providers which render unusual amounts of uncompensated care may well have the effect of perpetuating providers whose continuing existence is neither necessary nor desirable. Initiatives to increase access for the medically indigent should be directed toward increasing the purchasing power of the poor, so that they may buy services in an open system, subjecting such providers to the test of the marketplace.

The mandating of benefits, whether by their value to society or by type of provider, may appear sensible and even desirable. Quite aside from the limitations mandates place upon the prerogatives of the purchaser, we view them as essentially dangerous because they separate the beneficence of the mandating body from the obligation (or even the ability) to pay for that beneficence. They may and sometimes do inhibit the carrier's ability to work with providers to reduce the cost of services. And they motivate purchasers to self-insure to avoid the added costs created by mandates, thus diminishing the community's insurance pool and its ability to cover individuals who are not members of employee groups and whose experience, typically, is more expensive than groups'.
Submitted by Bernard R. Tresnowski

Comments of the American Nurses' Association are directed to Chapter V of the Health Policy Agenda, *Ensuring Quality.* Specifically ANA's remarks pertain to the section *Authority of State Licensure/Disciplinary Boards.* Recommendations in this section call for full and extensive disciplinary powers for state licensing/disciplinary boards within constitutional limits and urge that boards be granted immunity for actions performed in good faith. While ANA concurs with the premise put forth in these recommendations we do not believe that they should be interpreted in any manner to sanction the restriction of competitive behaviors between and among competent health care professionals and disciplines.

Regulatory activity is essential to society because it continues to attest to the accountability of statutorily recognized professions to deliver safe and competent services to the public. In fact, recent and growing concerns about professional malpractice and an increasing fear of health professionals to participate in disciplinary activities because of potential litigation firmly support a call for stepped up regulatory efforts by state licensing/disciplinary boards. Unfortunately, some regulatory boards have engaged in anticompetitive conduct, aimed at restricting legitimate competition rather than policing professional incompetence.

ANA maintains that state regulatory boards of one professional group should have no authority over the actions of another professional group. Decisions by licensing/disciplinary boards must continue to address competency and should not result in the restriction of the ability of professionals to provide services to the public in their areas of practice.

Summary

Regulatory boards play a key role in assuring that all health care professions remain accountable for the delivery of safe competent and cost-effective services. However, efforts by regulatory boards to restrict unreasonably the practice of competent professionals will limit accessibility of affordable health care options.
Submitted by Eunice R. Cole, R.N.

The Health Policy Agenda for the American People (HPA) is an ambitious and complex task on behalf of medical care policy in the United States. The American Public Health Association (APHA) joined the HPA as a member of the steering committee only after the first phase of the project was completed. By then, the principles guiding the HPA and the issues to be addressed in the process were already well established. As a result, much of the foundation on which the recommendations rest, if not many of the specific recommendations, are inconsistent with APHA goals and policies.

APHA has three major concerns:

☐ the limited scope of the project: its focus on medical issues rather than the health of people;

☐ the lack of vision: the HPA relies too heavily on the rhetoric and concepts of the status quo, proposing only incremental changes, rather than reaching toward innovative long-range solutions to our problems;

☐ the value orientation: the emphasis on efficiency and cost constraint without balanced attention to equity of access and quality of care.

Scope:

The HPA is mislabeled. It is an agenda for "medical care" rather than for "health" of the American people. The bulk of the report deals with such issues as biomedical research (Chapter VII), technology development, assessment and dissemination (Chapters II, III, and VI), professional education (Chapter I), and the organization, delivery, and financing of health care services (Chapters III and VI). It deals with individual physician/patient relationships rather than with the health of the people or of society.

This is most evident in the recommendations related to health information and education (Chapter IV). The focus is largely on an inadequate individual one-to-one approach rather than a more appropriate community, population-based approach. Health education, fitness, and sports medicine is not the sum and substance of health promotion and prevention. Health promotion encompasses mental, physical, environmental, social, as well as emotional dimensions of health in an integrated mechanism focused on communities and populations, as well as, individuals.

This emphasis on the medical aspects of individual health, omits essential public health policy issues. We know that increased longevity in the United States, and in other developed countries, is largely due to improvements in the environment, nutritional status of the population, and prevention of disease rather than medical care. This evidence is given little or no recognition in the HPA. Consequently, even if all the HPA recommendations were implemented, they would have minimal impact on health status of the American people.

Vision:

While the plan of the HPA was to provide an agenda into the 21st century for the health of the American people, it has fallen far short of this vision. The HPA has failed to critically assess the effects of current reliance on the market place and competition as the resource allocation force in health care. Much of the analysis contained in the HPA that deals with the delivery, financing, and regulation of health services (Chapters III, IV, and VI) is quite selective in support of market-oriented recommendations, rather than an objective analysis of all the research and data that is available.

The market is inherently inequitable, a fact not addressed in the HPA. There is little recognition in the HPA report that while the market delivers health services to those who can pay, (i.e., those with adequate insurance coverage,) those who cannot pay, (45 million people at risk of medical indigency) get inferior care or no care at all. The result is that HPA proposes maintaining a two class system of health care in the United States, based on ability to pay.

Values:

The HPA relegates government's role to protection of the market and filling of gaps. The professions are delegated control of quality of care and price of services. APHA policy, on the other hand, places central trust and reliance on the people: individually as consumers and patients, and the public collectively as the community, state, and federal government.

While accepting the pluralistic nature of our current health care system, APHA is strongly supportive of a positive leadership role for government in health care as desirable and essential to ensuring public health and safety, quality and equity, as well, as efficiency and cost containment.

It is difficult to quarrel with many of the specific HPA recommendations, taken out of context. Who can *a priori* oppose more support for medical research? But HPA uncritically recommends that the federal government should provide annual increases of 10% in its support of biomedical research (Chapter VII). There is also a set of recommendations proposing the continued use of billions of dollars from Medicare, Medicaid, and private health insurance to subsidize medical education (Chapter I). On the other hand, Chapters III and VI, speak of rationing health care, insist on greater cost-sharing by patients as the principal means of cost containment, and propose options that would cut back on Medicare. Only three recommendations in Chapter III speak of access to health care: individual freedom of choice of providers; public and private charity for indigents; and ethics committees deciding on access to technology. The imbalance is also obvious from the relatively greater attention devoted to thorough analysis and discussion of industry-university cooperation in support of biomedical research, while much less is devoted to an inadequate discussion of access to health care by indigent persons.

In its chapter on the cost effective payment system, the HPA suggests that every American citizen should have access to a basic benefit package. This would seem to suggest that the HPA is agreeing that the American public has a basic right to health care. On the other hand, the basic benefit package is viewed largely as a private sector insurance mechanism, it has not been defined, and assignment of responsibility for meeting this guarantee is largely avoided.

Conclusion:

Implementation of this unbalanced policy agenda would continue to divert scarce resources toward professionally desired ends (research, technology) rather than toward enhancing the health of people.

APHA supports as a goal for the American people a national health program, providing universal coverage for all U.S. residents, with comprehensive services available as a right without restrictions on eligibility. Pending such a national health program, APHA supports public and private efforts that lead in the direction of such a program. Some of the recommendations in the HPA report lead in this direction, but as whole HPA falls far short of this kind of vision. The scope of the project is too limited, the vision short-sighted, and the values professionally self-serving. The American Public Health Association supports a more comprehensive view, a more comprehensive solution, and a balanced approach to considerations of equity and quality of care as well as efficiency of the health care system.

Submitted by Beverlee A. Myers, M.P.H.

The Business Roundtable believes that the participants and staff of the HPA should be highly commended for their efforts. The *Agenda* is, in most respects, workable and will, if followed, improve the quality and effectiveness of health care for the American people. However, there are four points which the Business Roundtable believes should be made regarding implementation of the policy proposals:

1. In various places the *Agenda* contemplates more direct federal government intrusion into the delivery of care than the Business Roundtable believes is necessary or efficient.

2. The *Agenda* seems to contemplate additional governmental mandating of the forms or level of employer health benefit programs. The Business Roundtable has serious reservations concerning the necessity and efficiency of additional governmentally mandated employer benefits.

3. The Business Roundtable believes that the *Agenda* should have addressed the issue of product liability as an important health care issue (refer to the Business Roundtable Tort Law Reform Policy Statement) and concurs with the general thrust of Comment and Dissent on this issue reported by HPA Work Group on Evaluation, Assessment and Control.

4. The Business Roundtable believes the *Agenda* has not properly positioned the importance of technology in providing quality health care to the American people. The Roundtable recognizes the vital role that technology plays in the maintenance and enhancement of quality medical care. In addition, the Roundtable believes that the *Agenda* is not explicit enough in explaining the role of the private sector, and health providers in encouraging a pluralistic system of technology assessment. The Roundtable believes that technology assessment is the concern of localities, institutions, individual providers, insurors and other payers, and the federal government's role should be minimized.

Submitted by Edgar G. Davis

The Department of Health and Human Services (DHHS) is pleased that the Health Policy Agenda (HPA) report presents a good, comprehensive statement of health policy, which in most cases is consistent with the general policies supported by President Reagan. In particular, we endorse the report's emphasis on individual responsibility and market competition.

Chapter I. Supplying the Professionals

"Financing Undergraduate Education for the Health Professions": DHHS agrees with the general thrust of the recommendations to provide broad-based support for undergraduate medical education, exclusive of the Federal government. However, contrary to the HPA recommendation that the Federal government continue its support of health professions education, it is Administration policy to discontinue programs in this area. This Federal policy is based upon recognition of an adequate supply, and a projected oversupply in some areas, of health professionals across the various disciplines.

"Quality Assurance Measures for Graduates of Foreign Health Professional Schools": The HPA recommends that all health care facilities should adhere to the same or equivalent licensing and credentialing requirements in their employment practices. This would imply some central or Federal role with which we would disagree. The Federal government has maintained a policy that individual States prevail in the determination of the criteria for credentialing health personnel, and that the licensure responsibility lies appropriately with each individual State. Resources available for health care vary significantly from State to State. Also, each State has its own unique health care needs. Similarly, some variation in credentialing criteria (consistent with quality health care outcomes) is needed across the various Federal health care systems.

We do not agree with Recommendations 11 and 12 in the section entitled *"Financing Clinical Graduate Education for the Health Professions."* Recommendation 11 states that "additional patient care costs associated with education programs should continue to be paid by Medicare and by insurance carriers." The examples provided are unneeded tests and supervisory faculty time. The Department's position is that

Medicare should not pay for unneeded services, and Medicare already recognizes supervisory faculty time as a reimbursable direct cost. Payment for additional patient care costs should either be borne by the education program of the facility or be part of the price of care provided. Medicare's (and other payers') obligations should be determined by their contractual agreement with the institution and/or the insured patient.

Recommendation 12 states in part that "teaching hospitals that engage in ... uncompensated care ... should be reimbursed by all payers in both the public and private sectors." Federal policy and Medicare law have been to limit Medicare's obligations to uncompensated deductible and co-payment amounts found to be uncollectible from patients. It is not proper for Medicare to fund care provided to patients who are not eligible for Medicare coverage.

Chapter III. Organizing the Resources

"Community Planning for the Delivery of Health Care Services": The HPA recommends that "government at all levels, as a provider, purchaser and consumer of health services, should play an integral role in the planning processes ... ensuring that government policies and/or regulations facilitate and not unduly restrict the planning process." While we cannot disagree with much of the text associated with this recommendation, we are compelled to issue a reminder that we do not believe there is a Federal role in the planning of health care resources at the community level. To the extent possible, resource planning should be a factor of market forces in a competitive environment. Any governmental responsibility for addressing resource development and deployment is a prerogative of the States and the local governments. We agree, of course, that any such planning activities should facilitate the efficient use of resources.

Chapter VI. Paying the Bill

"Quality Assessment and Utilization Review in Medicare": The implication of this recommendation is incorrect. Medicare has been supporting research and demonstrations concerning utilization review and quality assessment since the passage of

the 1972 amendments to the Social Security Act.

"Optional Supplemental Insurance": The HPA recommends that the basic Medicare package be supplemented by other resources, including private insurance. It should be recognized, however, that the *kinds* of supplements which pay Medicare's deductibles and normal coinsurance have had a substantial effect on Medicare utilization and spending since 1966. The private sector should develop additional and more effective options for beneficiaries to supplement the basic Medicare package. Individuals should be encouraged to place highest priority on those options which provide supplementation for long term care and other potentially catastrophic costs, instead of supplements which pay Medicare's deductibles or coinsurance for normally expected health care costs.

"Uniform Medicaid Standards for Eligibility, Benefits, and Payment Mechanisms": This recommendation overly stresses uniformity insofar as the terms and conditions for receiving Federal Financial Participation are concerned. The recommendation as phrased might hamper State abilities to manage Medicaid program expenditures and to bargain effectively with health service providers.

"Expansion of Medicaid to Include the Medically Indigent": This recommendation fails to consider the financial consequences of extending Medicaid to the noncategorically needy.

"Designing a Cost-Effective Payment System": In general, this section fails to encourage innovation and a more effective use of normal market forces in the health sector. Instead, it encourages resolution of the effective utilization of services to be worked out between third party payers and purchasers (Recommendation 146); between third party payers and individual providers (Recommendation 138); and standardization of benefits for both private health insurance plans and public programs that finance health care (Recommendation 141).

"Establishment of a Basic Benefit Package": This recommendation does not make clear why standardization is preferable to diversity. It cannot adequately be judged until the proposed follow-up group completes its work. Too rich a standard benefit package might hinder entry into the health care financing field and too scant a standard benefit package might hinder development of cost-effective delivery. Too rigid a standard benefit package might hinder competition between financial organizations. Also, it does not clearly establish why the same standard benefits should apply to both private and government plans.

"Options for Long-Term Care in the Basic Benefit Package": This recommendation implies that the medical aspects and social services aspects of long-term care can be distinguished legitimately and financed separately. This distinction is spurious, however. By most definitions, long-term care refers to a range of medical, health and social services for persons who, because of chronic illness or disability, need personal assistance in caring for themselves. The type and degree of services a person will need depends on the interplay of several factors, some of which are medical—degree of impairment, for instance; and some of which are social—personal living arrangements and the availability of family support systems, for example. Two persons with identical limitations in their capacity may require very different amounts of paid assistance or nursing home care, depending on the availability and capacity of informal caregiving arrangements. Thus, a financing system which ignores the social aspect of long-term care needs will be inherently inadequate for many individuals.

"Process for Determining Reimbursement from Third-Party Payors": The most important point in this discussion is that the justification for present laws which inhibit individual providers and third party payers from entering into contracts with each other and/or for collectively bargaining with each other should be seriously reassessed.

Chapter VII. Preparing for the Future through Research

While we enthusiastically endorse the HPA's strong support for Federal biomedical research, we suggest some restraint in the recommendations for increases in certain areas. For example, the recommendation for an annual increase in Federal funding of 10 percent (after inflation) for basic and applied biomedical research, as well

as the recommendation for Federal funding of 40 percent of the approved NIH and
ADAMHA grant applications are unrealistic and inconsistent with Federal budget policy.

The recommendation that NIH and ADAMHA should modify the renewal
grant application system by lengthening the funding period for grants that have received
high priority scores through peer review might not be a fair measure. We would suggest
an approach such as NIH's new merit awards program in which grant periods are
lengthened for investigators who have demonstrated an unusually good record of
accomplishment through several grant cycles.

Submitted by Robert B. Helms, Ph.D.

The Consumer Federation of America (CFA) is deeply concerned about the focus, emphasis and therefore a number of the specific recommendations of the Health Policy Agenda for the America People (HPA). CFA believes that health care policy should be based on a public, nationwide commitment to optimal health care that focuses on access to affordable, high quality care for all citizens and emphasizes public and private health promotion endeavors. Unfortunately, the HPA jeopardizes attainment of CFA's goals by placing unwarranted faith in the market mechanism to promote access to affordable, high quality care. Since CFA was asked to participate on the HPA steering committee after the HPA's principles and issues had been determined, CFA could not influence the overall thrust of the HPA process and therefore must dissent from the HPA's basic approach to solving health care problems.

CFA concurs in the dissenting views of the American Public Health Association and the American Association of Retired Persons. The HPA was built upon an anti-government bias and aimed at medical professionals' problems rather than peoples' health care needs.

In addition, the HPA process failed to provide ample consumer protection in issue areas where medical professionals' interests must be balanced against the concerns of other interest groups and the public interest. For example, consumers' interest in increased price competition among doctors and the public interest in protection of individuals' civil rights were damaged by the HPA's recommendation to provide broad legal immunity to members of state licensure/disciplinary boards.

Failure to enlist broader, more balanced participation in the HPA process led to ambiguities in recommendations, and the material supporting them, which may cause confusion. For example, imprecise use of technical legal terminology and inadequate representation from all facets of the legal profession led to HPA statements, assertions and recommendations that could be legitimately, but inappropriately interpreted as modifications of everything from constitutional to antitrust, labor, patent, tax and tort law.

Medical Malpractice

An overemphasis on doctors' complaints about our legal system led to HPA medical malpractice recommendations that could be interpreted as proposals to restrict the rights of individuals injured through inappropriate health care delivery. CFA believes these recommendations are meant to provide a no-fault addition to our current tort system, and CFA remains convinced that individuals injured as a result of medical negligence should be allowed to recover all their losses through the tort system. Had the legal profession and other interest groups been more thoroughly represented in the HPA, such confusion may have been averted.

Consumers' Role in Health Care Decisions

CFA believes that consumers must be allowed to play an active role in the health care decisions that affect them. While the HPA endorses consumer information in health care matters, it does not provide workable approaches to accomplish this result. Simply telling consumers to learn more or urging health care providers to divulge information and open up their decision making process will not provide the level of consumer participation that the HPA describes as essential to make its market-oriented recommendations successful. CFA believes that unless the HPA's consumer information and participation recommendations become a way of life in our health care system, the marketplace will not function to meet HPA's goals.

Basic Benefits Package

Despite CFA's concerns about the fundamental shortcomings in the HPA process described above, CFA supports a number of the HPA recommendations and endorses the HPA's consensus building process. The HPA recommendation that a basic benefit package should be provided to all Americans, with a commitment of public funding where the private marketplace fails to ensure provision of basic benefits, represents a major step forward for American health care policy. Without this HPA commitment, CFA would not have been able to participate in the HPA process.

Conclusion

To the extent that significant policy recommendations—like this commitment to quality health care through a guaranteed basic benefits package—overcome the substantial philosophical differences of the HPA participants, the HPA consensus building process has been successful. CFA believes the HPA should be viewed as a first step in the development of a nationwide dialogue about the health care needs of the American people.

Submitted by Gene Kimmelman

The U.S. Chamber is privileged to have had the opportunity to participate in this monumental project. The Chamber strongly supports this private-sector effort to develop a consensus for debate and a comprehensive framework for the current and future debate on major health policy issues. We commend those individuals and organizations that gave so generously of their time and resources to the Health Policy Agenda.

As noted in the Preface, the Chamber's participation and support for this project should not be deemed as an endorsement of, or opposition to, any specific policy recommendation or the accompanying rationale.

The Chamber believes that product liability is a significant issue that should have been included in the final proceedings of the Health Policy Agenda. Accordingly, the Chamber concurs with the statement on product liability filed by the Work Group on Evaluation, Assessment and Control.

The Chamber limits its "Statement of Comment and Dissent" to this issue because of our concern that detailed objections would detract from the "consensus" approach used to develop the recommendations and rationale. Further, the absence of a comment about a specific recommendation mistakenly could be deemed to indicate support for such recommendation or mistakenly be perceived as a lack of interest in the recommendation or denigration of its importance.

Submitted by Frederick J. Krebs

Chapter I

Under the recommendations on *financing clinical graduate education* for the health professions, we believe more emphasis should be placed that all payors should share *equitably* in the cost of medical education, so long as such costs are included in hospital patient charges.

Under the section on *boundaries of scope of practice,* we have concerns with the following recommendation:

□ *Recommendation 32: Third Party Payment Programs for Services.* This recommendation leaves unaddressed the issue of different payment levels for the same services provided by various health professionals. Further, payments to any category of health professionals has the potential to increase costs without a corresponding decrease in the level of services provided for costs overall.

Chapter II

We view the *definition of a health care facility* as a description and does not provide enough specification to allow insurers to satisfactorily implement their contractual responsibilities. The definition would have implications in the administration and interpretation of health insurance contracts.

Chapter III

Under the section on to ensure an adequate system for *planning and the delivery of health care services* we have concerns with the following recommendation.

□ *Recommendation 59: Community Planning for the Delivery of Health Care Services.* This recommendation is inconsistent with HIAA policy which calls for support of federal and state comprehensive health planning legislation.

Under the section to ensure the appropriate *transfer of technology* in the health care delivery system, we have concerns with the following recommendations:

□ *Recommendation 66: Third Party Payor Role in Diffusion and Regionalization of Technology.* We believe it is impractical for payors to encourage regionalization through their payment decisions, and a more systematic approach is required.

□ *Recommendation 67: Third Party Reimbursement for New Technologies.*

We believe this recommendation has clear anti-trust implications and appropriate legal clearance would be necessary to implement these recommendations.

□ *Recommendation 68: Health Care Facilities and the Acquisition of Health Care Technology.* HIAA policy in this area calls for a structured planning process to address various issues, e.g., to identify unnecessary duplication of costly technologies in facilities.

□ *Recommendation 69: Third Party Payor Support for Technological Innovation and Clinical Research.* We favor the approach that clinical research should be funded by the federal government. If funded by third party payors it could substantially increase health insurance premiums with no assurance it would reduce premiums in the future.

Chapter IV

Under the section on *information and education* for effective health promotion and health care utilization, we have concerns with the following recommendation:

□ *Recommendation 87: Third-Party Payors' Responsibilities for Health Promotion and Health Care Utilization.* We are concerned that the recommendation can be interpreted to support mandated benefits. (See comments on designing a cost effective payment system, under Recommendations 141-145.)

Chapter V

Under the section on *quality assurance in health care,* we have concerns with the following recommendations:

□ *Recommendation 107: Third-Party Payors and the Quality of Care in Health Care Facilities* Although we recognize the intent of this recommendation, carriers are not in the position to structure their reimbursement because of the lack of data on "quality of health care."

□ *Recommendation 110: Variations in Practice Patterns.* We support the promotion of national standards of care rather than utilization patterns accommodating economic considerations.

□ *Recommendation 112: Quality Assurance and Data Collection* This recommendation should be broadened to address the need for hospital charge and financial information, as well as utilization or quality assurance data.

Chapter VI

Under the section on *designing a cost effective payment system,* we have concerns with the following recommendations:

□ *Recommendation 135: Information on Professions, Licensure, Treatment Outcomes, and Prices* This recommendation, as well as the entire chapter, does not address the need for state health care management information systems in order for payors and consumers to identify cost effective and utilization efficient providers. We support the creation of mandated, uniform systems at the state level for the collection, analysis, and distribution of health care charge and utilization data, through a data disclosure board or commission. All hospitals should be required to submit specific utilization and charge data elements. The data would be displayed by hospital, by diagnosis and by payor category which would permit comparisons in the average length of stay, rate of admission and total charges broken by daily service and ancillary service charges. Only with these data systems in place, will purchasers of health care services have sufficient information to make knowledgeable decisions.

Further, the need for comprehensive health care management information systems is critical to all efforts aimed at health care payment reform including prospective payment, competition, utilization review and other marketplace options. Aggregation of comparable health care charge and utilization information as well as financial information, on a community-wide basis, will permit the identification of problems within the health care system, evaluation of options or solutions, and monitoring of the effectiveness of a broad spectrum of cost containment programs.

□ *Recommendation 141: Establishment of a Basic Benefit Package; Recommendation 142: Provision for Catastrophic Coverage in the Basic Benefit Package; Recommendation 143: Options for Long-Term Care in the Basic Benefit Package; Recommendation 144: Recipient Cost Sharing in the Basic Benefit Package; Recom-*

mendation 145: The Role of Healthy Lifestyles in a Cost-Effective Payment Program; We are concerned with the implication embodied in these recommendations, that policyholders would lose the freedom to select the characteristics of benefit programs to meet their needs. As long as these recommendations do not imply mandating of such benefits, we do not oppose these recommendations. However, HIAA opposes the proliferation of such benefits through government mandate.

□ *Recommendation 147: Role of Providers in a Cost-Effective Payment System* Regarding the recommendation on payment differentials, the HIAA supports the concept that discounts granted by hospitals be economically justified and not result in cost shifting to other payors.

Overall, this section relies exclusively on a competitive, deregulated system in order to control the rate of escalation in health care costs and utilization. However, competitive strategies, in addition to being unproven as a total approach to a cost effective payment system, leave an unanswered agenda regarding access, growing uncompensated care, underfunding of teaching hospitals and cost shifting. Hospital prospective payment programs in a number of states are currently dealing effectively with these issues. Therefore, future directions suggest cost effective systems at the state level which integrate regulatory and competitive approaches.

Under the section on the *role of government* in health care, we have concerns with the following recommendations:

□ *Recommendation 150: Restructuring of Medicare Funding.* Under *Options for Increasing Revenues,* HIAA opposes the taxation of employer contributions to health insurance.

□ *Recommendation 159: Regulation of Self-Funded Health Benefit Plans.* HIAA's position is to support the utilization of a tax code approach or incentive approach to guarantee participation by employers in risk pooling arrangements at the state level.

□ *Recommendation 160: Public and Private Coverage for Preventive Child Health Services.* (See comments on designing a cost effective payment system, under Recommendations 141-145.)

Submitted by James L. Moorefield

Chapter VII. Preparing for the Future through Research

The recommendations on the availability of human resources for biomedical research (recommendations 165-173) appears incomplete because of a lack of specific discussion of human resources for research in the behavioral sciences. Behavioral abnormalities, including substance abuse, are a major health problem facing the Nation. For many years the principle diagnosis associated with admission to VA medical care facilities has been mental disorder.[1] That category of principle diagnosis includes various types of substance abuse. The percentage exceeds by a small amount those diagnoses for disorders of the circulatory system, neoplasms, digestive system disorders, and disorders of the respiratory tract. The Veterans Administration has recognized this need and developed specific programs to encourage training in clinical research among physicians, nurses, and associated health professionals involved in treatment of patients with behavioral disorders.

The problem is larger than that faced by the microcosm of the Veterans Administration as identified in a recent report from the Institute of Medicine on Research on Mental Illness and Addictive Disorders[2] which notes in part "current ADAMHA funding mechanisms do not meet the needs of physicians who want research training, despite a serious lack of medical researchers to study mental and addictive disorders." — "In addition, more and better research opportunities are needed for physicians during residency." — "Both low stipends and programmatic restrictions of such positions are incompatible with the realities of most residency training programs."

This statement is substantiated by analysis of the history of NIMH research training support between FY 1977 and FY 1985. During that period, total support dropped (in inflation adjusted dollars) from 17.8 million to 8.9 million dollars or $\frac{1}{2}$ during the eight year period.

A 1985 Report of the Institute of Medicine on Personnel Needs and Training for Biomedical and Behavioral Research[3] separates the training of physician researchers including psychiatrists and the training of behavioral scientists, including clinical psychologists, sociologists, and anthropologists.

That report notes in part that "there has been an increase both absolute and relative to other areas, in the number of Ph.D.s who identified themselves as clinical psychologists and the number of new Ph.D. degrees being granted in that field. From the standpoint of the Federal Government's research program in the behavioral sciences, this trend is cause for some concern since most clinical psychologists work outside the academic center and many do not contribute to the research effort." The committee went on to note that "the number of non-clinical psychologists with post-doctoral appointments fell to its lowest level since the committee began monitoring these data. While some of these shifts may be due to sampling fluctuations the change could signal an important decline in research potential." The study goes on to point out that the total enrollment in behavioral sciences in both the graduate and undergraduate level have declined steadily since 1976.

In the section on the clinical sciences, the report notes that important changes have taken place in the way that medical schools are financing their operations and that there now is more emphasis on revenue generating patient care and relatively less on research. In addition, although physicians are applying for research grants at the same rates as they did in the 1970s, they are having less success in obtaining them. Finally, they note that "the Committee believes that more newly hired clinical faculty members should have some research training if the professional schools are to maintain their clinical research capability."

Specific concern in psychiatry was reflected in a recent paper in the *American Journal of Psychiatry*[4] noting that as clinical research in psychiatry has grown, the need for a growing pool of skilled clinician researchers has become increasingly recognized. Compared with positions in other specialties, psychiatrists and academic positions have less training in research and devote less time to it, which is reflected in a growing concentration of research funds from the National Institute of Mental Health in just a few medical school departments. The authors of this article suggest a four-point program to improve the situation. They further note that Federal spending on mental health research should be more than its current level of 0.5% of direct health costs for mental disorders.

The plea of this statement is to increase the number of researchers focusing attention on mental disorders and substance abuse without regard to the orientation or discipline. Research training budgets at the present time for NIMH, NIDA, and NIAA are low, approximating 17.5, 1.5, and 1.5 million dollars respectively, and have been virtually unchanged during the past decade.

The message to those reading this statement is that a specific area of research that needs attention, if the health needs of the American people are to be met, is the increased training of researchers in the behavioral sciences.

Submitted by David M. Worthen, M.D.

---

[1] Veterans Administration Annual Report 1985; [2] Institute of Medicine, "Research on Mental Illness and Addictive Disorders: Progress and Prospects," October 1984; [3] Institute of Medicine, "Personnel Needs and Training for Biomedical and Behavioral Research," 1985 Report; [4] Burke, J.D., Pincus, H.A., Pardes H.: The Clinician-Researcher in Psychiatry. *Am J Psychiatry* 143:8, August 1986.

While the *Agenda* adequately addresses the issue of professional liability in tort law as it relates to health policy for the future, we are concerned that it fails to address the health policy need to reform tort law as it relates to product liability. The issues were extensively discussed and pertinent recommendations were developed by the HPA Evaluation, Assessment, and Control Work Group.

Although not unanimous, the clear consensus of the Work Group is that the omission of the discussion and recommendations developed for the important issue of product liability represents a serious misunderstanding of the impact of the continuation of current tort law on future health care.

Current trends in liability law threaten the availability and cost of high quality medical products. Similar problems exist in many other areas of manufacturing. The inappropriate application of legal theories, a proliferation of law suits involving medical products, rising liability insurance costs and, in come cases, the unavailability of insurance are all factors contributing to the current product liability climate which raise the cost of today's products and reduce incentives to innovate with new products to improve and extend health care.

The present array of state laws governing product liability and the unpredictability created by varying interpretations of those laws serve as disincentives to product manufacturers. State-by-state variations in law create confusion for both manufacturers and consumers in assessing liability. In addition, a product manufacturer may be held liable for an individual's injuries even though the manufacturer is not found to have been negligent in the product's design, manufacture, or marketing.

Uniform federal product liability legislation should be enacted to clearly delineate the rights and responsibilities of both manufacturers and consumers. Such legislation should restore the fault principle wherein injuries would be compensable by a manufacturer only when a clear determination of negligence by that manufacturer is ascertained within a reasonable period of time after an injury. State of the art and foreseeability of possible injury should be defenses. Where products are closely regulated — as drugs and devices are by the FDA — there should be at least a presumption of proper product design and warnings if the product and its marketing comply with applicable government standards.

Advances in medical science and in health care technology may foster high, and sometimes unrealistic, public expectations regarding health care. Therefore there should be an increase in public education efforts to warn consumers of risks involved in the use of medical products and to address the deleterious effect of product liability litigation on the availability of medical products. There should also be continuing development of incentives for individuals to purchase health, disability, and other forms of insurance which would compensate for unexpected and untoward injuries not resulting from another's wrongful act, including those that may be sustained from the use of medical products. In addition, public welfare programs should compensate for such injuries to those justifiably not covered by private insurance.

Product manufacturers *should be held fully liable* for illness or injury attributable to *negligence* in a product's design, manufacture, or marketing. Injured individuals in such circumstances should receive full and adequate compensation from such manufacturers. However, the high number and cost of suits against manufacturers of medical products under current law has already forced manufacturers to remove beneficial products from the market and has threatened product innovation. Legislative changes, increased public education, and adequate private and public insurance are necessary to combat the present adverse product liability climate.

Submitted by Robert M. Vanecko, M.D.

The following section lists all 159 principles categorized by the Work Groups in which they were developed. The order in which the Work Groups appear represents the progression of health care as it moves from a scientific base (Medical Science), to the transmittal of knowledge (Education), to the application of knowledge (Health Resources; Delivery Mechanisms and Processes), to evaluation and payment (Evaluation, Assessment, and Control; Payment for Service).

Commitment to Medical Science

1-1. Biomedical research is essential to the continued improvement in the health of the American people.

1-1a. The productivity of biomedical research is dependent on continuing and long-range support. The nation must be willing to commit itself to the long-range goals of research to achieve future medical advances.

1-1b. The success of biomedical research is dependent on a population of highly trained and productive investigators. The federal government and the private sector must continue to encourage and support the growth, development, and maintenance of this corps of researchers.

1-1c. Funding of biomedical research in the United States should be the responsibility of both the public and private sectors.

1-1d. The federal government has the primary responsibility for assuring the viability of the nation's biomedical research effort. In matters of funding, the federal government has the primary responsibility for the support of basic biomedical research. The federal government also has a significant role in the funding of applied research.

1-1e. Private industry support of biomedical research is essential. Private industry has applied research as its major focus, but it also must play a significant role in basic research.

1-1f. The continued support of philanthropic foundations and voluntary health agencies for important and innovative biomedical research should be encouraged.

1-1g. University and other health-related institutions carry a primary responsibility for the conduct of basic and applied biomedical research and for the training of investigators. Continuing long-term support of this role by these institutions, by agencies that fund them, and by the public is essential.

1-1h. The goals and priorities of biomedical research appropriately are set by many funding organizations and institutions.

1-1i. The peer review system for research support has proved successful. It must be maintained with continuing strong support.

1-1j. Mechanisms to encourage and support innovative research and research into new and compelling problems of health care should be assured.

1-1k. Mechanisms to facilitate the timely application by industry of new discoveries and knowledge to health care should be encouraged.

Freedom of Scientific Inquiry

1-2. The freedom of scientific inquiry in biomedical research must be preserved.

1-2a. The acquisition of new knowledge should not be limited by concerns regarding the potential application of that new knowledge.

1-2b. It is proper that the conduct of scientific research be regulated to the extent necessary to protect the public interest and the rights of the individual.

Development and Evaluation of Health Care Technology

1-3. The biomedical research community must be free to follow promising, new, or unexpected leads and to apply the knowledge so derived toward the development and improvement of health care technology.

1-4. Ongoing assessment is essential to the assurance and improvement of the safety, efficacy, and conditions of use of the nation's new and existing health care technology. This information should be widely disseminated to health professionals and the public.

1-4a. The research and health communities must continue to participate in the assessment of new and existing health care technologies. Assessment should be impartial and broadly representative.

1-4b. Assessment of health care technology must be based on valid scientific evidence and expert technical opinion. A funding mechanism for accomplishing this assessment must be identified.

Communication in Medical Science

1-5. The free exchange and dissemination of new knowledge must be preserved.

1-5a. Open and expeditious sharing of research results within the biomedical research community is essential to the orderly, efficient advancement of biomedical knowledge and health care technology.

1-5b. Methods to assure the timely and accurate communication of the results of biomedical research to health professionals are essential to the continued improvement in the nation's health.

1-5c. The public should be informed about the nature of biomedical research and its outcomes. To encourage realistic expectations, knowledgeable support, and appropriate adoption of research findings, it is essential that public presentation through any medium be accurate and in perspective.

1-5d. Marketing and promotional strategies must assure an accurate and balanced presentation of the benefits and risks of products and technologies to be used in health care.

Ethics in Biomedical Research

1-6. Public trust in the nation's science rests on the integrity of the scientific community. Personal honesty and adherence to established ethical guidelines are prime obligations of each investigator.

1-7. In conducting research, the rights, welfare, and safety of the participants must be protected.

1-7a. In overseeing the conduct of research, institutional review boards or comparable bodies perform a function essential to the protection of research subjects and to the advancement of medical science.

1-8. Progress in medical science and the development of new therapies rest on the appropriate use of animals in research. The scientific community has an obligation to exercise high standards of care and humane treatment of all animals used in research.

1-9. The scientific community has an obligation to consider the societal impact of research advances. When issues of broad social import arise, the scientific community should take leadership to assure that such issues are evaluated by interdisciplinary groups that consider the biological, medical, ethical, and legal aspects of the problem.

Access to Education for the Health Professions

2-1. Health care professionals, including practitioners, educators, and research scientists are essential for the health care needs of the American people.

2-1a. Individuals intending to enter the health professions should undertake a general preparatory education in the arts, humanities, and social sciences, as well as in the biological and physical sciences. Admissions criteria for programs of education for the health professions should be structured to encourage general preparatory education.

2-1b. Preparation for entry into the health professions begins early in an individual's education; at every stage, personal integrity, an attitude of inquiry, and academic excellence are essential.

2-1c. Access of education for the health professions should be available to qualified persons without regard to race, sex, or ethnic background.

2-1d. Programs of education for the health professions should actively seek to enroll and to retain qualified students from underrepresented groups.

Content and Administration of Programs of Education for the Health Professions

2-2. The faculty and administration of programs of education for the health professions should be sensitive to standards set by the professions, to the expectations of potential employers, and to changing needs of society.

2-2a. The professions, educational institutions, and society at large share in the responsibility to assure that teachers and research scholars are prepared for and available for health professions education.

2-2b. Institutions engaged in education for the health professions should assure that their faculty maintain competence.

2-2c. Excellence in teaching should be an explicit goal of programs of health professions education.

2-2d. Decisions concerning the content of a program of education for the health professions should be the responsibility of the faculty. In exercising this responsibility, faculty should be sensitive to the concerns of the public, of accrediting bodies, of licensing authorities, of certifying agencies, and of the professions. The basic responsibility of faculty for determining educational content should be respected.

2-2e. Requirements for admission, promotion, and graduation in programs of education for the health professions should be determined by the faculty providing instruction. Principles of due process must be followed when promotion or graduation is denied.

2-2f. In graduate education for the health professions, professional organizations, including accreditation bodies, share responsibility with faculty for determining the content of education. Final responsibility for content remains with the faculty.

2-2g. Education for the health professions should promote an attitude of inquiry. The presence of research and other scholarly activities in the educational environment is an important means of promoting this attitude.

2-2h. Programs of education for the health professions should provide both the theoretical basis for the practice of the profession and a variety of appropriate, supervised practical experiences.

2-2i. General professional education should precede specialty education in the health professions.

2-2j. Faculty supervision in programs of education for the health professions should assure effective patient care and patient safety while providing increasing supervised responsibility for patient care.

2-2k. Those persons engaged in programs of education for the health professions should learn to work effectively with health professionals in other disciplines. Interdisciplinary learning experiences are an important means to this end.

2-2l. Programs of education for the health professions should provide for teaching cost-effective health care at the undergraduate, graduate, and continuing education levels.

Financing Education for the Health Professions

2-3. Continued excellence in education for the health professions requires long-term, adequate financial support.

2-3a. Financial support of education for the health professions should be shared by the public sector, the private sector, and students through tuition.

2-3b. Financial assistance should be available to enable qualified students with limited financial resources to enter the health professions.

2-3c. Funding from both public and private sectors should be provided for support of libraries and other information systems as fundamental and essential components of higher education.

Graduate Education for the Health Professions

2-4. Graduate education (education beyond the professional degree or certificate) for the health professions should be directed toward preparing specialists, educators, and research scientists.

2-4a. Programs of graduate education for health professionals are essential.

2-4b. Payments are justified to persons enrolled or otherwise participating in graduate education.

2-4c. The number of positions in graduate education should depend on the demonstrated ability of programs to provide education that meets standards acceptable for accreditation. The number of positions at the graduate level should be free from centralized regulatory control and should be allowed to adjust in response to changing circumstances.

2-4d. There should be a mix of graduate programs sufficient to provide education in all specialty fields.

Continuing Professional Education

2-5. Throughout their careers, health professionals should assume the responsibility to develop and enhance their knowledge, skills, and attitudes. The health professions should continue their efforts to assure the continuing competence of practitioners.

2-5a. New knowledge and the need to improve skills require that health professionals be involved in continuing education.

Accreditation of Programs of Education for the Health Professions

2-6. Accreditation should assure that all programs of education for the health professions meet acceptable standards. Principles of due process must be followed in accreditation procedures.

2-6a. Accreditation should be based on an assessment of the quality of an educational program, and should not be directed toward controlling the number of persons admitted to the practice of a profession.

2-6b. Accreditation should be the responsibility of nongovernmental bodies that include representatives of the lay public, the educational community, and the health professions.

2-6c. The cost and administrative involvement required in the accreditation process should be minimized: the quality and effectiveness of the system must be assured.

Health Manpower

3-1. The supply and distribution of health manpower should be determined by the health care needs of the people to be served, consistent with the availability of resources, avoiding harmful excesses and shortages.

3-1a. Decisions regarding the supply and distribution of health professionals must be a shared responsibility.

3-2. A qualified health professional should manage and coordinate an individual's health care as a shared responsibility with that individual (or his or her representative).

3-2a. Specific health care services should be provided by professionals who possess the training and competence to provide safe, effective, and appropriate health care.

3-2b. Information on professional qualifications of health professionals should be communicated to individuals in a manner enabling informed, cost-effective choices of the source of care.

3-3. The American public should have the assurance of qualified health professionals.

3-3a. The national origin of health professionals should not be a criterion for restricting entry into training or obtaining appropriate credentials.

3-3b. National mechanisms should evaluate and accredit foreign schools that graduate health professionals who seek postgraduate training or practice in the U.S.

Health Care Facilities

3-4. The number, type, and location of health care facilities should be determined by the health care needs of the people to be served, consistent with the availability of resources, avoiding harmful excesses and shortages.

3-4a. Funds must be adequate to encourage development and maintenance of needed health care facilities in appropriate locations.

3-4b. The determination of the services to be provided at local health care facilities must be shared by health care providers, those that pay for health care, and appropriate public, private, and professional regulatory mechanisms.

3-4c. A health care facility, through its governing board, should be held accountable for development of its facilities and services, with community need being the principal priority.

3-5. Once a facility's range of services has been defined, each health care facility should choose the specific services it wishes to provide and who should provide the services.

3-5a. Individuals should be able to choose their source of care within the limits established by the health care facility.

3-5b. The division of responsibility among health professionals within a health care facility should be determined at that facility on the basis of what is most conducive to safe, effective, and appropriate patient care.

3-6. The primary purpose of health care facilities should be to serve community needs by delivering health care.

3-6a. Those facilities with the capacity to do so should not neglect their role in education of health care personnel and in research.

3-6b. All health care facilities and health professionals should fulfill their social responsibility for delivering high quality health care to those without the resources to pay.

3-6c. Financing mechanisms and the regulatory environment should promote incentives for health care facilities to fulfill their primary purpose.

3-7. Each health care facility should be accredited, certified, or licensed by those organizations whose approvals are vital to help assure that the facility meets acceptable, recognized standards.

3-7a. Accreditation, certification, and licensing procedures should be conducted in a coordinated and cost-effective manner.

3-7b. Organizations that accredit, certify, or license health care facilities should base their decisions on a set of clearly stated standards and criteria that are relevant to the facility's mission.

3-8.   The use and distribution of health care technology should be determined by the health care needs of the people to be served, consistent with the availability of resources, avoiding harmful excesses and shortages.

3-8a. The incorporation of any technology in a given health care setting should be governed by the ability to use the technology safely, effectively, efficiently, and legally.

3-8b. The individual health care facility or health professional should be responsible for controlling the use of technology, for sharing expensive technology, and for cooperating in regionalization.

3-8c. Ethical issues should be considered in all applications of health care technology.

3-9.   Technology should be used in the care of patients solely to achieve potential meaningful benefit in health or quality of life.

3-9a. The choice of appropriate technology should be made by the responsible health professional; such technology should be utilized only with the informed consent of the patient.

3-9b. The individual health professional is obligated to utilize health care technology in accordance with professional standards and the clinical needs of the patient; third-party payors should limit their reimbursement to utilization that meets professional standards.

4-1.   The American people should be collectively responsible for the assurance of access to necessary health care for every individual, regardless of ability to pay.

4-2.   Individuals should have the freedom to choose from among the health care delivery mechanisms available to them.

4-3.   Innovation in health care delivery mechanisms should be encouraged and allowed to develop freely.

4-4.   Health care delivery mechanisms should be regularly evaluated.

4-5.   Health care providers and purchasers of health care have the mutual responsibility to make the most efficient and effective use of available health care resources; develop and promote safe and healthful life styles for all Americans; and encourage active participation by individuals in the planning and implementation of their health care.

4-6.   Interactions of the medical and legal systems should encourage efficient and effective use of health care resources.

4-7.   The successful administration and management of health care delivery programs require the knowledgeable participation of physicians and other health care professionals for such programs to function at the most effective level.

4-7a. Research concerning the effectiveness of methods of health care delivery should be encouraged.

4-7b. Financing for health services research should be recognized as an appropriate component of the cost of health care.

Health Promotion and Disease Prevention

4-8.   Health care professionals and other providers of health services should assume a major responsibility for the preparation and provision of educational information, incentives, and services to individuals and the public to promote health and prevent disease and disability. Representatives of government, industry, labor, and educational and philanthropic organizations should participate in these efforts. Emphasis should be given to preventive services for pregnant women, and infants and children.

4-9.   Individuals have a personal responsibility to seek out and act on information that promotes a healthful lifestyle for themselves and those for whom they are responsible and should be given incentives for the pursuit or continuation of such conduct.

4-10. Employers should utilize their unique opportunity and responsibility to promote health and prevent disease and disability by taking every reasonable step to provide a safe and healthful workplace consistent with the nature and inherent risks of the employment activity; fully informing employees, their representatives, and government agencies of workplace hazards; and promoting workplace practices and personal behavior that enhances the health of their employees.

4-11. Health professionals, in conjunction with scientists and representatives of industry, government agencies, and philanthropic organizations, should inform the public of environmental factors that influence their health. Further, research should be supported to identify, correct, and prevent present and potential environmental hazards and to stimulate their correction or elimination.

First Contact/Continuing, Referral/Consultation, and Specialized Care

4-12. Development of health care delivery mechanisms should be a collaborative effort of health care providers, those that pay for health care, and appropriate public, private, and professional regulatory mechanisms.

4-13. Delivery of health care is a shared responsibility of fully licensed physicians and other appropriately licensed or credentialed health care professionals who possess the training and competence to provide safe, effective, and appropriate health care.

4-14. Individuals have a right and a responsibility to participate knowledgeably in the planning and implementation of their own health care.

4-15. Individuals should have a free choice in the selection of an appropriate health care provider within an available health care delivery mechanism.

4-16. Individuals should be informed by those involved in the delivery of and/or payment for health care about appropriate and cost-effective utilization of the health care system.

4-17. Individuals have the responsibility to provide payment or to cooperate in another payment mechanism for the health care they receive.

4-18. Health care professionals should provide or guide their patients to the appropriate level of services and assure continuity of care when a referral is made.

4-19. When resources are finite, decision mechanisms should be available for the application of equitable criteria to determine that limitations should be imposed on the scope and intensity of care to be provided.

Long-Term Care

4-20. The provision of long-term care services should be based on a demonstrated need for care.

4-21. Long-term care should be provided in a setting appropriate to the individual's capabilities, needs, and preferences, and under the supervision of a qualified health care provider.

4-22. Individuals and their families have a responsibility to help provide for their long-term care in the home or other appropriate setting.

4-23. Payment mechanisms and benefit design should offer options for long-term care and should provide incentives for the use of the most appropriate setting and level of care.

Professional Jurisdiction

5-1.   Health professionals should educate the public regarding their scope of practice and the appropriateness of various treatment modalities. Patients should be able to choose a health care professional based on individual social, economic, personal, and other preferences.

5-2.   Health care institutions and their professional staffs should ensure the coordination, continuity, and quality of health care for all their patients.

Licensure

5-3.   A health profession or occupation should be licensed if the practice of that profession or occupation by persons who have not shown themselves to be competent and qualified to deliver health care services would pose a risk to the life, health, or safety of the public.

5-3a. Individual states should set the standards for licensure, but should cooperate with each other and with the appropriate professional groups to ensure that each state's requirements and implementation procedures best serve the goal of protecting the public health, safety, and welfare.

Professional Liability

5-4.   The primary responsibility of health care professionals should be the provision of high quality appropriate medical care by the most efficient available means.

5-4a. There should be fair and adequate compensation for injuries that occur as a result of deviations from acceptable levels of professional and institutional care.

5-4b. There should be fair and adequate compensation for injuries by medical products that fail to meet appropriate standards.

Certification

5-5.   Health professions specialty certification should be a voluntary procedure representing recognition by professional peers of education, achievement, and advanced training, and should not be required by state government authorities for licensing.

5-6.   Hospital medical staffs should broadly review each applicant's formal training and areas of demonstrated competency in considering applicants for staff privileges, rather than relying exclusively on certification.

Informing Patients

5-7.   Health care professionals have the responsibility to communicate with patients in a frank and informative manner that encourages both informed decision making by patients and a relationship of trust between patients and professionals.

5-8.   Informed consent to diagnostic procedures and treatment should include the following elements: ensuring of the patient's right of self-determination; the legal capacity as well as the actual ability of the patient or his/her representative to give consent to the particular procedure or treatment; disclosure of the purpose and the potential effects on the patient of the procedure or treatment and alternatives to permit an informed decision; and the voluntary decision of the patient regarding the procedure or treatment. The duty and responsibility for providing the information to be disclosed and for obtaining the informed consent should rest with each individual who initiates or directs the procedures involved in the particular case.

Peer Review

5-9.   Health care professionals in all fields should engage in peer review whenever the quality or efficiency of patient care can be enhanced by the process. The various health care professions should coordinate their efforts to facilitate one another's peer review programs and to avoid duplication.

5-10. Professional peer review should be the responsibility of each profession, a responsibility that should be exercised voluntarily.

5-10a. Judgments relating to quality and utilization review should be made by professional peers, especially when such review is mandated.

5-11. Professional peer review should promote high quality of care and should encourage economy of resources in the delivery of health care.

5-12. Maintaining confidentiality is primarily the responsibility of individual health care providers. Confidential information should be released only with the patient's or the legal representative's consent; in any event, no more information should be disclosed than is necessary for the particular, stated purpose in the consent.

5-12a. Third parties to whom information has been released should respect and protect the patient's interests and privacy. Patients should be informed if additional disclosures by third parties are anticipated without prior consent.

5-12b. Access to patient information for research and educational purposes should be available to appropriate individuals and agencies without compromising confidentiality.

5-12c. Health care professionals and institutions that maintain patient records should develop reasonable procedures to allow patients access to the information in their individual patient records.

5-12d. Procedures for the evaluation, control, and reimbursement of health services should protect the health care provider's legitimate need for confidentiality and due process.

5-12e. Defined, reportable diseases and unusual clinical phenomena that may affect the public health should be reported in confidence to the responsible public agencies.

Professional Judgment

5-13. Professional judgment should be an integral component of high quality care.

5-14. Professional judgment should be responsive to professional standards of care.

5-15. Professional judgment should be subject to review by peers to ensure that high quality, cost-effective care is delivered, in light of individual circumstances and conditions.

Professional Standards and Government Regulation

5-16. Government regulation within the health care delivery system is appropriate when it is necessary to protect the public health and safety or to ensure accountability for health care expenditures. Such regulation should give full and reasonable consideration to established professional standards.

5-17. The public health and safety require the establishment, implementation, and enforcement of professional standards to ensure high quality health care within the limits of available resources.

5-18. Primary responsibility for the establishment and implementation of professional standards should rest with the health care professions and institutions.

5-19. Applications of standards in the care of individuals should be based on the exercise of competent professional judgment.

Ethics

5-20. Health care practitioners should function according to codes of ethics that take into account traditions of the profession, moral values of society, and developments in science and medicine. Codes of ethics should be in addition to requirements of the law and the dictates of personal conscience.

5-21. Adherence to a code of ethics mandates that health care decisions by professionals not be made for the purpose of personal or institutional economic gain.

5-22. Codes of ethics should preserve and enhance patients' dignity and respect patients' rights to self-determination.

5-23. Health policy decisions should be based on medical, scientific, economic, and ethical criteria that preserve personal well-being, while assuring equitable access to care.

Determination of Payment and Expenditures

6-1. The financing and delivery of health care services should evolve through a process such that a pluralistic system is assured; price is determined through the interactions between individual recipients of care and providers or their agents; benefits for reimbursement of health care services are determined through the interactions of purchasers, payors, and their beneficiaries; individuals are responsible to provide payment or to cooperate in another payment mechanism for the care they receive; society pays for needed health services for those without the resources to pay; and regulation is sufficient to assure fair competition and access to health care services.

6-2. A market process should determine the balance between expenditures on health care (aggregate and per capita) and those for other goods and services.

Cost-Effective Health Care

6-3. Payment systems and benefit design should encourage the cost-effective use and delivery of health services while maintaining high quality care.

6-4. Government spending and taxing policies should encourage efficient production and consumption of health services.

6-5. Payment systems and benefit design should encourage the use of preventive services and the promotion of health.

6-6. New and existing health care technologies should be evaluated for safety, efficacy, and economic impact to be eligible for payment system coverage.

Individual Choice of Provider

6-7. Payment systems and benefit design should offer some options that allow individual choice of provider or delivery mode.

6-8. Payment systems and benefit design should encourage continuity of care.

Payment for Terminal Care

6-9. Payment systems for care of the terminally ill should emphasize concern for the quality of life.

Payment for Long-Term Care

6-10. Payment systems and benefit design should offer options for long-term care and should provide incentives for the most appropriate setting and level of care.

Education and Research

6-11. Payment systems should help support health professions education and some forms of research.

Material in this report was developed on the basis of policy proposals that were prepared by the Work Groups, reviewed by the Advisory Committee, and approved by the Steering Committee. The policy proposals contain background and statistical information, and can be found in the Reference Report. This guide has been prepared to enable the reader to cross-reference material in this report to material in the Reference Report.

For each chapter, the title of the policy proposal and the originating Work Group are listed. Because of overlapping content, policy proposals may appear under more than one chapter heading.

Chapter	Policy Proposal	Work Group
I. Supplying the Professionals	Financing Undergraduate Education for Health Professionals	Education
	Financing Clinical Graduate Education for the Health Professions	Education
	Enrollment and Retention of Minorities and Other Underrepresented Groups in the Health Professions	Education
	Educating Competent and Caring Practitioners in the Health Professions	Education
	Maintaining the Professional Competence of Practitioners in the Health Professions	Education
	Quality Assurance Measures for Graduates of Foreign Health Professional Schools	Health Resources
	Health Professionals: Boundaries of Practice	Health Resources
	Supply of Health Professionals	Health Resources
	Distribution of Health Professionals	Health Resources
	Qualifications of Health Professionals	Evaluation, Assessment, and Control
II. Providing the Technology and Facilities	Moral and Ethical Issues in the Application of Technology	Health Resources
	Allocation of Privileges to Use Health Care Technology	Health Resources
	Role of Cost in Availability of Technology	Health Resources
	Definition of Health Care Facility	Health Resources
	Health Care Facilities: Licensure	Health Resources
	Health Care Facilities: Supply and Distribution	Health Resources
	Resource Allocation and Access to Health Care	Delivery Mechanisms and Processes
III. Organizing the Resources	Communication between the Health Care Community and the Public	Medical Science
	Technology Transfer	Medical Science
	Role of Cost in Availability of Technology	Health Resources
	Allocation of Privileges to Use Health Care Technology	Health Resources
	Planning and Development of the Health Care Delivery System	Delivery Mechanisms and Processes
	Resource Allocation and Access to Health Care	Delivery Mechanisms and Processes

Chapter	*Policy Proposal*	*Work Group*
IV. Communicating Health Information	Communication between the Health Care Community and the Public	Medical Science
	The Response of Programs of Health Professions Education to Public Needs	Education
	Health Information and Education	Delivery Mechanisms and Processes
	Patient Health Care Decision-Making	Evaluation, Assessment, and Control
	Patient Health Care Information	Evaluation, Assessment, and Control
V. Ensuring Quality	Evaluation of Health Care Technology	Medical Science
	Health Care Facilities: Quality of Care	Health Resources
	Health Professionals: Boundaries of Practice	Health Resources
	Role of Cost in Availability of Technology	Health Resources
	Health Services Research and Evaluation	Delivery Mechanisms and Processes
	Quality of Health Care	Evaluation, Assessment, and Control
	Quality Assurance	Evaluation, Assessment, and Control
	Qualifications of Health Professionals	Evaluation, Assessment, and Control
	Professional and Societal Responsibility Regarding Patient Injury	Evaluation, Assessment, and Control
	Ethical Considerations in Health Care	Evaluation, Assessment, and Control
VI. Paying the Bill	Health Professionals: Boundaries of Practice	Health Resources
	Resource Allocation and Access to Health Care	Delivery Mechanisms and Processes
	Qualifications of Health Professionals	Evaluation, Assessment, and Control
	Design of a Cost-Effective Payment System	Payment for Service
	The Role of Government in Health Care	Payment for Service
VII. Preparing for the Future through Research	Availability of Funding For Biomedical Research	Medical Science
	Availability of Human Resources for Biomedical Research	Medical Science
	University-Industry Cooperative Ventures	Medical Science
	Ethical and Societal Implications of Biomedical Research	Medical Science
	The Use of Animals in Biomedical Research	Medical Science
	Communication between the Health Care Community and the Public	Medical Science

The following glossary was developed to provide clarity and consistency in the way selected terms were used in the Health Policy Agenda reports. The numbers at the end of definitions refer to the reference used in developing the definition.

Accreditation

A system for recognizing the credibility of educational institutions and professional programs affiliated with those institutions for a level of performance, integrity, and quality which entitles them to the confidence of the educational community and the public they serve. (13)

Applied Biomedical Research

Research directed toward the attainment of targeted objectives (e.g., development of a particular drug) through the application of existing knowledge to the solution of specific problems. (17)

Basic Biomedical Research

Research with the acquisition of knowledge as its objective. Basic biomedical research seeks greater knowledge and understanding of the physical, chemical, and functional mechanisms of life processes and disease. (17)

Beneficiary

An individual protected against certain present and future health care expenses by private or public programs. (22)

Benefit

A sum of money provided in an insurance policy payable for certain types of loss, or for covered services, under the terms of the policy. The benefits may be paid to the insured or on the insured's behalf to others. (12)

Biomedical Research

The formal quest for the acquisition of knowledge in the life and behavioral sciences and the formal investigation of the application of that knowledge for the advancement of preventive, palliative, curative and rehabilitative medicine and, thus, for the promotion and improvement of the health of people. (17)

Certification

The procedure for formal recognition of the qualifications of an individual in a professional or occupational field by an established group of professional peers applying predetermined standards. (1)

Competent

Duly qualified; answering all requirements; having sufficient ability or authority; possessing the requisite natural or legal qualifications. (4)

Confidentiality

Status given to a practitioner-patient communication in order to prevent unauthorized intrusions in the delivery of care and to protect the patient's right of privacy. (21)

Consumer

A person who may receive or is receiving health services. (12)

Continuing/Continuity of Care

Care received by a patient over time from a single health professional or from multiple but related health professionals (i.e., those practicing in a group), or coordination of care when referral is necessary. (11)

Continuing Education

Any education or training which serves to develop, maintain, or increase the knowledge, interpretive and reasoning proficiences, applicable technical skills, professional performance standards, or ability for interpersonal relationships that a health professional uses to provide the services needed by a patient or the public. (18)

Cost-effective

The activity which requires the least cost to produce a desired effect, or provides the greatest effect for a given level of cost. (6)

Credentialing

The recognition of professional or technical competence. The credentialing process may include registration, certification, licensure, professional association membership, or the award of a degree in the field. (12)

Delivery Mechanisms

Entities within the health system for delivering care e.g., private practitioner, HMO, hospital outpatient department, etc. (20)

Equitable

Impartial or reasonable in judgment or treatment. (6)

Faculty

The body of persons responsible for instruction and administration in educational programs. For purposes of this report, faculty is limited to persons with formal appointments. (18)

Government

The organization, machinery, or agency through which a political unit exercises authority and performs functions and which is usually classified according to the distribution of power within it. For purposes of this report, local, state and federal levels are included in the term "government" unless the term is modified. (14)

Graduate Education

Education beyond the professional degree or certificate, e.g., in medicine or nursing. (18)

Health

A state of physical and mental well-being and not merely the absence of disease or infirmity. (16)

Health Care

Those services provided by or under the direction of a qualified health professional for the maintenance of health and the prevention, diagnosis, or treatment of illness, injury, or disability. (19)

Health Care Facility

A formally organized and legally constituted entity that arranges or contracts for the provision of health care and shares public accountability for the quality, accessibility, and costs of such care with the health professionals who provide or direct the care. (19)

Health Education

The process of providing learning experiences which favorably influence understandings, attitudes, and conduct in regard to individual and community health. (7)

Health Care Provider(s)

Health care facility or health care professional or group of health care facilities or health care professionals that provide health care services. (2)

Health Care Setting

A location where health care is rendered. (20)

Health Care Technology

A set of techniques, drugs, equipment and procedures used by health care professionals in delivering health care to individuals, and the systems within which such care is delivered. (8)

Health Manpower

Those professionals who provide health services, whether as individual practitioners or employees of health care facilities. (12)

Health Professional

While this term has no consistent or agreed upon meaning, the following are a number of usual components of professionalism: formal education and examination are required for membership in the profession; certification or licensure is required for membership, reflecting community sanction or approval; there exist regional or national professional associations; there is a code of ethics governing the activities of individuals in the profession; there is a body of systematic scientific knowledge and technical skill required; and the members function with a degree of autonomy and authority. (12)

Health Services Research

Research concerned with the organization, financing and administration, effects or other aspects of health services, rather than with human biology and disease and its prevention, diagnosis, and treatment. In a sense, health services research concerns itself with the form and biomedical research with the content of medicine. (12)

Informed Consent

An act which supports the patient's right to self-determination and respect for personal autonomy in making voluntary decisions, based on the current state of knowledge, regarding a proposed procedure or treatment. (9)

Institutional Review Board

A group of at least five individuals with varying backgrounds which reviews protocols for clinical research studies conducted in a particular institution. The board must assure the acceptability of proposed protocols in terms of safety of human subjects, scientific merit, and adherence to applicable laws and regulations, institutional policy and relevant standards of professional conduct and practice. Most importantly, the board must assure that the investigator obtains the informed consent of participants and safeguards their rights and welfare. (17)

Licensure

The granting of permission by an agency of government to individuals to engage in a given profession or occupation. (21)

Long-Term Care

A range of medical, health, and/or custodial services for individuals who have lost some capacity for self-care due to a chronic or terminal illness or condition, and who are expected to need care for an extended period. (20)

Market Process

A process whereby decentralized, individual decision- making determines fees/charges, payment system benefits, and utilization. (22)

Medical Care

The provision by a physician of services related to the maintenance of health, prevention of illness, and treatment of illness or injury. (2)

Outcome of Care

A measure of the quality of medical care in which the standard of judgment is the attainment of specified end results, or outcomes. Outcomes of medical care are measured with such parameters as improved health, lowered mortality and morbidity, improvement in abnormal states, and patient satisfaction. (12)

Patient

A person who receives a health care service from a provider. (2)

Payment System

The method or methods by which providers or patients are paid. (22)

Peer Review

The process by which peers assess the quality and appropriateness of the care provided to patients by other peers; it encompasses both quality assurance and utilization review. (3)

Physician

A person who, having been regularly admitted to a medical school duly recognized in the country in which it is located, has successfully completed the prescribed course of studies in medicine and has acquired the requisite qualifications to be legally licensed to practice medicine. (3)

Preceptorship

The position of a preceptor or instructor; a tutorship. (18)

Prevention

Primary, those activities undertaken to prevent the occurrence of disease or illness; secondary, those activities undertaken after disease can be detected, but before it is symptomatic; tertiary, those activities undertaken to prevent the progression of symptomatic disease or illness. (10)

Private Sector

Nongovernmental entities including for-profit and non-profit organizations and individuals. (15)

Professional Judgment

The decision of a practitioner as to a recommended course of treatment based on the practitioner's diagnosis, training, experience, and skill, and on what is best for the individual patient under the circumstances. (21)

Professional Liability

Obligation of providers or their professional liability insurers to pay for damages resulting from the providers' acts of omission or commission in treating patients. The term is sometimes preferred by providers to "medical malpractice" because it does not necessarily imply negligence. It is also a term which more adequately describes the obligations of all types of professionals, e.g., lawyers, architects and other health providers, as well as physicians. (12)

Professional Standards

Patterns of practice developed by practicing professionals which take into account national as well as local variations in a particular professional practice; professionally developed expressions of the range of acceptable variations in health care. (12)

Public Sector

Government at the federal, state, and local levels. (17)

Quality of Care

A level of performance or accomplishment that characterizes the health care provided. Ultimately, measures of the quality of care always depend upon value judgments, but there are ingredients and determinants of quality that can be measured objectively. These ingredients and determinants have been classified by Donabedian into measures of structure (e.g., manpower, facilities), process (e.g., diagnostic and therapeutic procedures), and outcomes (e.g., case fatality rates, disability rates, and levels of patient satisfaction with the service). (5)

Regionalization

Efforts by individual facilities within a health care service area to share their services or technology with other facilities. (19)

Regulation

A principle, rule or law designed to control or govern behavior; may be voluntary or mandatory; includes self-regulation. (6)

Specialized Care

The health care provided to patients with complex medical and surgical problems by specialized providers in technologically sophisticated support facilities. (20)

Technology Transfer

An evolutionary process that encompasses translation of the results of biomedical research into the development of new technology and the subsequent availability, diffusion, and widespread use of technology in the health care system. (17)

Terminally Ill

(An exact definition is difficult because often a patient can only be identified as terminally ill in retrospect.) Patients who, according to the opinion of a licensed medical practitioner, have a life expectancy of six months or less due to disease or a medical condition for which there is no known cure. (22)

Third-Party Payor

Any organization, public or private, that pays or insures health or medical expenses on behalf of beneficiaries or recipients (e.g., Blue Cross and Blue Shield, commercial insurance companies, Medicare and Medicaid). (22)

1. American Board of Medical Specialties: *Annual Report and Reference Handbook, 1982.* Evanston, Illinois.

2. American Hospital Association: *Hospital Administration Terminology.* Chicago, 1982.

3. American Medical Association: *Proceedings of the House of Delegates.* Chicago, 1970-1983.

4. Black HC (ed): *Black's Law Dictionary,* revised ed 4. St. Paul, Minnesota, West Publishing Company, 1968.

5. Last JM (ed): *A Dictionary of Epidemiology.* New York, Oxford University Press, 1983.

6. Morris W (ed): *American Heritage Dictionary,* ed 2. Boston, Houghton Mifflin, 1982.

7. National Education Association and American Medical Association, Joint Committee on Health Problems in Education: *Health Education: A Guide For Readers and a Text for Teacher Education.* Washington, D.C., 1961.

8. Office of Technology Assessment, Congress of the United States: *Development of Medical Technology: Opportunities for Assessment,* Stock 052-003-00217-5. Government Printing Office, 1976.

9. President's Commission for the Study of Ethical Problems in Medicine and Biomedical and Behavioral Research: *Making Health Care Decisions.* Government Printing Office, 1982.

10. Report of the Departmental Task Force on Prevention: *Disease Prevention and Health Promotion: Federal Programs and Prospects,* publication DHEW (PHS) 79-55071B. U.S. Department of HEW, Government Printing Office, 1978.

11. Roos LL, Roos NP, Gilbert P, Nicol JP: Continuity of care: Does it contribute to quality of care? *Medical Care,* February, 1980.

12. Subcommittee on Health and the Environment of the Committee on Interstate Foreign Commerce: *A Discursive Dictionary of Health Care,* publication 59-8920. U.S. House of Representatives, Government Printing Office, 1976.

13. The Council on Post-Secondary Accreditation: *The Balance Wheel for Accreditation.* Washington, D.C., July, 1983.

14. *Webster's New Collegiate Dictionary.* Springfield, Massachusetts, G & C Merriam Company, 1981.

15. Weisbrod B: Private Goods, Collective Goods: The Role of the Non-Profit Sector, in Clarkson KW, Martin DL (eds): *Economics of Nonproprietary Organizations.* Greenwich, Connecticut, Jai Press Inc, 1980.

16. World Health Organization: Constitution of the World Health Organization, Basic Document, ed 15. 1961.

17. Medical Science Work Group of the Health Policy Agenda.

18. Education Work Group of Health Policy Agenda.

19. Health Resources Work Group of the Health Policy Agenda.

20. Delivery Mechanisms Work Group of the Health Policy Agenda.

21. Evaluation, Assessment, and Control Work Group of the Health Policy Agenda.

22. Payment for Services Work Group of the Health Policy Agenda.

Medical Science Work Group

Chairman

Richard T. F. Schmidt, M.D. (1982-1986)

Members

W. Daniel Barker

John R. Beljan, M.D.

Christopher Bladen

Hollis G. Boren, M.D.

Alice Chenault, M.D.

Bradford Cohn, M.D.

Jack P. Connelly

Marian Craighill, M.D.

Joe M. Crosthwait, M.D.

J. Richard Crout, M.D.

Ezra Davidson, M.D.

Herschel Douglas, M.D.

Tommy N. Evans, M.D., FACOG

Saul J. Farber, M.D.

Cpt. Peter A. Flynn, MC, USN, M.D.

Lawrence M. Gartner, M.D.

Robert S. Gordon, Jr., M.D.

Charles D. Hollis, Jr., M.D.

Jeffrey P. Koplan, M.D., M.P.H.

Robert D. Langdell, M.D.

Henri R. Manasse, Jr., Ph.D.

William L. Martz, M.D.

John L. Melvin, M.D.

Doris H. Merritt, M.D.

John H. Moxley, III, M.D.

John B. Nettles, M.D.

Frederick W. Pairent, Ph.D.

Nola J. Pender, Ph.D., R.N.

Vivian Pinn-Wiggins, M.D.

Ellen Pryga

William R. Robinson, M.D., M.P.H.

Joseph Seitchik, M.D.

Steve S. Sharfstein, M.D.

Greg Shipp, M.D.

David B. Skinner, M.D.

Alan Varley, M.D.

A. Carl Verrusio, D.D.S.

James E. Youker, M.D.

Primary Secretaries

R. Mark Evans, Ph.D. (1986)

William McGivney, Ph.D. (1982-1986)

Education Work Group

Chairman

Louis J. Kettel, M.D. (1982-1986)

Members

Jeanne F. Arnold, M.D.

Thomas D. Aschenbrener

David C. Broski, Ph.D.

Rose Marie Chioni, R.N., Ph.D.

Robert H. Christofferson, D.D.S.

Jordan J. Cohen, M.D.

Patrick J. V. Corcoran, M.D.

J. Lee Dockery, M.D.

Cindy L. Dyles

Lorene R. Fischer, R.N., M.A.

Robert D. Gibson, Pharm. D.

Robert Graham, M.D.

Jeffrey L. Houpt, M.D.

Eric R. Hubbard, D.P.M., M.S.Ed.

Gerald Hughes, M.D.

Kathleen Jennison, M.D.

Melvyn F. Jordan

James H. Lucien, III, M.D.

Mary McDermott, Ed.D., R.N.

Russell Miller, M.D.

Jack R. Pickleman, M.D.

James A. Pittman, Jr., M.D.

Edward James Potchen, M.D.

Robert R. Prentice, M.D.

Barbara Quaintance

Frank A. Riddick, Jr., M.D.

Mario V. Santangelo, D.D.S.

Raymond Alan Shelton, M.D.

Ned Smull, M.D.

Eugene L. Staples

Edward J. Stemmler, M.D.

Cpt. Marjorie A. Swetonic, NC, USN

Randy L. Teach, Ph.D.

Robert E. Windom, M.D.

David M. Worthen, M.D.

Primary Secretary

Arthur Osteen, Ph.D. (1982-1986)

Health Resources Work Group

Chairman

Sister Irene Kraus (1982-1986)

Members

Frank K. Abbot, M.D.

Kathryn Allen

Donald C. Ames, M.D.

Carolyn Baum, M.A., OTR

Lt. Col. Randy S. Blansett, USAF, MSC

Herbert W. Browne

Kenneth Clemens, D.D.S.

V. Agnes Davidson

Roy R. Deffebach, M.D.

Frank Delay

Keith Denkler, M.D.

William F. Donaldson, M.D.

Rhetaugh G. Dumas, Ph.D.

William A. Fogarty, M.D.

Sidney M. Ford

Evangeline R. H. Franklin, M.D.

Donald H. Hanscom, M.D.

Kevin F. Hickey

Nat E. Hyder, Jr., M.D.

William J. Jacoby, Jr., M.D.

Clarice Jones, M.S.W.

Doris C. Jones, R.N.

Joseph A. Leveque

Thomas M. Marchant, III

John E. Marshall, Ph.D.

Frederick T. Merchant, M.D.

Warren H. Pearse, M.D.

Richard P. Penna, Pharm.D.

Henry B. Peters, O.D.

Maurice F. Rabb, M.D.

William J. Reals, M.D.

Frank A. Riddick, Jr., M.D.

Frank Samuel

Malcolm O. Scamahorn, M.D.

Steven Sieverts

Scott Y. Sittler

Bruce Steinwald

W. Jack Stelmach, M.D.

Michael J. Sullivan, M.D.

Alvin R. Tarlov, M.D.

Samuel Wright

Primary Secretaries

Nicholas Griffin (1985-1986)

Douglas E. Hough, Ph.D. (1982-1985)

Delivery Mechanisms and Processes Work Group

Chairman

William R. Felts, M.D. (1982-1986)

Members

Cheryl Austein

Judith Barr

Leslie Bond, M.D.

P. M. Breaud, D.D.S.

Michael-Anne Browne, M.D.

Thomas K. Bullen, C.P.A., J.D.

Carlton Carpenter, Jr., M.D.

Barbara E. Chick, M.D.

Douglas Cocks, Ph.D.

George E. Collentine, M.D.

Michael E. Ervin, M.D.

Alvin B. Grant

Glenn M. Hackbarth

William J. Haskins

Kenneth O. Johnson, M.D.

Olga Jonasson, M.D.

Jonathan D. Klein, M.D.

John A. Knote, M.D.

Martin E. Liebling. M.D.

Douglas D. Lind

Ruth W. Lubic, Ed.D., R.N.

Joseph L. Moore

Dorothy Olson

Paul Q. Peterson, M.D.

Leonard Riggs, Jr., M.D.

Fredric L. Sattler

Donald A. Senhauser, M.D.

Roy W. Skoglund, M.D.

Henry F. Twelmeyer, M.D.

Peyton E. Weary, M.D.

Mary Wilkin

Ronald L. Williams

George T. Wolff, M.D.

Primary Secretary

Barry S. Eisenberg (1982-1986)

Evaluation, Assessment, and Control Work Group

Chairman

Robert M. Vanecko, M.D. (1982-1986)

Members

Karl H. Anderson

Charles N. Aswad, M.D.

George B. Beranek

Alexander M. Capron, Ph.D.

William Chase, M.D.

Frank E. Conrad, M.D.

Kathryn Derbonne

Herbert Derman, M.D.

Lawrence Deyton

Seymour Diamond, M.D.

John W. Eckstein, M.D.

John Farrington, M.D.

Palma E. Formica, M.D.

William M. Gallagher

Bryant L. Galusha, M.D.

Norma J. Goodwin, M.D.

Daniel Gordon, D.D.S.

Robert L. Hare, M.D.

William Harper

Paul D. Hofmann

Harold E. Jervey, Jr., M.D.

John S. Klyop, M.S.

Norma M. Lang, Ph.D.

Diane Bolay Lawrence

Robert W. Love, Jr., M.D.

William E. Mayer, M.D.

Robert E. McAfee, M.D.

Fred Merchant

Joel E. Miller

Joseph D. Millerick, M.D.

George Mitchell, M.D.

John C. Nelson, M.D.

Michael Nieder, M.D.

Paul A. Nutting, M.D.

Charles F. O'Donnell, M.D.

Beverly C. Payne, M.D.

Mary Jo Reilly

Joan Mary Roberts, M.D.

Grant V. Rodkey, M.D.

Robert E. Roush, Ed.D., M.P.H.

Eli Sorkow, M.D.

Paul M. Starnes

John Virts, Ph.D.

Cyril C. Wiggishoff, M.D.

David T. Williams

Primary Secretaries

Shirley D. Rivers, J.D. (1986)

Louis Goodman, Ph.D. (1982-1986)

Payment for Service Work Group

Chairmen

Donald K. Crandall, M.D. (1984-1986)

Joseph T. Painter, M.D. (1983-1984)

John J. Ring, M.D. (1982-1983)

Members

Theodore Allison

Cary E. Ashley

Glenn Austin, M.D.

Allan Beigel, M.D.

Cheryl L. Birchette-Pierce, M.D.

Peter Carlin

Douglas Cocks, PhD

Stephen N. Collier, Ph.D.

Roger C. Day

Joseph DiStasio, D.D.S.

Merlin K. Duval, M.D.

Richard H. Edgahl, M.D.

Robert B. Edmiston, M.D.

Robert S. Flom, M.D.

John J. Freysinger

Donald R. Gronewold

Fred Hannett

Robert Hatch

Ada K. Jacox, Ph.D., R.N.

John E. Joyner, M.D.

Luke Kramer

Deborah Lewis-Idema

Edward A. Lichter, M.D.

Robert B. Maxwell

Deborah McGregor, M.D.

Joseph D. McKean, Jr., M.D.

Kathleen Means

Sam A. Nixon, M.D.

James G. Nuckolls, M.D.

David M. Reed, M.D.

Michael A. Riddiough

Alex Scott, M.D.

Robert H. Shackelford, M.D.

R. Frances Smith

Robert A. Songe, M.D.

John K. Springer

Michael Wall

William G. Williams

Louis R. Zako, M.D.

Al Zamberlan

Raymond C. Zastrow, M.D.

Primary Secretaries

Christopher A. Damon, J.D. (1986)

Jack Werner, Ph.D. (1982-1986)

Susan E. Adelman, M.D.

Paul R. Ahr, Ph.D., M.P.A.

R. William Alexander, M.D.

William S. Apple

Beverly W. Armstrong, M.D.

Marc Baltzan, M.D.

James D. Barger, M.D.

Lewellys F. Barker, M.D.

Anne L. Barlow, M.D.

Robert J. Becker, M.D.

Maurice Q. Bectel

Bruce Bennett, Ph.D.

John S. Bennett, M.D.

Joe D. Bentz, M.D.

Robert Bernstein, M.D.

Charles E. Bickham, Jr., M.D.

Dan Billmeyer, M.D.

Jay Binder

Donald R. Bjornson, M.D.

Morton D. Bogdonoff, M.D.

Walter M. Bortz, II, M.D.

Robert M. Boughton, M.D.

Charles W. Bradley, D.P.M.

Richard V. Bradley, M.D.

Billie K. Brady

Thomas H. Browning, M.D.

Genevieve S. Burk, M.D.

Stanley L. Burns, M.D.

John J. Byrne, D.D.S.

David B. Carmichael, Jr., M.D.

Carlton L. Carpenter, Jr., M.D.

Steven Carter

Ann B. Catts, M.D.

John Henry Clark, M.D.

Edwin M. Cohn, M.D.

Bruce H. Colligen

Euta M. Colvin, M.D.

John P. Conomy, M.D.

John J. Corbett, M.D.

Carl J. Cornelius, Jr., M.D.

John P. Coughlin, M.D.

Thomas B. Dameron, Jr., M.D.

Brinton T. Darlington, M.D.

Frank Delay

G. Roy Diessner, M.D.

Charles K. Donegan, M.D.

Honorable Winfield Dunn, D.D.S.

William H. Eaglstein, M.D.

Richard D. Eberle, M.D.

Allen S. Edmonson, M.D.

James B. Eskridge, III, M.D.

Edwin C. Evans, M.D.

John T. Farrar, M.D.

Stuart L. Fischman, D.D.S.

William J. Frable, M.D.

Marian Frerichs, R.N., Ed.D.

Rhonda Friedman, Sc.D.

John Glasson, M.D.

Richard V. Grant, Ph.D.

William Walter Greaves, M.D.

Norton J. Greenberger, M.D.

Glenn Gullickson, M.D., Ph.D.

Charles M. Hair, M.D.

Val Halamandaris

Joseph N. Hamm, M.D.

C. Richard Harper, M.D.

William J. Haskins

J. Rhodes Haverty, M.D.

John W. Heizer, M.D.

Ronald E. Henderson, M.D.

Robert E. Henkin, M.D.

Lee C. Hess, M.D.

Joseph C. Hillman, M.D.

Melvin D. Hoffman, M.D.

Donald Honath, M.D.

Richard L. Hughes, M.D.

Joseph M. Jenkins

William E. Jobe, M.D.

Robert P. Johnson, M.D.

William W. Johnston, M.D.

Melvin Jordan

George H. Kamp, M.D.

Donald M. Keith, M.D.

Gerald C. Kempthorne, M.D.

I. Lawrence Kerr, D.D.S.

Jacquelyn Kinder, Ed.D.

William H. Kirby, Jr., M.D.

James F. Knapp, M.D.

John A. Knote, M.D.

Robert J. Kramer, M.D.

Burton Krimmer, M.D.

Edward J. Krol, M.D.

Raymond A. Kuthy, D.D.S.

Gene P. Lewis, D.D.S., M.P.H.

Howard L. Lieberman, M.D.

George Gerald Lindesmith, M.D.

Michael Lockshin, M.D.

James H. Lucien, III, M.D.

Bruce C. Lushbough, M.D.

John J. Lynch, M.D.

Douglas W. MacEwan, M.D.

W. Richard Marsh, M.D.

John L. Melvin, M.D.

Paul S. Metzger, M.D.

William A. Millhon, M.D.

Jack Moyers, M.D.

RADM Melvin Museles, MC, USN

Robert J. Musselman, D.D.S., M.S.D.

Wil B. Nelp, M.D.

John B. Nettles, M.D.

Sam A. Nixon, M.D.

Richard C. Oliver, D.D.S.

Peter Orris, M.D.

Edward M. Osetek, D.D.S.

John R. Page, M.D.

Henry B. Peters, O.D.

Stewart J. Petrie, M.D.

S. Baird Pfahl, Jr., M.D.

H. William Porterfield, M.D.

William T. Powers, M.D.

Hormoz Rassekh, M.D.

Richard J. Reitemeier, M.D.

C. David Richards, M.D.

Michael A. Riddiough

Neopito L. Robles, M.D.

Hugh Rohrer, M.D.

Rod J. Rohrich, M.D.

Andrew C. Ruoff, III, M.D.

Peter H. Sayre

William L. Scharringhausen, P.D.

John F. Schlegel, Pharm.D., M.S.Ed.

Rev. Robert W. Schlicht, CFACNHA

Ronald E. Schmid

Bert B. Schoenkerman, M.D.

James R. Scholles, O.D., J.D.

William Shadburn, M.D.

Harry Shannon, M.D.

Donald T. Sheridan

G. Thomas Shires, M.D.

Howard D. Slobodien, M.D.

Lowell R. Smith, M.D.

Roland T. Smoot, M.D.

Herbert Sohn, M.D.

Bruce Farrell Sorensen, M.D.

Bruce E. Spivey, M.D.

Frank E. Staggers, M.D.

Goodwill M. Stewart, M.D.

George B. Strumpf

J. H. Sunderbruch, M.D.

Bill T. Teague, MT(ASCP) SBB

F. Warren Tingley, M.D.

Bartholomew J. Tortella, M.D., MTS

Carl E. Trinca, Ph.D.

Theodore S. Vanderveen, M.D.

Robert M. Vanecko, M.D.

Donald G. Vidt, M.D.

Harold M. Visotsky, M.D.

Bernard M. Wagner, M.D.

Frank B. Walker, M.D.

Anderson J. Ward, Ph.D.

David G. Welton, M.D.

Douglas C. Wendt, D.D.S.

Stuart A. Wesbury, Jr., Ph.D.

W. Leonard Weyl, M.D.

Laurens P. White, M.D.

John Allen Whitesel, III, M.D.

Arnold Widen, M.D.

Morris J. Wizenberg, M.D.

Eugene F. Worthen, M.D.

Frank R. Wrenn, M.D.

Victor M. Zink

Aerospace Medical Association

American Academy of Allergy and Immunology

American Academy of Dermatology

American Academy of Facial Plastic and Reconstructive Surgery, Inc.

American Academy of Family Physicians

American Academy of Neurology

American Academy of Occupational Medicine

American Academy of Ophthalmology

American Academy of Oral Pathology

American Academy of Orthopaedic Surgeons

American Academy of Otolaryngology— Head and Neck Surgery, Inc.

American Academy of Pediatrics

American Academy of Pediatric Dentistry

American Academy of Periodontology

American Academy of Physical Medicine and Rehabilitation

American Association for the Advancement of Science

American Association for Thoracic Surgery

American Association of Blood Banks

American Association of Clinical Urologists, Inc.

American Association of Colleges of Nursing

American Association of Colleges of Pharmacy

American Association of Endodontists

American Association of Foundations for Medical Care

American Association of Neurological Surgeons

American Association of Oral and Maxillofacial Surgeons

American Association of Orthodontists

American Association of Pathologists, Inc.

American Association of Public Health Dentists

American Association of Public Health Physicians

American Association of Retired Persons

American Board of Medical Specialties

American College of Allergists

American College of Cardiology

American College of Chest Physicians

American College of Emergency Physicians

American College of Gastroenterology

American College of Health Care Administrators

American College of Healthcare Executives

American College of Hospital Administrators

American College of Nuclear Medicine

American College of Nuclear Physicians

American College of Obstetricians and Gynecologists

American College of Physicians

American College of Preventive Medicine

American College of Radiology

American College of Surgeons

American College of Utilization Review Physicians

American Dental Association

American Gastroenterological Association

American Geriatrics Society

American Group Practice Association

American Hospital Association

American Laryngological, Rhinological, and Otological Society, Inc.

American Medical Association

American Medical Association Auxiliary

American Medical Association Medical Student Section

American Medical Association Resident Physicians Section

American Medical Women's Association

American Nurses' Association, Inc.

American Occupational Medical Association

American Optometric Association

American Orthopaedic Association

American Pharmaceutical Association

American Podiatry Association

American Psychiatric Association

American Psychological Association

American Public Health Association

American Red Cross

American Rheumatism Association

American Roentgen Ray Society

American Society for Therapeutic Radiology and Oncology

American Society of Abdominal Surgeons

American Society of Allied Health Professions

American Society of Anesthesiologists

American Society of Cataract and Refractive Surgery

American Society of Clinical Pathologists

American Society of Clinical Pharmacology and Therapeutics

American Society of Cytology

American Society of Gastrointestinal Endoscopy

American Society of Internal Medicine

American Society of Plastic and Reconstructive Surgeons, Inc.

American Urological Association, Inc.

Arizona Medical Association

Association of American Medical Colleges

Association of Life Insurance Medical
Directors of America

Association of Military Surgeons of
the U.S.

Association of State and Territorial
Health Officials

Blue Cross and Blue Shield Association

Business Roundtable

California Medical Association

Canadian Medical Association

College of American Pathologists

Colorado Medical Society

Committee on Allied Health Education
and Accreditation

Congress of Neurological Surgeons

Connecticut State Medical Society

Consumer Federation of America

Council on Employee Benefits

Federation of American Hospitals

Federation of Prosthodontic Organizations

Federation of State Medical Boards

Florida Medical Association, Inc.

Group Health Association of America

Hawaii Medical Association

Health Insurance Association of America

Idaho Medical Association

Illinois State Medical Society

Indiana State Medical Association

International College of Surgeons—
U.S. Section

Iowa Medical Society

Kansas Medical Society

Kentucky Medical Association

Louisiana State Medical Society

Maine Medical Association

Massachusetts Medical Society

Medical and Chirurgical Faculty of the
State of Maryland

Medical Association of Georgia

Medical Association of the State
of Alabama

Medical Group Management Association

Medical Society of New Jersey

Medical Society of the District of Columbia

Medical Society of the State of New York

Medical Society of Virginia

Michigan State Medical Society

Minnesota Medical Association

Mississippi State Medical Association

Missouri State Medical Association

Montana Medical Association

National Academy of Science

National Association for the Advancement
of Colored People

National Association of Chain Drug Stores

National Association of Home Care

National Association of Insurance
Commissioners

National Association of Rehabilitation
Facilities

National Association of Retail Druggists

National Association of State and Mental
Health Program Directors

National Conference of State Legislatures

National HomeCaring Council

National League of Nursing

National Medical Association

National Organization on Disability

National Urban League, Inc.

Nebraska Medical Association

North Carolina Medical Society

North Dakota Medical Association

Ohio State Medical Association

Oklahoma State Medical Association

Oregon Medical Association

Pennsylvania Medical Society

Pharmaceutical Manufacturers Association

Radiological Society of North America

Rhode Island Medical Society

Society for Investigative
Dermatology, Inc.

Society of Medical Consultants to
the Armed Forces

Society of Nuclear Medicine

Society of Thoracic Surgeons

South Carolina Medical Association

South Dakota State Medical Association

Specialty and Service Society

State Medical Society of Wisconsin

Teamsters Local 380 Benefit Funds

Tennessee Medical Association

Texas Medical Association

U.S. and Canadian Academy
of Pathology, Inc.

U.S. Chamber of Commerce

U.S. Department of Defense

U.S. Department of Health and
Human Services

Utah State Medical Association

Vermont State Medical Society

Veterans Administration

Washington State Medical Association

West Virginia State Medical Association

Wyoming Medical Society

Index

Health Care Facilities
    acquisition of health care technology
        by, 71
    certificate-of-need laws, 62
    definition, 41, 51, 52
    delineating clinical privileges, 28
    establishment of ethics committees at,
        121
    federal role in supply and distribution
        of, 57
    inpatient facilities, skilled service units,
        special units, 52
    interagency accreditation structure, 107
    licensure of, 42, 53
    notification to state boards regarding
        disciplinary actions, 117
    principles to govern licensing, 55
    procedures to evaluate quality of care
        at, 106
    providing, 41
    public information on quality of care
        in, 108
    responsibility in transfer of technology,
        68
    responsibility to serve community
        needs, 57
    risk management programs at, 106
    role in allocation of privileges to use
        technologies, 48, 49
    supply and distribution, community,
        regional and state roles in, 56
    supply and distribution of, 42, 56
    voluntary accreditation in ensuring
        quality of care, 105
    voluntary accreditation of, 106

Health Care Professions
    allied professionals in research training
        programs, 161
    allied, reporting obligations for, 118
    certification program should be
        continued, 111

Health Care Professions *(con't)*
    determination of prices by health care
        providers, 134
    identification of "deficient"
        practitioners, 111
    increased use of allied health
        professionals in Medicare, 143
    individual professional responsibility in
        transfer of technology, 68
    information needed to make health
        care decisions, 133
    interjurisdictional transfer of licensure
        and disciplinary information, 118
    joint patient treatment decision-making
        involving ethical considerations, 120
    jurisdictional disputes increasing, 10
    licensure, certification and
        accreditation and supply of
        professionals, 34
    notification of disciplinary action to
        state boards, 117
    process for determining reimbursement
        from third-party payors, 135
    qualifications of professionals, 109
    qualifications of professionals and
        quality assurance, 102
    quality assurance is responsibility of,
        103
    reporting potential grounds for
        disciplinary action, 117
    responsibilities for health promotion
        and care, 86
    responsibilities in allocation of
        privileges to use technologies, 48
    responsibility for patient's health care
        and use of technology, 45
    responsibility of professional in health
        care decision-making, 89
    responsibility of professionals to obtain
        informed consent, 89
    role of providers in cost-effective
        payment system, 138
    seeking health information from
        professionals, 83

Health Care Professions *(con't)*
    self-regulation, 114
    shared responsibility with patient
        concerning health care, 81
    students role in research conduct, 172
    "truth in advertising" and health care
        providers, 87
    variations in practice patterns, 108

Health Care Services
    access to, 64, 65
    designating and using surrogate
        decision-makers, 90
    evaluation of government regulations
        affecting, 150
    funding for the planning of, 63
    informed consent and decision-making
        in, 89
    innovative and cost-effective,
        encourage development of, 63
    keeping duplication at a minimum, 105
    organizing resources for, 60
    providing for, 8
    research and evaluation, 125
    research and its use in national health
        policy development, 125
    research data and information,
        dissemination of, 127
    research, funding for, 126
    research, priorities for, 126
    roles of public and private sectors in
        ensuring access to, 65

Health Education
    communicating health information, 81
    evaluation of efforts, 88
    health providers role in, 86
    health information and, 82
    in health professions curricula, 87
    in occupational setting, 83
    in schools, 88
    on quality of health care, 104
    private support for, 88

Health Education *(con't)*
    public information on quality of care
        in health care facilities, 108
    state and local educational agency
        support for, 87
    third-party payors' responsibilities for
        health promotion and care, 87

Health Maintenance Organizations
    new health care delivery mechanism,
        62
    new health care facilities, 51
    support for undergraduate education,
        12

Health Manpower
    achieving an equitable distribution of
        health professionals, 34
    data on distribution of professionals
        relative to unmet needs, 34
    supply and distribution of professionals,
        32, 33
    supply and distribution of professionals
        and needs of underserved groups,
        34

Health Planning
    at community level, 60, 62
    community planning for needs of
        special populations, 64
    history of, 62

Health Policy
    involvement of faculty and
        administrators in determining, 96
    national, health services research and
        its use in development of, 125

Hill-Burton Act
    health planning, 62

Home Care Services
    community planning for, 64
    new health care setting, 41, 51, 52
    options for, in basic benefit package,
        136
    supply and distribution of, 56